Practical Primer of
Clinical
Neurology

Practical Primer of Clinical Neurology

William W. Campbell, MD, MSHA
Department of Neurology
Walter Reed Army Medical Center
Washington, DC

Rhonda M. Pridgeon, MD
Neurology Service
DeWitt Army Community Hospital
Ft. Belvoir, Virginia

LIPPINCOTT WILLIAMS & WILKINS
A Wolters Kluwer Company
Philadelphia · Baltimore · New York · London
Buenos Aires · Hong Kong · Sydney · Tokyo

Editor: Elizabeth Nieginski
Development Editor: Bridget Hilferty
Managing Editor: Marette Magargle-Smith

Copyright © 2002 Lippincott Williams & Wilkins

351 West Camden Street
Baltimore, Maryland 21201-2436 USA

227 East Washington Square
Philadelphia, PA 19106

The publisher is not responsible (as a matter of product liability, negligence or otherwise) for any injury resulting from any material contained herein. This publication contains information relating to general principles of medical care which should not be construed as specific instructions for individual patients. Manufacturers' product information and package inserts should be reviewed for current information, including contraindications, dosages and precautions.

Printed in the United States of America

Library of Congress Cataloging-in-Publication Data

ISBN # 0-781-72481-3

The publishers have made every effort to trace the copyright holders for borrowed material. If they have inadvertently overlooked any, they will be pleased to make the necessary arrangements at the first opportunity.

To purchase additional copies of this book, call our customer service department at **(800) 638-3030** or fax orders to **(301) 824-7390**. International customers should call **(301) 714-2324**.

02 03
1 2 3 4 5 6 7 8 9 10

To Rose, Rhonda, Robbie, my children and everyone who
has helped me along the way.

And especially to Harold Collings and Don Abbott; without them
I may never have discovered one of medicine's best
kept secrets—Neurology.

William W. Campbell

To my parents, James and Margaret Pridgeon,
for their unfailing love and support.

Rhonda M. Pridgeon

Preface

Clinical neurology texts used by junior trainees tend to suffer from various disadvantages. If short and concise, they lack the rich detail that makes neurology a fascinating subject. If very detailed, they are too long to read during the usual neurology rotation. Most lack the sort of practical information that is really useful in day-to-day life on the neurology ward. When asked by students to recommend a text to use, we have been hard-pressed to find one that did not suffer from these disadvantages. Our attempts to fill the void in medical student neurology teaching materials resulted in the creation of a homemade manual, which, after about 10 years of use, has evolved into this book. We found that students wanted practical information, a review of neuroanatomy, guides to performing and interpreting the neurologic examination, clinical information, and enough detailed material to "pass the test."

We have tried to create a book specifically for medical students and junior house staff. Most medical students in the United States rotate on neurology for only 1 month, in either the third or fourth year. They need a book that can be read and assimilated during that time period. Junior neurology house staff may also find the book useful as an early review while getting started with their training. They are just learning neurology, and most full-sized treatises contain too much esoterica and not enough practical clinical information for the beginner. Furthermore, few of the standard texts contain much basic science.

To accommodate different needs, we have used a hypertext format, with basic information in the main body of the text but with more advanced, optional information set aside in "Enrichment Boxes." The main body of the text stands alone and the enrichment boxes need not be read unless the student would like additional information. Those who are interested may read the fine print, but the discussion holds together without it.

We begin with a brief overview of clinically relevant neuroanatomy and neurophysiology. Most students have not given much thought to these topics since the first year. More than most medical disciplines, neurology requires a familiarity with basic science. These sections are optional. Within them, advanced material is segregated into enrichment boxes. We have tried to include only clinically relevant basic science, with the relevance judged by clinicians (i.e., us) rather than by clinically naive PhDs.

We have tried to make the book reader friendly: concise, well organized, usefully illustrated, and well indexed. We have tried to exclude anything not having immediate clinical relevance. We have emphasized a practical clinical approach, describing a screening neurologic examination rather than a complete examination, and emphasizing differential diagnosis and major principles of disease. We have deliberately given short shrift to treatment for several reasons. Medical students do not make the primary therapeutic decisions. It is more important for them to learn the principles of neurologic diagnosis. When they become responsible for treatment, the treatments will likely have evolved from now, and current information should be sought.

Contents

How to Make the Most of Your Neurology Rotation

Neurologic complaints and disorders are common, and are encountered in every field of medicine. It has been estimated that 30% of patients seen in a primary care setting have a neurologic illness, a neurologic complaint, a neurologic complication of a medical illness, or a neurologic complication of drug therapy. For most medical students, the basic clerkship is the total formal exposure to neurology for their career. Not even this minimal amount of training is required in some institutions. The rotation is usually for 1 month. Learning is sometimes hampered by "neurophobia," and the overwhelming and sometimes intimidating amount of information to be absorbed in such a short time, like medical school in general. Then, to add further stress, there is the specter of an evaluation looming at the end. The following section provides counsel and guidance regarding how to learn neurology, how to take good care of your patients, and how to make a good impression on those who evaluate you.

General Guidance

One of the most important things you can learn this month is how to do a competent neurologic examination. Watch your resident and attending physician examine patients at every opportunity. Have someone who is knowledgeable watch you do a neurologic examination on a patient and critique your technique. Examine a patient with the resident or attending physician. Practice neurologic examinations on your fellow students, spouse, significant other, neighbor, or whoever else is willing. Ask someone to critique your write-ups as well, if this is not already a requirement.

A central consideration is that you as a medical student have major responsibility for patient care. This is the crux of any ward rotation. It is not only the driving force behind learning medicine, but is also an integral part of the socialization process whereby medical students become members of the fraternity of physicians. This responsibility includes the patients assigned to you, the other patients on your team, and the patients you are covering on night or weekend call. You must have a continuous knowledge of all of the relevant details regarding each and every one of your patients. This means an intimate familiarity with their chart, scans, laboratory results, electrodiagnostic studies, and physical examination findings at all times. Take responsibility for having your patients ready for presentation to the attending physician. It is not acceptable under any circumstances to claim ignorance of any aspect of your patient's case. Even worse than claiming ignorance is fabrication of information. Habitual perpetrators are inevitably discovered, and nothing has more adverse consequences on a student's evaluation and reputation.

Avoid a myopic outlook with a narrow focus only on your own patients. It is perfectly acceptable to see, examine, and learn from patients not assigned to you personally. Do not wear blinders. Examine other students' patients whenever possible, especially to see abnormal physical findings. Take advantage of seeing "classic" examples of anything or patients with interesting neurologic findings. If you adopt a provincial perspective when one of your colleagues is caring for a patient with abdominal pain and neuropathy, you may miss the only opportunity of your professional career to see a patient with porphyria.

Arrive at the hospital early to better care for your patients. It is best to beat your resident and attending physician to the hospital; with some residents and attending staff this is difficult to do. Stay until your work is done. Students arriving late and bailing out early leave a bad impression. Do not disappear. Do not be a phantom. Answer pages promptly. At the end of the day, check out to the person covering your patients regarding anything that needs to be followed up. Never leave more than minor, routine work on your patients for those providing night coverage. The night coverage people are responsible for emergencies and very sick patients, not for ensuring that routine daily work on your stable patients is completed. Follow up the results of emergent laboratory tests or procedures before you leave.

You should perform a full history and general and neurologic examinations on each new patient, including transfers from other services. Never "dry lab" your examination by copying someone else's note. Never engage in chart wars (acrimonious, contentious, or insulting remarks written in the patient's record). Do not dump work on your colleagues, or try to steal their thunder by telling the attending staff the study results or news on their patients. Enter orders whenever possible.

As a medical student, do not be overly concerned with learning the details of treatment. Before you have primary responsibility for therapeutic decisions, treatments will have changed. Focus your learning on differential diagnosis, general principles of neurologic disease, broad therapeutic concepts, and the examination. Learn what constitutes a real neurologic emergency and when to call for help. The Internet is a ready source of the latest information about treatments. Table 1–1 lists useful Web sites. In addition, the associations for many diseases, such as Alzheimer or Parkinson disease, host Web sites with professional areas that have up-to-date information on therapy.

Different attending and house staff may excel at teaching different things. Some are good at didactics, whereas others can effectively guide students through procedures or question them in a way that leads to better understanding. Still others excel as role models, or at hands-on instruction. Rare individuals can do all of these things. Do not undervalue any of these styles; take advantage of the strengths of your mentors rather than complaining about their imperfections. Remember that everyone can teach you something. Try to develop a thick skin, especially if your resident or attending physician is one of those people who loses his temper easily, yells, or verbally abuses his underlings. These people are encountered in every walk of life, and generally have to be endured. Try not to be one of them when your time comes.

Maintain good relations with the nurses and ancillary medical personnel. Do not underestimate their knowledge and professionalism. Failure to do so may make your working life unnecessarily difficult.

Evaluations

Your evaluation is based on many factors, which usually include performance in direct patient care, tending to ward duties, presentations, attendance, and how well you honor your responsibilities. Evaluators are usually impressed by students who aggressively pursue their own education. There is a natural tendency to look favorably on students who seem to have an interest in the evaluator's field. This leaning is difficult to fabricate, and attempts to do so are usually transparent. Clarify what is expected of you. Avoid asking, "How am I doing?" Ask instead, "What or how can I do better?"

You must demonstrate your expertise, knowledge, and capabilities in the setting of rounds. It is imperative to speak up if you know the

TABLE 1–1.   A SELECTION OF USEFUL WEB SITES FOR RAPID REFERENCE

Best general search engines for medical information (in approximate order of speed and efficiency)

www.google.com

www.altavista.com

www.alltheweb.com

www.lycos.com

www.cyber411.com

Neurology metasites with many links to other sites

www.neuroland.com

www.neuroguide.com

www.neuropat.dote.hu

www.toddtroost.com/mylinks2000.html

General clinical neurology information

www.merck.com/pubs/mmanual

www.emedicine.com/neuro/contents.htm

www.neuropat.dote.hu/signs.htm

neuro-www.mgh.harvard.edu

www.ninds.nih.gov/health_and_medical/disorder_index.htm

www.nlm.nih.gov/medlineplus/brainandnervoussystem.html

www.vnh.org/FSManual/07/SectionTop.html

www.vnh.org/GMO/01Contents.html#Neurology

www.vh.org/Providers/ClinRef/FPHandbook/14.html

Neuroanatomy

www.neuropat.dote.hu

anatomy.uams.edu

Neuromuscular disease

www.neuro.wustl.edu/neuromuscular*

Neurologic examination

www.medinfo.ufl.edu/year1/bcs/clist/neuro.html

www.vnh.org/FSManual/07/02GeneralNeurol.html

Neuro-ophthalmology

cim.ucdavis.edu/eyes[†]

www.richmondeye.com/md.htm[†]

www.wfubmc.edu/neurology/lectures

(*continued*)

TABLE 1-1. A SELECTION OF USEFUL WEB SITES FOR RAPID REFERENCE (*Continued*)

www.revoptom.com/handbook/section6.htm

Neuropathology

www.neuropat.dote.hu

Neuroradiology

www.med.harvard.edu/AANLIB/home.html†

rad.usuhs.mil/rad/edu/edu.htm

Stroke

www.strokecenter.org/prof

Rare diseases

www.raredisease.org

rarediseases.info.nih.gov/ord

www3.ncbi.nlm.nih.gov/Omim

www.irsc.org/rare.htm

---

*This site has concise printable "wallet Web sites."

†There are wonderful interactive areas for learning about abnormal eye movements and pupils.

†This interactive site is great for learning the difference between T1 and T2 weighting for magnetic resonance imaging.

answer to a question being posed. There is no other way for your attending physician to know what you know. Being overly quiet, shy, and diffident leaves your attending physician in the dark and without much of an impression of you at evaluation time. Few attending staff persist long at dragging information out of bashful students; the meek will not inherit the good grade. On the other hand, you should behave diplomatically and remain tactful and polite. Do not blurt out the answer, even if you know it, when the question has been directed at one of your colleagues. If you are rude, obtrusive, and domineering, you will lose on personality points, despite your fund of information. As a rule, "roundsmanship" is a civilized, scholarly game. However, in some institutions, being abrupt and aggressive may be the norm, in which case you may have to do as the Romans do.

The Daily Routine

The day-to-day routine on most ward rotations consists of varying combinations of rounds, clinics, conferences, ward work, procedures, and reading. Attend all conferences unless one of your patients requires your urgent attention. Attend the outpatient clinics to which you are assigned. In the era of managed care, many of the patients who were once cared for in the hospital are now seen in the clinic, and some of the most interesting cases are to be found in the outpatient setting. There are advantages and disadvantages to learning neurology by seeing a large proportion of clinic patients, but the situation is not likely to change. Many of the same principles apply as for an inpatient service: taking advantage of seeing other student's patients, practicing the examination, and so forth. If caught in a queue waiting to present, use the time to read or do the sort of ward work that only requires a phone and computer.

Procedures

The major procedure for students to learn on the neurology rotation is the lumbar puncture. Make every effort not to let the month end without doing at least one. Be sure to review any available imaging studies before doing a lumbar puncture.

Reading

For more detailed information, try to read something about each of your patient's conditions in a full-sized internal medicine or neurology textbook. Another approach is to read a recent review paper or the proceedings from a clinical pathological conference on each major clinical problem you encounter. Table 1–1 lists useful Web sites for obtaining information quickly on various topics. The site *www. neuroland.com* is especially helpful. It contains brief notes on many common neurologic diseases, up-to-date information on therapy, and numerous links to other neuroscience Web sites. The search engine at *www.google.com* can find almost anything, including esoteric medical information, in nothing flat. It handily won our "search-off," which compared various common search engines for the ability to rapidly retrieve medical arcana.

Rounding

There are different types of rounds, including individual rounds, work rounds, attending rounds, teaching rounds, and check-out rounds. Attending rounds and teaching rounds, sometimes done separately, are where much of the formal teaching transpires.

BEFORE ATTENDING ROUNDS

Make your own preliminary work rounds before your team makes work rounds and certainly before attending rounds occur. Adequate prerounding often requires early arrival at the hospital. Prerounding includes a review of all of your patients' charts (including nurses' notes), orders, laboratory tests, overnight radiologic studies, and morning examination. This should be done on intensive care unit patients first, then on floor patients. Gather any relevant new information (x-ray and laboratory results, change in patient status, or new complaints); and try to formulate plans for diagnosis or management, as appropriate. Discuss the patient's status with your resident. Practice your initial patient presentation with the resident. On days after the initial workup, do a focused neurologic examination on each of your patients every day. Pay particular attention to any changes from previous examinations. Do a focused medical examination; listen to heart and lungs, check for deep venous thrombosis, and examine any other relevant areas, depending on the medical situation. It is not generally necessary to do a complete general or neurologic examination on every patient every day, but areas of potential problems or concerns should be assessed. A major rule is that there should never be ugly surprises for the attending physician on rounds, such as finding a patient comatose, herniating, with high fever, or in respiratory distress. Such unpleasant discoveries reflect poorly on the student who should have prerounded. You are much better off to find these bombshells yourself.

Prerounding as a team allows you to practice presentations and to ask questions in a setting that is often less intimidating than that of attending rounds.

DURING ATTENDING ROUNDS

Be there on time. Find out how your neurology attending physician likes to be presented to. The verbal presentation should generally be a pithy synopsis. Wean yourself away from looking at your write-up while presenting, and never succumb to the temptation to read your write-up aloud as your presentation on rounds. Take advantage of every opportunity to present. Practice, practice, practice. Try to locate a copy of *The Effective Scutboy* by RA Harrell and GS Firestein, 3rd edition, New York, Appleton and Lange, 1988 (out of print but check your library), and read the sections on how to present and how to do a write-up. You must attain proficiency or the house staff will take over. If asked a question to which you do not know the answer, admit that you do not know. Do not make up anything. If possible, have the actual computed tomography scan or magnetic resonance imaging films on hand to show the attending physician. Avoid side conversations, especially at the patient's bedside.

AFTER ATTENDING ROUNDS

Complete any new tasks that the attending physician has assigned. Write your daily note, or amend your prerounds note as necessary. On individual patients, keep a workup summary sheet with important laboratory and x-ray results on the chart. Include the date the test was ordered, the date the test was done, and the test results. (This can be a great time-saver during rounds and for the person dictating the discharge summary.) Check back with any patient whose condition was discussed at the bedside to be sure that nothing was said that is causing the patient concern or distress.

Suggestions For Patient Care

1. **Always read the old chart.** Reading the old chart may save you time and the patient unnecessary testing if a previous workup has been done for the presenting problem. It is important to put the current episode of care in context. Except for emergency cases, the patient has been admitted for a reason that somehow ties into events that have gone before and will come after.
2. **Read the nurses' notes.** Often nurses' notes contain vital information that is not verbally passed on to the physician (or they may contain comments that you may not agree with). Also read progress notes by ancillary medical personnel, medical consultants, and other physicians who may have seen your patient in the middle of the night for acute problems. Comment on or acknowledge their observations (in a polite and appropriate manner) in your note.
3. **Periodically review standing orders.** A review of standing orders should be done at least once per week, probably more often on recently admitted or very ill patients, or on patients whose medical status has changed drastically.
   a. **Intravenous (IV) fluids.** Does the patient really need IV fluids? Is the amount of fluid or potassium she is getting appropriate? If a "nothing by mouth" order has been given, does she need IV multivitamins (and extra thiamine if there is a question of ethyl alcohol abuse)? Has her IV site been changed recently?
   b. **Devices.** Does the patient have a Foley or external catheter, a nasogastric tube, or restraints? Does he still need them?
   c. **Activity.** Are your activity orders up to date and appropriate? Does the patient still need to be at "bed rest"? If the patient's gait is unsteady, then his activity needs to be restricted.
   d. **Vital signs.** Do the patient's vital signs still need to be checked every 2 hours?

e. **Diet.** Are your dietary orders up to date? Is the patient getting adequate calories, nutrition, and fluids? Does she need a dietary or nutrition consult?

f. **Medications.** Review medication orders frequently; some medications may have become unnecessary in the time since admission, or the dose may be inappropriate. This is especially important in elderly patients. Review the medication list with possible drug interactions in mind.

Discharging Patients

1. Do not send home a patient who cannot swallow. He is likely to be readmitted with aspiration pneumonia, dehydration, malnutrition, or sepsis. Such a patient needs an evaluation by a speech pathologist; if it is likely that he will not be able to consume adequate calories or fluids or he is at risk for aspiration, then he probably needs a percutaneous endoscopic gastrostomy or jejunostomy. Try to avoid sending him home with a nasogastric tube; these devices often promote aspiration, are easily dislodged, are uncomfortable, and can cause damage to the nasal septum when left in place for long periods. Reevaluation can or should be done at intervals by a speech pathologist to determine if swallowing function has improved to the point that feeding tubes can be removed.

2. Do not send home a patient who cannot walk before ensuring that a full evaluation of her gait disorder has been done. Many patients admitted to the service are too ill for evaluation of gait; "gait not tested" is written on the chart. However, at some point, a gait evaluation should be done and documented on the chart. If the patient cannot walk or has a disorder of gait, the reason for it must be found. If the cause is found and is not treatable or does not need further workup, evaluation of gait needs to be done by a physical therapist. It is unwise to send a patient with unsteady gait home without the proper assistive devices; the patient and family need to be instructed about the patient's limitations.

3. Make sure the patient has adequate follow-up, both neurologically and otherwise. If the patient has diabetes, hypertension, cardiac disease, or other chronic conditions, he needs to be followed by an internist or family practitioner in addition to whatever neurologic follow-up he needs. In many cases, he should also be followed up by the referring physician, and a discharge summary should be sent to facilitate follow-up. Make sure the patient has enough medication to last him through to his clinic visit.

If the patient is on or has been recently placed on warfarin, he needs a timely clinic visit for follow-up. The patient also needs a timely follow-up to the neurology clinic or pharmacy clinic for anticonvulsant levels if he has been recently placed on anti-convulsants, if his medication dose has been recently changed, or if a medication has been added that interferes with the metabolism of the present anticonvulsants. Make sure the patient or caregiver understands the way the patient is supposed to take his medications. If the patient has been started on insulin in the hospital, make sure the patient or caregiver knows (and has practiced) how to administer it (or arrange for a home health visit).

4. Document laboratory and x-ray results in the record before discharge, either in the progress notes or on a special summary sheet. Never send the patient home or dictate the discharge summary by saying "Computed tomography scan (or magnetic resonance imaging or myelogram or arteriogram) results pending at the time of discharge." If it is necessary to send the patient home with laboratory, x-ray, or biopsy results pending, it is imperative that the results are followed up in a timely manner (*not* at the patient's 6-month follow-up visit).

Good luck.

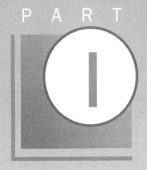

P A R T

1

Clinically
Relevant
Neuroscience

2

An Overview of Neuroanatomy

Introduction

Neuroanatomy is a complex and intimidating subject, quickly forgotten unless applied. It is nonetheless a major underpinning of the practice of clinical neurology. This chapter provides an overview of some of the clinically relevant neuroanatomy used when caring for patients. Clinical perspective is provided as often as possible. This discussion is intended as a review, and assumes some prior familiarity with the topic. Some of the more detailed information has been included in the Enrichment Boxes. Table 2–1 at the end of the chapter provides a summary description of the functional and clinical manifestations of damage to various structures of the nervous system.

The Skull

The skull is composed of several large bones and myriad complexly articulated smaller bones (Figure 2–1). The major bones are the frontal, temporal, parietal, occipital, and sphenoid; all are joined by suture lines. The major sutures are the sagittal and coronal, but there are numerous others. Sometimes sutures close prematurely, before the skull has completed growth, producing one of several distinctive varieties of malformed and misshapen skulls, depending on the sutures involved.

The *frontal bone* contains the frontal sinuses. The *temporal bone* has two parts: the thin squamous portion that forms the temple, and the thick petrous part that forms the floor of the middle fossa. The squamous part contains the groove of the middle meningeal artery and may be easily fractured, sometimes producing epidural hematoma. The petrous pyramids have their apices pointed medially and their thick bases pointed laterally; deep within are the middle and inner ear structures, the internal auditory meatus, the facial canal with its genu, and the air cells of the mastoid sinus. Fractures through the petrous bone

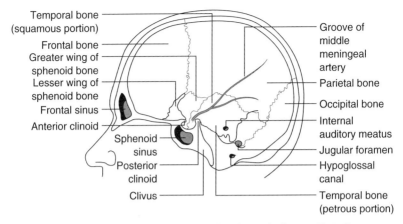

FIGURE 2–1. ■ Interior view of the skull showing the major bones. Note the groove of the *middle meningeal artery* crossing the squamous portion of the *temporal bone;* fractures here can lead to epidural hematoma.

may cause hemotympanum (i.e., blood in the middle ear cavity), hearing loss, or facial nerve palsy.

The *sphenoid bone* has greater and lesser wings, and contains the sella turcica. The greater wings form the anterior wall of the middle fossa, and the lesser wings form part of the floor of the anterior fossa. The greater and lesser wings attach to the body of the sphenoid; buried within is the sphenoid sinus cavity. The best way to appreciate the anatomy of the sphenoid bone is to look at it in disarticulated isolation, when the wings become obvious. The sella turcica makes up a saddle-shaped depression in the body of the sphenoid. Neurosurgeons perform transsphenoidal hypophysectomy by drilling up through the nose and sphenoid sinus to snatch pituitary tumors from the sella turcica. Alongside the sella turcica lie the cavernous sinuses, through which travel the carotid arteries and several important cranial nerves.

The *occipital bone* makes up the posterior fossa and contains the confluence of venous sinuses (torcula herophili) and the foramen magnum.

The *clivus* makes up the anterior wall of the posterior fossa and ends superiorly by forming the posterior clinoid processes and dorsum sellae. The basilar artery and brainstem lie along the clivus. Sometimes a tumor, most often a chordoma, erodes the clivus and produces multiple cranial nerve palsies.

The interior of the skull is divided into compartments, or fossae. The anterior fossa contains the frontal lobes, which rest on the orbital plates. The cribriform plate lies far anteriorly, between the orbital roofs; when fractured during head injury, cerebrospinal fluid (CSF) rhinorrhea may ensue. The middle fossa contains primarily the temporal lobes, and several major cranial nerves run through the area. The posterior fossa contains the brainstem, cerebellum, and vertebrobasilar vessels. Except for cranial nerves I and II, all of the cranial nerves run through or exit from the posterior fossa.

Various structures pass into or out of the skull through the numerous foramina that pierce its base (Table 2–2). Pathologic processes may involve the regions of different foramina; the resultant combination of cranial nerve abnormalities permits localization (Enrichment Box 2–1).

The Vertebral Column

The vertebral column is composed of 7 cervical, 12 thoracic, and 5 lumbar vertebral bodies, plus the sacrum. The vertebral bodies are separated by intervertebral discs, which are composed of an outer fibrous ring, the annulus, and an inner gelatinous core, the nucleus pulposus (Figure 2–2). Discs desiccate and degenerate with the passage of time, causing no end of trouble and woe.

The vertebral bodies have posterior elements, which spread out to encircle the spinal cord and form the spinal canal (Figure 2–3). Extending backward from the vertebral body, with varying degrees of slant, are the pedicles. The pedicles end in a bony mass, which has

TABLE 2–2. MAJOR SKULL BASE FORAMINA AND THEIR CONTENTS*

Foramen	Contents
Cribriform plate	Olfactory nerves
Optic canal	Optic nerve, ophthalmic artery
Supraorbital fissure	III, IV, VI, ophthalmic V, superior ophthalmic vein
Rotundum	Maxillary V
Spinosum	Middle meningeal artery
Ovale	Mandibular V
Internal auditory meatus	VII, VIII, internal auditory artery
Jugular foramen	IX, X, XI, internal jugular vein
Hypoglossal	XII
Carotid canal	Carotid artery

*The Roman numerals refer to cranial nerves III through XII.

Skull foramina syndromes

Unilateral palsies of cranial nerves IX, X, and XI suggest a process near the jugular foramen, such as a glomus tumor. Unilateral palsies of CN III, CN IV, ophthalmic CN V, and CN VI suggest pathology near the cavernous sinus or superior orbital fissure. Unilateral palsies of CN VII and CN VIII indicate a process near the internal auditory meatus.

The intervertebral foramina

The intervertebral foramen is a passageway formed by the vertebral body anteriorly, pedicles above and below, and the facet mass and its articulation, the zygapophyseal joint, posteriorly. The uncovertebral "joints" (of Luschka), which are not true joints, are the points where the posterolateral surfaces of a vertebra come into apposition with neighboring vertebrae. Degenerative osteophytes projecting into the intervertebral foramen from the uncovertebral joints or the zygapophyseal joints may narrow it and cause radiculopathy. Sometimes a laminectomy is combined with a foraminotomy to remove such osteophytes.

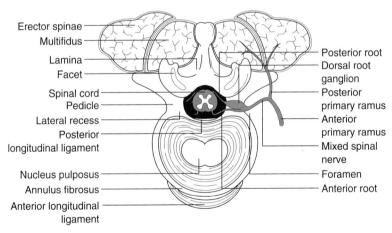

FIGURE 2–2. ■ Cross-section of a *vertebral body* with one pedicle cut away to show the contents of the *intervertebral foramen,* with the *dorsal root ganglion* lying in the midzone. The *posterior longitudinal ligament* is incomplete laterally, and disc ruptures tend to occur in a posterolateral direction. When a facet joint becomes enlarged because of osteoarthritis, the facet joint may encroach on the lateral recess, where the nerve root is entering the foramen. (Reprinted with permission from Campbell WW: *Essentials of Electrodiagnostic Medicine.* Baltimore, Williams and Wilkins, 1998, p 185.)

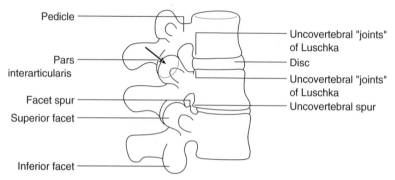

FIGURE 2–3. ■ Lateral view of the *cervical spine* showing the vertebral bodies separated by intervertebral discs, the pedicles merging into the facet joint with its superior and inferior facets, and the intervening pars interarticularis. The facets are oblique in the cervical region and more vertical in the lumbosacral spine. The *uncovertebral joints* are not true joints, but merely the opposing surfaces of the vertebral bodies. The uncovertebral processes may form osteophytes, or spurs, which then project into the foramen. (Reprinted with permission from Campbell WW: *Essentials of Electrodiagnostic Medicine.* Baltimore, Williams and Wilkins, 1998, p 184.)

smooth upper and lower surfaces (i.e., the superior and inferior articulating facets) and from which the transverse processes extend laterally. Extending backward from the facet masses are the laminae, which join in the midline to complete the circle. From the junction point of the laminae, the spinous process extends backward a bit further. To remove a herniated nucleus pulposus, the surgeon creates a laminectomy (i.e., a hole in the lamina) to remove the disc material.

The spinal nerves pass outward from the vertebral column through the intervertebral foramina (see Enrichment Box 2–1).

Meninges and Cerebrospinal Fluid Pathways

The meninges are composed of the dura mater, pia mater, and arachnoid (Figure 2–4). The pia mater is thin, filmy, and closely adherent to the brain and its blood vessels, extending down into all the nooks and crannies. The dura mater is thick and tough, and provides the substantive protective covering for the central nervous system (CNS). The arachnoid abuts the inner surface of the dura, and filmy strands that resemble a spider's web cross the subarachnoid space to join the arachnoid to the pia. Over the surface of the brain and spinal cord, the pia mater and the arachnoid are closely adherent and virtually inseparable; they often are referred to as essentially one membrane: the pia-

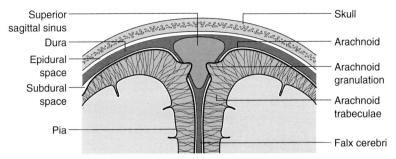

FIGURE 2–4. ■ The relationships among the skull, meninges, and superior sagittal sinus. The *epidural space* lies between the inner table of the skull and the dura; the *subdural space* lies between the dura and the arachnoid. Hematomas can occur in both locations. Aneurysmal hemorrhage occurs primarily into the subarachnoid space between the arachnoid and the pia mater. Cerebrospinal fluid circulates in the subarachnoid space and is reabsorbed into the superior sagittal sinus through the arachnoid granulations.

arachnoid or the leptomeninges. Traumatic and aneurysmal bleeding into the subarachnoid space is common.

A potential space exists between the dura mater and the arachnoid. Rupture of the delicate bridging veins may cause subdural hematomas to form in this space. Epidural hematomas may form between the outer dura mater and the skull, most often due to fractures of the temporal squamosa tearing the middle meningeal artery (see Figure 2–1).

THE VENTRICLES

The lateral ventricles are made up of a body and an atrium, or common space, from which extend the horns (Figure 2–5). The temporal horn extends forward into the temporal lobe, and the occipital horn extends backward into the occipital lobe. Within the atrium of each ventricle lies the CSF-forming choroid plexus. The two lateral ventricles come together in the midline, where they join the third ventricle. The foramen of Monro is the passageway between the lateral and third ventricles. Sometimes tumors form in the region of the foramen of Monro (most commonly a colloid cyst of the third ventricle) and obstruct CSF flow, causing hydrocephalus and positional headache.

The third ventricle is a thin slit lying in the midline between and just below the lateral ventricles. Anteriorly, it forms spaces, or recesses, above and below the pituitary gland. Posteriorly, the third ventricle creates a recess above the pineal gland. The third ventricle ends at the cerebral aqueduct (of Sylvius), which conveys CSF down to the fourth ventricle. The fourth ventricle is also a midline structure that has su-

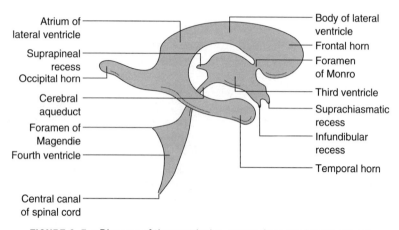

FIGURE 2–5. ■ Diagram of the ventricular system from the lateral aspect.

perior, inferior, and lateral extensions like narrow cul-de-sacs. The inferior extension of the fourth ventricle ends at the cervicomedullary junction and becomes continuous with the central canal of the spinal cord. The lateral recesses of the fourth ventricle contain small apertures (i.e., the foramina of Luschka) through which CSF empties into the subarachnoid space surrounding the brainstem. A midline aperture in the roof of the fourth ventricle (i.e., the foramen of Magendie) joins the fourth ventricle with the cisterna magna. Choroid plexus lies in the roof of the fourth ventricle.

Folds of dura mater separate the two hemispheres (the falx cerebri) and the middle fossa from the posterior fossa structures (the tentorium cerebelli) (Figure 2–6). With increased intracranial pressure, parts of the brain may herniate out of their normal compartments (Enrichment Box 2–2).

CEREBROSPINAL FLUID CIRCULATION

CSF is produced by the choroid plexus formations in the fourth ventricle and atria of the lateral ventricles. It percolates from the lateral ventricles, through the foramen of Monro, into the third ventricle, and from there down the aqueduct into the fourth ventricle. From the fourth ventricle, a small amount enters the central canal of the spinal cord, although the majority is discharged through the foramina of Luschka and Magendie into the subarachnoid cisterns surrounding the brainstem and cerebellum. There is continuous circulation between these basal cisterns and the spinal subarachnoid space all the way to the lumbosacral region. Eventually, CSF migrates into the subarach-

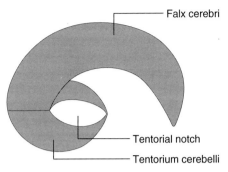

Falx cerebri

Tentorial notch

Tentorium cerebelli

FIGURE 2–6. ■ The *falx cerebri* is a leaf of dura mater that lies between the cerebral hemispheres. The *tentorium cerebelli* is a leaf of dura mater separating the posterior fossa from the middle fossa. The *tentorial hiatus* or *notch* is the opening in the tentorium containing the upper brainstem. With increased intracranial pressure, herniation of components of the cerebrum through the tentorial notch can occur.

noid space over the convexities of the hemispheres alongside the superior sagittal sinus. Arachnoid granulations jut into all of the venous sinuses, but mostly into the superior sagittal sinus. CSF passes through the granulations back into the venous blood. CSF production is continual. The entire reservoir of CSF contains 100–150 ml of fluid, and this amount is totally replaced about every 8 hours.

Very rarely, hydrocephalus is caused by overproduction of CSF, such as by a papilloma of the choroid plexus. Obstructive hydrocephalus is due to blockage of the CSF circulation within the ventricular system (see

ENRICHMENT BOX 2–2

Herniation syndromes

In patients with transtentorial herniation, supratentorial structures shift downward through the tentorial hiatus. In patients with subfalcial herniation, one hemisphere shifts under the falx to the opposite side. In patients with cerebellar tonsillar herniation, the tonsils move through the foramen magnum into the upper cervical spinal canal (see Figure 10–1).

Hydrocephalus

Obstructive hydrocephalus may result when the outlet foramina of the fourth ventricle fail to develop normally; the ventricle becomes massively dilated, creating a cystic structure in the posterior fossa (Dandy-Walker syndrome). In a deviation of obstructive hydrocephalus, congenital stenosis of the aqueduct of Sylvius may cause dilatation of the third and lateral ventricles with a normal-sized fourth ventricle.

Enrichment Box 2–2). Communicating hydrocephalus is caused by impaired circulation of the CSF after it leaves the ventricular system (e.g., from fibrosis and scarring of the basal cisterns because of meningitis) or by impaired function of the arachnoid granulations from subarachnoid hemorrhage. The impaired CSF circulation or decreased absorption transmits increased back pressure into the system, causing compensatory ventricular dilatation. Obstruction at the level of the fourth ventricular outlet foramina is referred to sometimes as a form of obstructive and sometimes as a form of communicating hydrocephalus.

BLOOD–BRAIN BARRIER

Early investigators noticed that when an animal's circulatory system was injected with various dyes, all of the body organs became stained except the brain. They postulated a blood–brain barrier (BBB) to explain this finding. Modern investigators have amply shown the accuracy of the observation. Depending on molecular weight, many compounds are excluded from entry to the CNS by the BBB. For this reason, many antibiotics cannot gain access to the CNS unless the meninges and the BBB are damaged by inflammation. Parkinson disease is treated with levodopa because the BBB excludes dopamine, the compound that is really needed.

Some areas of the CNS lack a BBB. The most clinically important area of the brain that lacks a BBB is the chemoreceptor trigger zone in the area postrema, in the floor of the fourth ventricle. Many drugs produce nausea and vomiting as a prominent side effect because they go directly to the area postrema and stimulate the chemoreceptor trigger zone.

The Thalamus

The thalamus serves as the quarterback of the CNS. It is a relay station that modulates and coordinates the function of various systems. The thalamus serves as a locus for integration, modulation, and intercommunication between various systems and has important motor, sensory, arousal, memory, behavioral, limbic, and cognitive functions. Understanding the general organization and function of the thalamus is important to understanding the workings of the brain. The thalamus is to the nervous system as acetyl coenzyme A is to intermediary metabolism: the point where everything converges. In fact, the word thalamus is from the Greek word for meeting place.

Except for olfaction, all of the ascending sensory tracts end in the thalamus, from which projections are sent to the cortex. The thalamus is sophisticated enough to allow crude appreciation of most sensory modalities. Only very fine discriminative sensory functions such as stereognosis, two-point discrimination, graphesthesia, and precise tactile localization require the cortex. Likewise, the thalamus integrates the motor system, receiving input from the "lower centers" of motor function (e.g., the basal ganglia and cerebellum) and relaying it to the motor cortex. The motor cortex in turns sends collaterals to the thalamus to keep it informed of what the cortex is doing. The thalamus also integrates function between the limbic system, emotional brain, and cortex; is important in arousal mechanisms; subserves important memory circuits; and has specialized relay nuclei for visual and auditory function.

The thalamus sits atop the brainstem. It is divided by internal medullary lamina into large nuclear groups (i.e., medial, lateral, and anterior), which are in turn divided into component nuclei (Figure 2–7). The intralaminar nuclei lie scattered along the internal medullary laminae, and essentially comprise a rostral extension of the brainstem reticular formation. The largest and most easily identified of these is the centromedian nucleus. These nuclei seem primarily concerned with arousal.

ANTERIOR AND MEDIAL NUCLEI

The internal medullary lamina diverges anteriorly, and the anterior nucleus lies between the arms of this Y-shaped structure. The anterior nucleus communicates with the mamillary bodies and the cingulate gyrus, and it is related to memory function (Enrichment Box 2–3).

The medial nucleus is a single large structure that lies on the medial side of the internal medullary lamina. Because its position is also slightly dorsal, it is usually referred to as the mediodorsal or dorsomedial (DM) nucleus. It sends or receives projections from the amygdala, olfactory and limbic systems, hypothalamus, and prefrontal cortex. The DM nucleus has vaguely understood functions related to cognition, judgement, affect, and memory. In patients with Wernicke-Korsakoff disease, lesions typically are located in the DM nucleus and

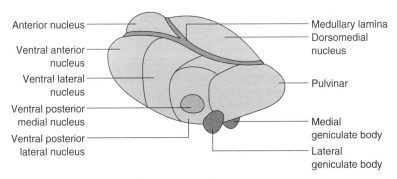

FIGURE 2–7. ▪ The thalamus, showing major nuclei. The internal medullary laminae fork anteriorly to enclose the anterior nucleus.

Anterior nucleus

The mamillothalamic tract ascends from the mamillary bodies bound primarily for the anterior nucleus. The anterior nucleus in turn sends its major output to the cingulate gyrus, so the anterior nucleus of the thalamus is a relay in the limbic system.

Dorsal tier nuclei

Dorsal tier nuclei consist of the lateral dorsal and lateral posterior nuclei and the pulvinar. The lateral posterior nucleus and the pulvinar have reciprocal connections with the occipital and parietal association cortex; they may play a role in extrageniculocalcarine vision or so-called "blindsight," with which completely blind people seem able to crudely localize and respond to visual stimuli.

Ventral tier nuclei

Ventral tier nuclei consist of the major sensory relay nuclei. Ventral posterior lateral (VPL) nuclei receive the termination of the lemniscal and anterolateral (spinothalamic) sensory pathways for the body and project in turn to the somatesthetic cortex (Brodmann areas 1, 2, and 3). Ventral posterior medial (VPM) nuclei serve the same function for the head. Lesions in VPL or VPM, most often strokes, sometimes produce the syndrome of thalamic pain. Patients affected have spontaneous, dysesthetic, often burning pain involving all or part of the contralateral body.

Ventrolateral nucleus

The ventrolateral (VL) nucleus receives input from the basal ganglia [globus pallidus (GP)] and cerebellum (dentate nucleus via superior cerebellar peduncle, the dentatothalamic tract). The VL then projects to the motor and premotor cortices. The motor cortex in turn projects into the striatum, which projects to the GP, which projects to the VL. It is thus via the VL that the basal ganglia and cerebellum influence motor activity.

in the mamillary bodies, and they are likely related to the characteristic memory defects.

LATERAL NUCLEI

In contrast to the straightforward anterior and medial nuclear groups, the lateral nuclear group is subdivided into several component nuclei. The major division is into the dorsal tier and the ventral tier (see Enrichment Box 2–3). In general, the lateral nuclei serve as specific relay stations between motor and sensory systems and the related cortex.

The ventral tier subnuclei of the lateral nucleus are true relay nuclei, connecting lower centers with the cortex and vice versa. The ventral posterior lateral (VPL) nucleus and ventral posterior medial (VPM) nucleus are the major sensory relay nuclei. The ventral lateral (VL) nucleus coordinates the motor system. Occasionally, neurosurgeons place selective, stereotactic lesions in the VL nuclei to treat movement disorders.

The geniculate bodies also are part of the ventral tier. The medial geniculate body receives the termination of the auditory pathways ascending through the brainstem and projects to the auditory cortex. The axons in the optic tract synapse in the lateral geniculate body, from which arise the optic radiations destined for the occipital lobe.

Sensory System

The sensory system includes somatosensory faculties, special senses (e.g., olfaction, taste, vision, and hearing), and unconscious sensory elements. The unconscious sensory systems monitor the position of the limbs in space and help regulate the internal environment. The conscious somatosensory system has two components: the position/vibration/fine touch system and the pain/temperature/crude touch system. Fine touch, position, and vibration sensations from the body are carried over the posterior column/medial lemniscus system. These sensations from the head and face are processed by the principal sensory nucleus in the pons. Pain and temperature sensations from the body are carried over the spinothalamic tracts, from the head and face over the spinal tract and nucleus of the trigeminal nerve (Figure 2–8).

Fine touch, position, and vibration sensation is carried over large, myelinated peripheral nerve fibers from joint capsules, tendon receptors, and pacinian corpuscles. Dorsal root ganglia contain unipolar cells, and the peripheral fibers are technically dendrites, although they usually are referred to as axons. The central processes (true axons) of the dorsal root ganglia cells enter the spinal cord via the posterior root, then turn upward in the ipsilateral posterior column. Fibers from the lumbosacral region aggregate near the midline, and fibers from successively more rostral regions stack up in a progressively more lateral position, producing somatotopically organized lamination (Figure 2–9). All of the fibers below approximately the eighth thoracic vertebra (T8) are grouped together in the fasciculus gracilis; analogous fibers above T8 form the fasciculus cuneatus (see Figure 2–9). Understanding the somatotopic organization of the sensory tracts is important for appreciating certain phenomena seen in diseases of the spinal cord, such as sacral sparing (preservation of sensation in a saddle distribution when there is sensory loss present below a certain spinal level).

Axons in the gracile and cuneate fasciculi synapse with second-order neurons in the gracile and cuneate nuclei at the cervicomedullary

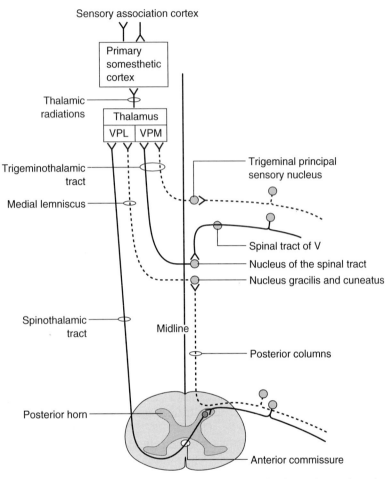

FIGURE 2–8. ■ The light touch, pressure, position, and vibration pathways from the body and face are indicated by the *dashed line;* the pain and temperature fibers from the body and face are indicated by the *solid line.* Fibers from these various sources ultimately converge on the ventral posterior nuclei of the thalamus, which projects via the thalamic radiations to the primary sensory cortex in the postcentral gyrus. V = trigeminal; VPL = ventral posterior lateral; VPM = ventral posterior medial.

junction. The second-order neurons sweep anteriorly as internal arcuate fibers, cross the midline, and accumulate in the medial lemniscus (ML). Somatotopic organization is maintained (Enrichment Box 2–4). The lemniscal fibers are joined by analogous fibers subserving facial sensation, which have decussated after synapsing in the trigeminal principal sensory nucleus in the pons. These fibers all terminate in the

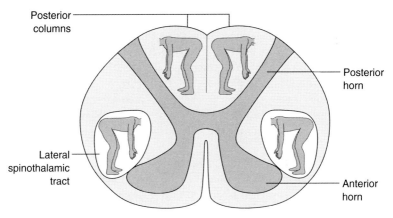

Posterior columns

Posterior horn

Lateral spinothalamic tract

Anterior horn

FIGURE 2–9. ■ The posterior columns and the lateral spinothalamic tracts are both somatotopically organized, but the lamination scheme is opposite in the two systems. In the posterior columns, the sacral fibers are mostly medial; in the spinothalamic tracts, the sacral fibers are mostly lateral. Recall that analogous head and face sensory fibers are not carried by either of these systems.

thalamus, from which the thalamocortical radiations project to the somatosensory cortex.

Fibers subserving pain and temperature arise mostly from free nerve endings in the periphery and travel over small myelinated and unmyelinated axons to enter the spinal cord through the posterior root. These fibers synapse near the substantia gelatinosa of the pos-

ENRICHMENT BOX 2–4

Medial lemniscus

In the medial lemniscus (ML), the head is represented most posteriorly at the medullary level (like a little person standing up). The ML ascends the brainstem, moving from a vertical, paramidline position gradually to a horizontal position (little person sits, then lies down), and finally migrating to lie far lateral at the midbrain level (little person in Trendelenburg position).

Anterolateral system

In the past, anatomists thought the anterior spinothalamic tract carried crude touch and the lateral spinothalamic tract carried pain and temperature sensations. Current evidence suggests that all of these modalities are carried in both tracts, so the lateral and anterior spinothalamic tracts are now sometimes lumped together as the anterolateral system (ALS) or the ventrolateral system.

terior gray horn, then cross the midline in the anterior white commissure to gather into the lateral spinothalamic tract. Lowermost fibers (i.e., sacral and lumbar) entering first are displaced progressively more laterally by subsequently entering fibers, producing somatotopic lamination the reverse of the posterior columns. In the spinothalamic tracts, the sacral fibers are most lateral; in the posterior columns, the lowest fibers are most medial (see Figure 2–9). Some fibers from this system enter the anterior spinothalamic tract (see Enrichment Box 2–4).

The spinothalamic fibers ascend the spinal cord and brainstem in a lateral position. They are joined in the rostral brainstem by the laterally migrating lemniscal fibers, so that ultimately all the fibers subserving somatosensory function run together on the last leg to the thalamus.

Pain and temperature fibers from the face enter the pons through the gasserian ganglion, then descend in the spinal tract of the fifth cranial nerve to varying levels, where they synapse on neurons in the adjacent nucleus of the spinal tract. These second-order neurons decussate and form the trigeminothalamic tract, which is snug against the ascending spinothalamic and lemniscal fibers.

In the upper lateral midbrain, all the somatosensory fibers begin to converge: the ML has moved laterally to lie near the spinothalamic fibers, and these are then joined by the ascending trigeminothalamic fibers. These all proceed to the thalamus, through which they are relayed up to the somatesthetic cortex (see Enrichment Box 2–3).

Motor System

The chief executor of the motor system is the precentral gyrus. It receives input for coordination and control from the premotor and supplementary motor areas of the cortex, the basal ganglia, and the cerebellum. The corticospinal (pyramidal) and corticobulbar tracts arise from the precentral gyrus, descend through the corona radiata, and enter the posterior limb of the internal capsule (Figure 2–10). The internal capsules merge in their descent with the cerebral peduncles, which form the base of the midbrain. In the pons, the descending motor fibers intermingle with crossing pontocerebellar fibers bound for the middle cerebellar peduncle to form a lattice-like network comprising the basis pontis. Enrichment Box 2–5 summarizes the major connections of the motor system.

Corticobulbar fibers terminate in the lower brainstem on cranial nerve nuclei and other structures. Corticopontine fibers, originating from cortical areas other than the precentral gyrus, synapse with pon-

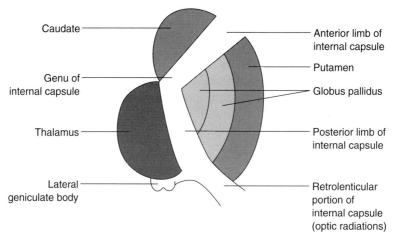

Caudate

Genu of
internal capsule

Thalamus

Lateral
geniculate body

Anterior limb of
internal capsule

Putamen

Globus pallidus

Posterior limb of
internal capsule

Retrolenticular
portion of
internal capsule
(optic radiations)

FIGURE 2–10. ■ The relationships between the internal capsule, basal ganglia, and thalamus. *Corticobulbar fibers* innervating the face and head lie near the genu of the capsule; *corticospinal fibers* lie more posteriorly. The retrolenticular part of the capsule lies posterior to the lentiform nucleus and carries the optic radiations.

ENRICHMENT BOX 2–5

The motor cortex gives rise to the *descending corticospinal tract,* which preferentially innervates contralateral distal muscles and certain pyramidal muscles. It also sends fibers to the *ipsilateral red nucleus* and to the *pontine nuclei.* The pontine nuclei project to the contralateral cerebellum via the *middle cerebellar peduncle.* The contralateral cerebellum in turn projects to the contralateral red nucleus via the *superior cerebellar peduncle,* which decussates in the midbrain. The red nucleus gives rise to the *rubrospinal tract,* which immediately decussates and descends to provide a facilitatory input to the flexor muscles, primarily of the upper extremity. The cerebellum also sends input to the *ipsilateral vestibular nuclei,* which give rise to the *vestibulospinal tract,* which provides facilitatory input to the ipsilateral extensor muscles.

The cerebellar hemispheres influence ipsilateral muscles. The mechanism for this is a double crossing of the projection to the contralateral red nucleus, which in turn decussates back to the same side as the cerebellar hemisphere. The vestibulospinal input remains ipsilateral throughout.

The cerebral motor cortex on one side and the cerebellar hemisphere on the opposite side act in concert to control the arm and leg on a given side of the body. They communicate to coordinate the control by projections from the cerebrum to the pontine nuclei, which project to the contralateral cerebellum, which projects back to the cerebrum on the original side via the decussation of the dentatorubrothalamic tract.

tine nuclei, which then give rise to fibers projecting to the contralateral cerebellum through the middle cerebellar peduncle.

Corticospinal fibers aggregate again into compact bundles, the pyramids, in the medulla (Figure 2–11). At the level of the caudal medulla, 90% of the pyramidal fibers decussate to the opposite side and descend throughout the spinal cord as the lateral corticospinal tract. Approximately 10% of the corticospinal fibers descend ipsilaterally in the anterior corticospinal tract and decussate at the level of the local spinal synapse. Pyramidal fibers preferentially innervate certain lower motor neuron groups (Enrichment Box 2–6).

Descending motor system fibers send collaterals to many other structures to help control and coordinate movement (see Enrichment Boxes 2–3 and 2–6). Other centers and pathways important in motor function include the substantia nigra (SN), rubrospinal tract, and vestibulospinal tract (Figure 2–12). The physiology of the motor system is discussed in more detail in Chapter 3.

Cerebral Hemispheres

The two hemispheres are divided by the interhemispheric fissure, within which lies the falx cerebri. Deep in the fissure run branches of the anterior cerebral artery. The central sulcus demarcates the frontal lobe from the parietal (Figure 2–13). The Sylvian, or lateral, fissure separates the temporal lobe below from the frontal and parietal lobes above. Deep in

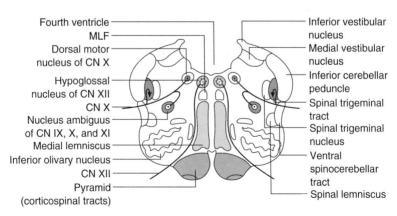

Fourth ventricle
MLF
Dorsal motor nucleus of CN X
Hypoglossal nucleus of CN XII
CN X
Nucleus ambiguus of CN IX, X, and XI
Medial lemniscus
Inferior olivary nucleus
CN XII
Pyramid (corticospinal tracts)

Inferior vestibular nucleus
Medial vestibular nucleus
Inferior cerebellar peduncle
Spinal trigeminal tract
Spinal trigeminal nucleus
Ventral spinocerebellar tract
Spinal lemniscus

FIGURE 2–11. ■ The medulla at midolivary level showing the *pyramids, olives, nuclei of the hypoglossal and ambiguus nerves, medial lemniscus, medial longitudinal fasciculus,* and *spinal tract of the trigeminal nerve.* (Modified with permission from Fix JD: *BRS: Neuroanatomy,* 2nd ed. Baltimore, Williams and Wilkins, 1995, p 147.) CN = cranial nerve; MLF = medial longitudinal fasciculus.

Distal muscles, especially hand muscles, receive more pyramidal innervation than proximal muscles. In the upper extremity, the wrist, finger, and elbow extensors and the external rotators and abductors of the shoulder are preferentially innervated. In the lower extremity, the foot and toe extensors and the knee and hip flexors receive more pyramidal innervation than their antagonists. This pyramidal distribution is important clinically, and is discussed in more detail in Chapters 5 and 6.

Although fibers from the motor cortex project downward through the internal capsule, they simultaneously send fibers to the caudate and putamen, which in turn project to the globus pallidus (GP). The major output of the basal ganglia is via the GP. Fibers project from the GP to the ventral lateral (VL) nucleus of the thalamus. VL also receives the dentatothalamic tract from the cerebellum. VL projects to the motor cortex, and thus serves to integrate these various motor functions.

The motor cortex and cerebellum are also part of a circuit. Corticopontine fibers convey impulses from the cortex onto pontine nuclei, from which pontocerebellar fibers project across the midline to enter the cerebellum via the contralateral middle cerebellar peduncle. The cerebellum in turn projects to the VL via the superior cerebellar peduncle, which decussates in the midbrain back to the appropriate side. VL in turn projects to the motor cortex to complete the circuit. The cerebellum also receives unconscious proprioception from muscle spindles and Golgi tendon organs via the spinocerebellar and cuneocerebellar tracts.

Cerebellar output is ipsilateral. The right cerebellar hemisphere receives input from the left cerebral cortex via the middle cerebellar peduncle and projects back to the left thalamus and motor cortex via the superior cerebellar peduncle. Therefore, both the left cerebral hemisphere and the right cerebellar hemisphere control movements on the right side of the body (see Figure 2–12).

The substantia nigra (SN) projects to the striatum and influences its activity. The rubrospinal tract descends from the red nucleus to the spinal cord, where it facilitates flexor muscle tone, primarily in the upper extremities. The vestibulospinal tract descends from the vestibular nuclei to the spinal cord, where it facilitates extensor tone. The premotor and supplementary cortices contribute by controlling the planning and preliminary preparation for movements that the primary motor cortex executes.

the depths of the Sylvian fissure lies the insula, and more superficially run branches of the middle cerebral artery. The landmarks separating the occipital lobe are vague and of no clinical consequence.

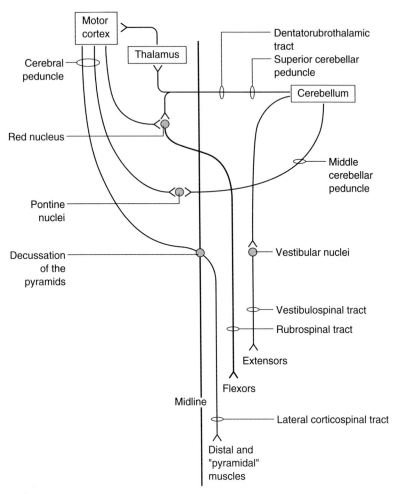

FIGURE 2–12. ■ Major connections of the motor system (see Enrichment Box 2–5).

FRONTAL LOBE

The frontal lobe contains a vast amount of tissue whose function is uncertain. Large lesions may occupy this "silent area" without producing any apparent clinical deficit. When dysfunction does occur, it involves abnormalities in behavior, judgment, and intellect.

The precentral gyrus, or motor strip, lies just anterior to the central sulcus (see Figure 2–13). Giant pyramidal neurons, or Betz cells, residing here give rise to the major descending motor pathways, the corticospinal and corticobulbar tracts. Anterior to the motor strip lie the premotor and supplementary motor regions. Other important structures

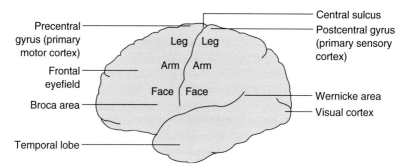

FIGURE 2–13. ■ Lateral view of a cerebral hemisphere showing the location of some major clinically important areas.

in the frontal lobe include the frontal eye fields and Broca area (Enrichment Box 2–7).

PARIETAL LOBE

The somatosensory cortex receives the thalamocortical sensory radiations from the VPL and VPM thalamic nuclei. Adjacent to the primary somatesthetic cortex lies the sensory association cortex. Parietal lobe lesions produce abnormalities of higher-level sensory functions, which require the association cortex (i.e., stereognosis, graphesthesia, two-point discrimination, and tactile localization).

The angular gyrus lies just at the posterior end of the Sylvian fissure

---

ENRICHMENT BOX 2–7

Lying anterior to the motor strip, the frontal eye fields are responsible for conjugate horizontal gaze to the contralateral side. Gaze palsies and deviations of different sorts are important clinical localizing signs. Patients with seizures originating focally in one frontal lobe may show tonic deviation of the eyes to the opposite side. With damage to one frontal eye field, as in an acute stroke, patients are unable to look to the opposite side; because of unopposed action by the intact fellow eye field in the other hemisphere, they often have gaze deviation toward the damaged hemisphere. The clinically important subject of gaze palsies and deviations is discussed in more detail in Chapter 7.

Lying in the inferior part of the dominant frontal lobe, Broca area subserves the motor, articulatory control of language. Patients with damage to Broca area have severely nonfluent speech with intact comprehension. Broca area is connected to Wernicke area by the arcuate fasciculus.

immediately adjacent to Wernicke area (see Figure 2–13). Dominant hemisphere lesions located here produce various combinations of anomic aphasia, agraphia, finger agnosia, and right–left confusion. Patients with nondominant parietal lobe lesions may display various forms of apraxia, hemi-inattention, hemineglect, and denial of disability, culminating in the amazing syndrome of anosognosia, in which patients deny owning their contralateral limbs.

TEMPORAL LOBE

At the posterior end of the Sylvian fissure lies the Wernicke area, essentially the sensory association cortex for the auditory cortex (transverse temporal gyri of Heschl). Patients with lesions here have Wernicke aphasia, characterized by lack of speech comprehension and fluent speech; their speech is devoid of content and often totally nonsensical (e.g., "word salad", jargon aphasia).

The structures of the medial temporal lobe, the uncus, hippocampus, and amygdala are important in memory and limbic lobe functions. The temporal lobe also contains fibers of the optic radiations. After synapsing in the lateral geniculate body, fibers from the lower retina (upper visual field) fan out far anteriorly in the temporal lobe before looping back and heading for the occipital lobe. These anterior fibers are referred to as Meyer's loop. Lesions in the anterior temporal lobe, most often tumors, may involve these fibers and produce as an early clinical manifestation a contralateral superior quadrantanopia ("pie in the sky", see Chapter 7).

OCCIPITAL LOBE

The occipital lobe contains the primary visual cortex, the calcarine cortex, and the visual association cortex (Figure 2–14). The visual cortex

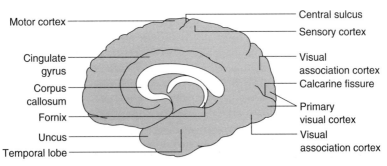

FIGURE 2–14. ■ Medial view of a cerebral hemisphere showing the location of some major clinically important areas.

receives the optic radiations, axons that arise from the neurons in the lateral geniculate body. The visual cortex is visuotopically organized, which can have localizing significance (Enrichment Box 2–8).

Corona Radiata

All of the assorted fibers coming to and proceeding from the cortex make up the fan-shaped corona radiata. It is easy to see how early CNS dissectors saw this profusion of fibers going in all directions as a "radiating crown" perched atop the internal capsule.

Internal Capsule

Fibers of the corona radiata funnel into and out of the internal capsule. Fibers ascending to and descending from the anterior frontal lobe run in the anterior limb. Progressively more posterior cortical areas use more posterior parts of the capsule. Corticobulbar fibers descending from the precentral gyrus occupy the genu. Corticospinal fibers were previously thought to lie in the anterior two-thirds of the posterior limb, but more recent work suggests they occupy a bundle more posteriorly. Thalamic radiations to and from the parietal lobe also occupy the posterior limb. The optic radiations are so far back, lying in the part of the capsule posterior to the lenticular nuclei, that they are said to run in the retrolenticular part of the capsule.

The internal capsule is frequently involved in cerebrovascular disease, especially small-vessel lacunar infarcts related to hypertension. Because all of the descending motor fibers are grouped compactly together, a single small lesion impairs the function in all of them and pro-

---

ENRICHMENT BOX 2–8

In the optic radiations, lower retinal fibers run forward in the temporal lobe before looping back; upper retinal fibers run in the deep parietal lobe. The optic radiations converge as they approach the occipital lobe, with the upper retinal (parietal) fibers contacting the upper bank of the cortex as the lower retinal (temporal looping) fibers contact the lower bank. In the visual cortex, macular fibers are most posterior; progressively more peripheral retinal fibers are progressively more anterior.

Lesions along the visual pathway produce different types of visual field defects, which are discussed in more detail in Chapter 7. The general localization rules are as follows: the more congruous a field cut, the more posterior the lesion; macular sparing indicates an occipital lesion; homonymous defects are postchiasmal; heteronymous defects are chiasmal; and uniocular defects are prechiasmal.

duces a pure motor hemiparesis with equal involvement of face, arm, and leg: the syndrome of capsular stroke.

Olfactory Pathways and the Limbic System

OLFACTION

The olfactory nerves are short structures that travel only the distance from the olfactory mucosa through the cribriform plate to synapse in the olfactory bulbs. The olfactory tracts arise from the bulbs and run along the inferior surface of the frontal lobe toward the optic chiasm. Just before termination, the tracts divide into medial and lateral olfactory striae. In the Y-shaped space between the striae lies the anterior perforated substance. The perforations are caused by the lenticulostriate arteries. The lateral olfactory striae project to the region of the hippocampus and amygdala, which in turn have connections with the limbic system.

Anosmia most often results from dysfunction of the olfactory epithelium related to viral infection or chronic sinus disease. Occasionally, the olfactory nerves are damaged traumatically, sometimes with an associated fracture through the cribriform plate. Anosmia is a common sequela of head injury.

LIMBIC SYSTEM

Components of the limbic lobe include the hippocampus, which lies deep in the medial temporal lobe and becomes continuous with the fornix; the mamillary bodies, which are part of the hypothalamus; the anterior nucleus of the thalamus; the cingulate gyrus; and the parahippocampal gyrus. These structures are connected in sequence in Papez circuit. The limbic system is phylogenetically old and is involved with emotion, behavior, memory, olfaction, and other hypothalamic functions. The limbic lobe is not so much a structurally separate entity as it is a functional system. It is sometimes involved in a peculiar syndrome called limbic encephalitis, which occurs most often as a paraneoplastic syndrome.

Hypothalamus

The hypothalamus makes up the walls and floor of the anterior third ventricle, stretching from the optic chiasm to the mamillary bodies. The infundibulum arises from the hypothalamus, connects it to the pituitary, and provides the conduit for releasing factors and neurotransmitters. Numerous nuclei make up the hypothalamus; the details are of little clinical importance. The regulation of thirst, serum osmolality, appetite, sexual function, body temperature, and some emotions resides in the hypothalamus. Lesions in the region may produce any number of aberrations of these functions (Enrichment Box 2–9).

Basal Ganglia

STRUCTURE

Basal ganglia terminology can be confusing, and it is not used very consistently. The caudate, putamen, and globus pallidus (GP) are all intimately related from an anatomic and functional standpoint, so the term corpus striatum is sometimes applied to the whole complex. The term *basal ganglia* includes these plus other related structures, such as the subthalamic nucleus, SN, and claustrum. Most clinicians use the term basal ganglia to refer to the caudate, putamen, GP, and SN.

The *caudate* (tailed) nucleus is composed of a head, body, and tail. The head is connected by gray matter bridges to the putamen and forms a prominent structure indenting the lateral wall of the lateral ventricle anteriorly. Loss of the head of the caudate, producing a square-shaped lateral ventricle, is a neuroradiologic sign of Huntington chorea. The body and progressively thinner tail of the caudate extend backward from the head and arch along just outside the wall of the lateral ventricle, ultimately following the curve of the temporal horn and ending in the medial temporal lobe in close approximation to the amygdala. The caudate is thus a long C-shaped structure with bulbous ends. The long, curving tail is the feature that gave the caudate its name.

The *putamen* is basically an extension of the caudate, separated by fibers of the anterior limb of the internal capsule. As the corticospinal and corticobulbar fibers descend from the primary motor strip, they pass between and intermingle with the gray matter bridges that con-

ENRICHMENT BOX 2–9

Clinical manifestations of hypothalamic dysfunction include hyperthermia, hypothermia, hyperphagia and obesity, anorexia and wasting, rage reactions, and sexual dysfunction. The more frequent of these include diabetes insipidus and hyperthermia due to hypothalamic failure in patients with severe central nervous system (CNS) pathology, such as head injury or intracranial hemorrhage (so-called central fever). In pediatric patients, precocious puberty sometimes results from hypothalamic disease.

nect the caudate and putamen. These heavily myelinated capsular fibers cause the caudate–putamen junction to look striped; hence the etymology of the term corpus striatum (striped body) to refer to the caudate and putamen. The putamen is a frequent site for hypertensive intracerebral hemorrhage.

The *GP* lies medial to the putamen and just lateral to the third ventricle. The putamen and GP together are shaped like a lens, hence the term lenticular nuclei (see Figure 2–10). The GP is separated from the caudate by the anterior limb and from the thalamus by the posterior limb of the internal capsule. Myelinated fibers running through this gray matter structure led to its name ("pale body").

The *SN* lies in the midbrain just posterior to the cerebral peduncle. It is divided into pars compacta and pars reticulata portions. In the pars compacta lie the prominent melanin-containing neurons, which give the region its dark color and its name.

FUNCTION

The caudate/putamen serves as the central receiving area of the basal ganglia. The majority of the output from the caudate/putamen goes to the GP. The GP is then responsible for most of the output; it is essentially the effector system of the basal ganglia. A host of motor abnormalities may occur with basal ganglia disease (Enrichment Box 2–10).

ENRICHMENT BOX 2–10

Globus pallidus

Efferent fibers from the globus pallidus (GP) travel through or around the intervening fibers of the internal capsule en route to the ventrolateral (VL) nucleus of the thalamus. The VL nucleus of the thalamus in turn projects to the motor cortex. Therefore, the important influences of the basal ganglia on motor function are exerted indirectly by connections via the VL nucleus to the motor cortex, rather than by a separate descending pathway.

Basal ganglia disorders

The most common basal ganglia disorder is Parkinson disease, which is manifested by hypokinesia (poverty of movement), bradykinesia (slowness of movement), rigidity, resting tremor, and impaired postural reflexes. Loss of the caudate mass is a neuroradiologic sign of Huntington disease, which is characterized by chorea. Athetosis and dystonia are other movement disorders that occur with basal ganglia disease.

Brainstem

GENERAL CHARACTERISTICS

Brainstem anatomy is quite important in clinical neurology. Brainstem syndromes are common and often confusing. The brainstem, throughout its length, is composed of three parts: tectum (roof), tegmentum (midportion), and base (Figure 2–15). In the midbrain, the tectum consists of the quadrigeminal plate. In the pons and medulla, the tectum devolves into nonfunctional tissue forming the roof plate of the fourth ventricle, the anterior medullary velum in the pons, and the posterior medullary velum in the medulla. The base is straightforward: descending corticospinal and corticobulbar fibers in different configurations. The tegmentum is where the action is. Running throughout the length of the tegmentum is the reticular core, a loose network of neurons with extensive connections and ramifications with most of the ascending and descending pathways; the reticular core terminates at the intralaminar nuclei of the thalamus. The reticular activating system is part of this loose network, and is responsible for controlling arousal. Running in the tegmentum are the long ascending and descending tracts (e.g., medial lemniscus, spinothalamic tract, rubrospinal tract). The motor and sensory nuclei associated with cranial nerves also reside in the tegmentum.

PRETECTUM

The pretectum is the short section of the far rostral brainstem sandwiched between the midbrain and the thalamus. It is the region subserving the pupillary light reflex (Enrichment Box 2–11). The pathways for upgaze run through the pretectum and adjacent midbrain; lesions in this area sometimes cause upgaze paresis or forced downgaze.

MIDBRAIN

The midbrain is composed of tectum, tegmentum, and base. The tectum is the quadrigeminal plate, and the base is the crus cerebri. There are two segmental levels with different characteristics.

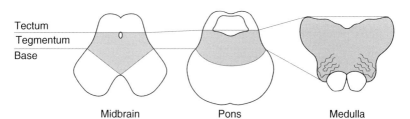

Tectum
Tegmentum
Base

Midbrain   Pons   Medulla

FIGURE 2–15. ■ Three levels of the brainstem showing what constitutes the tectum, tegmentum, and base at each level.

ENRICHMENT BOX 2–11

In the pretectum, collaterals from optic tract fibers synapse on interneurons, which in turn synapse on the nearby Edinger- Westphal subnucleus of the oculomotor nuclear complex in the midbrain. There is abundant crossing, explaining the direct and consensual features of the pupillary light reflex. Argyll Robertson pupils result from lesions in the pretectum or adjacent midbrain. Although classic for neurosyphilis, conditions such as multiple sclerosis and neurosarcoidosis may be more common causes in the modern era. So-called "tectal" pupils are large pupils with light near dissociation (see Chapter 7). The posterior commissure is a prominent tract across the pretectal area. Lesions in the vicinity of the posterior commissure characteristically produce sustained bilateral eyelid retraction and a staring expression (Collier sign).

Parinaud syndrome (upgaze paresis with retraction-convergence nystagmus on trying to look up, plus tectal pupils) is usually due to pressure on the pretectum. Pretectal/midbrain dysfunction from ballooning of the posterior third ventricle in obstructive hydrocephalus can cause a forced downgaze in infants (i.e., the setting sun sign).

Superior Colliculus Level

The functions of the superior colliculi are closely related to those of the pretectum. In addition, they subserve visual reflexes, tracking, and orienting behavior. In the tegmentum at this level the most prominent structure is the red nucleus, which gives rise to an important descending pathway, the rubrospinal tract (Figure 2–16). After decussating, the rubrospinal tract descends in the lateral funiculus of the spinal cord, lying just beside the pyramidal tract; it functions to facilitate flexor tone.

The third nerve nuclei lie in the midline anterior to the aqueduct, and send axons that stream through and around the red nucleus to exit in the interpeduncular fossa. The ML, which was in the midline in the medulla, has by now in its ascent moved out far laterally, and been joined by ascending fibers of the anterolateral (spinothalamic) system and trigeminothalamic tract. The medial longitudinal fasciculus (MLF) courses posteriorly in the midline, bound for the medial rectus subnucleus of the oculomotor complex. Lying in the area adjacent to the aqueduct is the superior cerebellar peduncle, the major efferent pathway from the cerebellum. The gray matter immediately surrounding the aqueduct is one of the characteristic sites for lesions in patients with Wernicke disease.

Anteriorly at this level, the base of the midbrain is composed of the crus cerebri, which consists of the SN and cerebral peduncle. The cere-

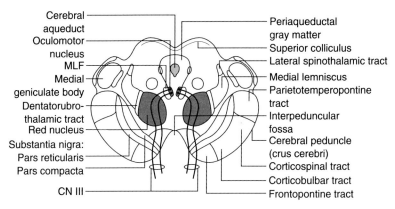

FIGURE 2–16. ■ The midbrain at the superior collicular level, showing the *oculomotor nucleus,* the *red nucleus,* and the *fibers of the third nerve* as they exit through the interpeduncular fossa. (Modified with permission from Fix JD: *BRS: Neuroanatomy,* 2nd ed. Baltimore, Williams and Wilkins, 1995, p 155.) CN = cranial nerve; MLF = medial longitudinal fasciculus.

bral peduncle is a direct continuation of the internal capsule and conveys mostly descending corticospinal and corticobulbar fibers. In the space between the peduncles (i.e., the interpeduncular fossa), the third nerve emerges. Vascular lesions at this level of the midbrain, primarily strokes, may cause Weber syndrome, which is third nerve palsy with a contralateral hemiparesis, a neurologic classic. The basilar artery divides into its terminal branches at the level of the upper midbrain. Vascular lesions in this location produce the "top of the basilar syndrome," in which evidence of midbrain dysfunction is prominent.

Inferior Colliculus Level

The inferior colliculus is a relay station in the auditory pathway; it receives fibers from the lateral lemniscus and sends fibers to the medial geniculate body, which in turn sends fibers to the auditory cortex. In the tegmentum at this level, the most prominent structure is the decussation of the superior cerebellar peduncle (Figure 2–17). These axons originated in the dentate nucleus and cross the midline bound for the contralateral VL nucleus of the thalamus. The superior cerebellar peduncle is, for all practical purposes, the dentatothalamic tract. The fibers dance in and around the red nucleus, completely obscuring it at this level. (The tract was once called the dentatorubrothalamic tract, until it became clear that most of the fibers passed through the red nucleus without synapsing, and the "rubro" was deleted in the lexicon).

The fourth nerve nuclei lie posteriorly just beneath the aqueduct.

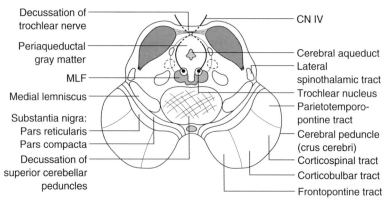

FIGURE 2–17. ▪ The midbrain at the inferior collicular level showing the decussa-tion of the *superior cerebellar peduncle,* the medial longitudinal fasciculus, and *fibers of the fourth nerve* as they exit through the tectum. (Modified with permis-sion from Fix JD: *BRS: Neuroanatomy,* 2nd ed. Baltimore, Williams and Wilkins, 1995, p 154.) CN = cranial nerve; MLF = medial longitudinal fasciculus.

The fourth nerve takes a highly aberrant course out of the brainstem, curving posteriorly to decussate in the tectum and exit through the dor-sal surface. The fourth is the only cranial nerve to cross and the only one to exit dorsally. The remainder of the tegmentum and base are es-sentially the same as at the superior collicular level.

PONS

At the level of the pons, the tectum consists of the nonfunctional ante-rior medullary velum. The base is rounded and protuberant (the "belly" of the pons) and consists of descending corticospinal and corticobulbar fibers admixed with crossing pontocerebellar fibers entering the middle cerebellar peduncle (Figure 2–18 and Enrichment Box 2–12). The tegmentum of the pons contains numerous important structures such as the cranial nerve nuclei and the pontine lateral gaze center. The major long tracts include the medial and lateral lemnisci and the MLF.

Near the midline in the gray matter lies the sixth nerve nucleus, around which loop seventh nerve fibers. Fibers of the sixth nerve exit straight out through the front of the pons, in the same manner as third nerve fibers exit the midbrain into the interpeduncular fossa. Fibers of the seventh nerve, which loop around the sixth nerve nucleus, are called the internal genu of the facial nerve. They form a bump in the floor of the fourth nerve called the facial colliculus, which is a promi-nent landmark for surgeons. The seventh nucleus lies more antero-laterally because of its branchial arch relationships.

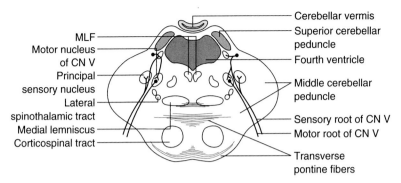

FIGURE 2–18. ■ The midpons, showing the cavity of the *fourth ventricle, trigeminal nucleus, medial longitudinal fasciculus, transverse pontine fibers,* and *cerebellar peduncles.* (Modified with permission from Fix JD: *BRS: Neuroanatomy,* 2nd ed. Baltimore, Williams and Wilkins, 1995, p 151. CN = cranial nerve; MLF = medial longitudinal fasciculus.

After circling the sixth nerve nucleus, facial nerve fibers exit the pons laterally (typical behavior for branchial arch–related nerves), cross the cerebellopontine angle (CPA) in company with the eighth cranial nerve, and disappear into the internal auditory meatus. When facial muscle weakness is present, its pattern is highly localizing (Enrichment Box 2–13).

The gasserian, or trigeminal, ganglion lies just beside the pons in a depression in the petrous ridge called Meckel cave. A large sensory and a smaller motor root join the ganglion to the pons. The motor fibers are derived from the trigeminal motor nucleus in the lateral pontine tegmentum and are destined for the nerve's mandibular division. Afferent fibers conveying light touch and pressure enter the

---

ENRICHMENT BOX 2–12

In the belly of the pons, descending corticopontine fibers synapse on pontine nuclei in the base. Axons from the pontine nuclei cross to the opposite side and enter the massive middle cerebellar peduncle (MCP) en route to the cerebellum. Efferent fibers from the cerebellum go to the ventral lateral (VL) nucleus of the thalamus and are relayed to the cortex, which then sends fibers to the pontine nuclei, forming a corticocerebellocortical motor control servoloop. The base of the pons is thus made up of a lattice created by descending corticospinal/bulbar fibers and crossing pontine nuclei/MCP fibers, within which lie scattered pontine nuclei.

ENRICHMENT BOX 2-13

The facial nucleus neurons supplying the upper face receive both crossed and uncrossed corticobulbar fibers, whereas those supplying the lower face receive only crossed fibers. Because of this residual innervation by the intact ipsilateral hemisphere, some or all of the strength of the upper face is preserved in patients with an upper motor neuron facial palsy. Pathology involving the facial nucleus or nerve fibers proper, however, has no sparing of the upper face. A central or upper motor neuron facial palsy is therefore characterized by weakness disproportionately more severe in the lower face; a peripheral or lower motor neuron facial palsy is characterized by equal and symmetric weakness of both lower and upper facial muscles.

principal sensory nucleus, which lies beside the trigeminal motor nucleus; there, they synapse and give rise to second-order neurons, which cross the midline on the way to the VPM thalamic nucleus. Fibers conveying pain and temperature enter the spinal tract of the trigeminal nerve, where they descend to various levels (depending on their somatotopic origin) and synapse in the adjacent nucleus of the spinal tract. The axons of second-order neurons cross the midline, aggregate as the trigeminothalamic tract, and ascend to VPM in nucleus of the thalamus with their traveling companions, the medial lemniscus and spinothalamic tracts.

Just within or adjacent to the sixth nucleus in the pontine paramedian reticular formation lies the pontine lateral gaze center, an important structure involved in horizontal conjugate gaze (Enrichment Box 2-14).

At the junction of pons and medulla, the eighth nerve enters far laterally after crossing the CPA. The cochlear component consists of fibers from the organ of Corti and the spiral ganglion of the cochlea, which synapse in the cochlear nuclei. From the cochlear nuclei a complex, crossed, and uncrossed ascending pathway with multiple nuclear relays arises. Most auditory fibers eventually ascend in the lateral lemniscus en route to the inferior colliculus, then to the medial geniculate and on to the auditory cortex in the temporal lobe.

The vestibular component consists of fibers from the vestibular ganglion, which synapse in one of the four vestibular nuclei. Fibers from these nuclei ascend and descend the brainstem and spinal cord as vestibulospinal tracts and as part of the MLF. The vestibulospinal tract is important in facilitating extensor muscle tone and is a counterbalance to the rubrospinal tract, which facilitates flexor tone.

ENRICHMENT BOX 2-14

Pontine lateral gaze center

Descending fibers from the contralateral frontal eye field synapse on the pontine lateral gaze center. On receiving a command to initiate lateral gaze, the pontine paramedian reticular formation activates the nearby sixth nucleus and simultaneously sends impulses up the medial longitudinal fasciculus (MLF) to activate the contralateral medial rectus subunit of the third nerve nucleus, thus producing coordinated conjugate lateral gaze. Patients with lesions in the area of the pontine paramedian reticular formation have a gaze palsy toward the lesion; a patient with a frontal eye field lesion cannot gaze contralateral to the lesion. A lesion of the MLF produces inability to adduct the involved eye on horizontal gaze (i.e., an internuclear ophthalmoplegia).

The lateral medulla

The inferior cerebellar peduncle is a prominent structure arising from the lateral aspect of the medulla and receiving fibers from the ascending spinocerebellar tracts as well as from the olive. The nucleus ambiguus lies deep in the tegmentum anterolaterally, in a position analogous to that of the seventh nucleus in the pons, again because of its branchial arch innervation relationships. From the nucleus ambiguus, motor fibers exit laterally to enter both the ninth and tenth nerves. The dorsal motor nucleus of the vagus nerve, which supplies the vagus nerve with its autonomic component, sends fibers laterally to join with the exiting ambiguus fibers. The solitary tract lies lateral to the dorsal motor nucleus of the vagus nerve and receives entering taste fibers from the facial and glossopharyngeal nerves. Descending in the reticular core are sympathetic fibers destined for the intermediolateral gray column of the thoracic and lumbar cord.

MEDULLA

In the medulla, the tectum again consists of nonfunctional tissue in the roof of the fourth ventricle, the posterior medullary velum. The base consists of the medullary pyramids, which are in the process of decussating (see Figure 2–11).

The tegmentum of the medulla is conveniently divided into medial and lateral portions, especially because of the differences in blood supply. The medial medulla contains the medial lemniscus in a vertical midline position (like a little person standing up) with the MLF capping it posteriorly. The hypoglossal nerve nucleus lies in the midline and projects axons that exit anteriorly in the groove between the pyramid and the olive. The olive is a prominent, wrinkled structure lying just posterior to the pyramids. Neurons in the olive project axons that cross the midline to enter the contralateral inferior cerebellar peduncle.

The lateral medulla contains the spinal tract and nucleus of the trigeminal nerve; ascending spinothalamic (anterolateral system) fibers run nearby. Other important structures in the lateral medulla include the inferior cerebellar peduncle, nucleus ambiguus, dorsal motor nucleus of the vagus, solitary tract, and descending sympathetic fibers (see Enrichment Box 2–14).

The lateral medullary (Wallenberg) syndrome is the most common brainstem stroke. It is caused by ischemia of the posterior inferior cerebellar artery (PICA), which supplies the lateral medulla (either from PICA or, more commonly, vertebral artery disease). The clinical manifestations of Wallenberg syndrome directly reflect the anatomy of the region.

Cerebellum

The cerebellum has the task of bringing finesse to the motor system. Lesions of the cerebellum do not cause weakness but rather loss of the ability to gauge and regulate the rate, range, and force of movement. Cerebellar lesions produce ataxia, a composite term clinically connoting tremor, incoordination, impaired rapid alternating movements, impaired balance, and difficulty with gait.

Anatomically, the cerebellum is divided into three lobes: anterior, posterior, and flocculonodular, each of which has a vermis and hemisphere portion. Clinicians usually divide it into the hemispheres, which are responsible for appendicular coordination; the anterior vermis, which is responsible for gait functions; and the flocculonodular lobe (or vestibulocerebellum), which is concerned with vestibular function. The clinical manifestations of disease in the flocculonodular lobe are difficult to separate from the invariably accompanying vestibular findings, primarily nystagmus. Isolated flocculonodular lobe dysfunction is usually caused by ependymomas and medulloblastomas in children. The vermis lies in the midline and subserves midline functions such as sitting and walking. Disease in the vermis may have no clinical signs other than gait ataxia, which is the situation in alcoholic cerebellar degeneration that characteristically affects the anterior, superior vermis.

The bulk of the cerebellum is made up of the phylogenetically new hemispheres. These are concerned with coordinating movement and providing fine motor control to the extremities. The modulatory influence of the cerebellar hemispheres is achieved by linking their output with continuous sampling of the position of the limbs in space, mediated by the spinocerebellar tracts (Enrichment Box 2–15).

ENRICHMENT BOX 2–15

To coordinate cerebellar function, large myelinated muscle spindle and Golgi tendon organ afferents travel to the cerebellum via the spinocerebellar tracts and enter primarily through the inferior cerebellar peduncle. This information is processed in the hemispheres and influences the activity of Purkinje cells in the deep midline (primarily dentate) nucleus. The Purkinje cells send axons via the superior cerebellar peduncle (SCP) to the contralateral ventrolateral nucleus of the thalamus, which in turn projects to the motor cortex. Descending cortical fibers then synapse on pontine nuclei in the basis pontis, which in turn send axons via the middle cerebellar peduncle (MCP) to the cerebellar hemispheres. Other descending corticomotor fibers actually execute the task at hand. The cerebellum can thereby communicate the need for fine adjustment of movement to the cortex, and the cortex can take corrective action while simultaneously informing the cerebellum of the extent of the correction so that further adjustments can be made.

Cranial Nerves

OLFACTORY NERVE

The olfactory nerve (CN I) is described under the LIMBIC SYSTEM.

OPTIC NERVES

The optic nerves (CN II) are formed by axons of retinal ganglion cells, which exit the eye through the lamina cribrosa, acquire a myelin sheath, travel through the posterior orbit and optic canal, and emerge from the optic foramina to join at the chiasm. Fibers from the temporal retina continue into the ipsilateral optic tract, whereas fibers from the nasal retina decussate and enter the contralateral optic tract.

The macula lutea is the fixation point and site of greatest visual acuity and color perception. The projection of the macula to the optic nerve is massive, and macular fibers make up approximately 90% of all optic nerve fibers. Because of this preponderance of macular fibers in the optic nerve, early signs of optic nerve disease reflect macular function: impaired color vision, impaired acuity, and central scotoma. Further details regarding the optic nerve are found in Chapter 7.

OCULOMOTOR NERVE

The third cranial nerve (CN III) arises from the oculomotor complex in the midbrain and conveys motor fibers to extraocular muscles, as well as parasympathetic fibers to the pupil and ciliary body. It exits the midbrain in the interpeduncular fossa, travels between the posterior cerebral and superior cerebellar artery, and runs alongside the posterior communicating artery. Third nerve palsy is a classic and important sign of posterior communicating aneurysm. The nerve travels through the cavernous sinus, where it has important relationships with the carotid artery, ascending pericarotid sympathetics, and cranial nerves four, five, and six. After exiting the cavernous sinus and passing through the superior orbital fissure, the third nerve innervates the medial rectus, inferior oblique, and superior and inferior recti. Long ciliary nerves swerve off to the ciliary ganglion, from which short ciliary nerves arise to innervate the iris and ciliary body.

TROCHLEAR NERVE

The fourth nerve (CN IV) arises from the trochlear nucleus at the level of the inferior colliculus, and travels backward and around to decussate and exit through the tectum (see Figure 2–17). The nerve winds around the brainstem from its exit in the tectum, then runs forward, passes through the cavernous sinus in proximity to the oculomotor nerve, traverses the superior orbital fissure, and enters the orbit to supply the superior oblique. Despite having the longest intracranial course of any cranial nerve, it is seldom injured. Fourth nerve palsy produces difficulty with depressing the adducted eye.

TRIGEMINAL NERVE

Motor fibers of the trigeminal nerve (CN V) arise from the motor nucleus in the midpons, exit laterally, pass through the gasserian ganglion, and travel with the mandibular sensory branch to exit the skull through the foramen ovale. Trigeminal motor fibers innervate the masseter, temporalis, and pterygoid muscles.

Sensory trigeminal fibers arise from the ophthalmic, maxillary, and mandibular divisions supplying the face. Ophthalmic fibers enter the skull via the superior orbital fissure, and maxillary fibers enter through the foramen rotundum; both pass through the cavernous sinus before joining the ganglion. The mandibular fibers enter through the foramen ovale, and just nip the posterior end of the cavernous sinus before entering the ganglion. For the central connections of the trigeminal nerve, refer to the section on the BRAINSTEM.

ABDUCENS NERVE

The cells of origin of the abducens nerve, CN VI, lie in the pons near the pontine lateral gaze center. Axons pass forward through the substance of the pons, weaving among descending corticospinal fibers, and exit anteriorly. The sixth nerve climbs up the clivus; traverses the cavernous sinus in company with the third, fourth, and fifth nerves; then passes through the superior orbital fissure and enters the orbit to innervate the lateral rectus muscle. The abducens nerve has a lengthy peripheral course, which likely is the reason for its proneness to injury. Sixth nerve palsies occur with increased intracranial pressure, after head injury, after lumbar puncture, with structural disease in the middle or posterior fossa, and for numerous other reasons (see Chapter 7). Many remain unexplained. Sixth nerve palsies are the most common and classic of all false localizing signs: they are nonspecific and bear no necessary anatomic relationship to the CNS pathology producing them.

FACIAL NERVE

Axons of the facial nerve (CN VII) arise from the facial nucleus in the pontine tegmentum (see BRAINSTEM); travel backward, up and around the sixth nerve nucleus (internal genu); then cross the pons to exit laterally. In the company of the eighth nerve, the facial nerve crosses the CPA, enters the internal auditory meatus, and travels along the internal auditory canal. It parts company with the eighth nerve and curves down and away at the external genu, which is also the location of the geniculate ganglion. After traversing the remainder of the petrous bone, the seventh cranial nerve exits through the stylomastoid foramen, turns forward, passes under the parotid gland, and ramifies into upper and lower divisions to supply the muscles of facial expression and provide taste sensation to the anterior two-thirds of the tongue.

The most common disorder by far of the facial nerve is Bell palsy (Enrichment Box 2–16).

VESTIBULOCOCHLEAR NERVE

The cochlear portion of CN VIII arises from the spiral ganglion, which occupies the center of the cochlea. Auditory stimuli activate hair cells in a frequency-dependent manner. Nerve fibers supplying the hair cells are the peripheral processes of bipolar neurons lying in the spiral gan-

---

ENRICHMENT BOX 2–16

Sometimes preceded by vague pain behind the ear, patients with Bell palsy develop total peripheral facial paralysis (i.e., involving the upper and lower face equally). They are unable to close the eye; liquids and saliva may drool from the affected corner of the mouth. Depending on the relationship of the lesion to the geniculate ganglion, to the takeoff of the chorda tympani, and to the takeoff of the branch to the stapedius, patients may note loss of taste sensation on the ipsilateral anterior two-thirds of the tongue, as well as dryness of the eye or hyperacusis.

glion. The central processes of these neurons form the auditory nerve, which follows a direct course through the internal auditory canal and across the CPA to enter the brainstem at the pontomedullary junction.

The vestibular nerve arises from the vestibular (Scarpa) ganglion. The peripheral processes of bipolar neurons receive impulses from the utricle, saccule, and three semicircular canals, and the central processes convey these impulses through the vestibular portion of CN VIII. Tucked between CN VII and CN VIII is the nervus intermedius, the primary component of which is the chorda tympani, which subserves taste sensation.

GLOSSOPHARYNGEAL NERVE

The nucleus ambiguus sends axons via the glossopharyngeal nerve (CN IX) to innervate the pharyngeal plexus. The functions of the glossopharyngeal and vagus are inseparable in this regard. Taste fibers from the posterior third of the tongue and parasympathetics are present as well. In company with CN X and CN XI, the nerve exits the skull through the jugular foramen.

VAGUS NERVE

The vagus nerve (CN X) also carries motor fibers from the nucleus ambiguus to the palate, pharynx, and larynx. In addition, a heavy input occurs from the dorsal motor nucleus of the vagus nerve conveying parasympathetic fibers to innervate viscera of the thorax and abdomen. The vagus nerve also carries visceral afferents and taste fibers.

ACCESSORY NERVE

The accessory nerve (CN XI) has two parts. The spinal portion arises from lower motor neurons in the upper cervical cord, exits laterally rather than through the anterior root (branchial arch behavior again), runs upward to enter the skull through the foramen magnum, and ascends to the jugular foramen. These fibers ultimately innervate the sternomastoid and trapezius muscles. The cranial portion of the accessory nerve really is more akin to cranial nerves IX and X than to the spinal portion of CN XI. It arises from the nucleus ambiguus, exits laterally, joins the spinal root for a short stretch, then quickly turns off to join cranial nerves IX and X. It innervates intrinsic muscles of the larynx.

HYPOGLOSSAL NERVE

The hypoglossal nerve (CN XII) arises from motor neurons in the hypoglossal nucleus, exits the medulla in the groove between the pyramid and the olive, leaves the skull through the hypoglossal foramen, and runs forward to innervate the genioglossus. Paresis of the genioglossus causes the tongue to deviate toward the weak side.

Spinal Cord

The spinal cord begins at the cervicomedullary junction and ends at the conus medullaris. The general organization is the same throughout, but there is some variability in detail at different segmental levels. The cord and vertebral column are of different lengths because of different fetal growth rates, so there is not absolute concordance between cord levels and vertebral levels. This discrepancy grows more significant at more caudal levels (Enrichment Box 2–17; Figure 2–19).

The anterior roots convey motor and autonomic fibers into the peripheral nerve. They join the posterior root just distal to the dorsal root ganglion to form the mixed spinal nerve (see Figure 2–2). In the thoracolumbar region, white and gray rami connect the spinal nerve to the paravertebral sympathetic chain.

Posterior roots bear ganglia composed of unipolar neurons. The roots are made up of the central processes of these neurons. The ganglion lies in the intervertebral foramen in close proximity to the anterior root.

Motor neurons innervating skeletal muscle (e.g., alpha motor neuron, skeletomotor neuron) and muscle spindles (e.g., gamma motor neuron, fusimotor neuron) lie in the anterior horn. Each skeletomotor neuron innervates a population of muscle fibers: its motor unit.

The substantia gelatinosa caps the posterior horn (Figure 2–20). Second-order neurons for the spinothalamic system originate primarily from the areas adjacent to the substantia gelatinosa. At the base of the posterior horn lies the nucleus dorsalis, or Clarke column, which contains second-order neurons for the posterior spinocerebellar tract.

In the thoracic and upper lumbar regions, lying laterally in an intermediate position between the anterior and posterior horns, is the intermediolateral gray column, which contains sympathetic neurons. Their axons project through the anterior horn and out the anterior

---

ENRICHMENT BOX 2–17

Nerve roots exit through the foramen above like-numbered vertebrae from C1 to C7. The "extra" C8 root ruins the scheme, exits below C7, and sets the pattern of root exit below like-numbered vertebra that is followed down the rest of the vertebral column.

The conus lies at approximately the L2 level. Vertebral levels below this have had to "drag" the corresponding nerve roots down, forming the cauda equina.

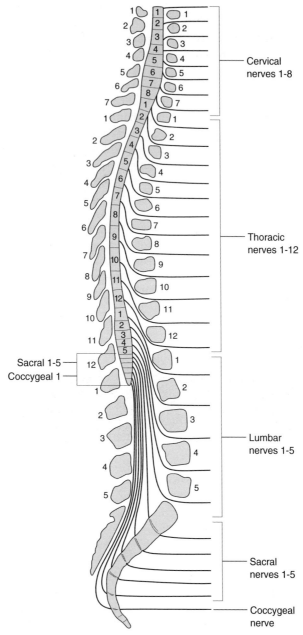

FIGURE 2–19. ■ The relation of segments of the spinal cord and spinal nerves to the vertebral column. The spinal cord ends at the level of the L1–L2 vertebral bodies; lumbar punctures are done below this level. The long trailing roots from the lower cord segments make up the *cauda equina*.

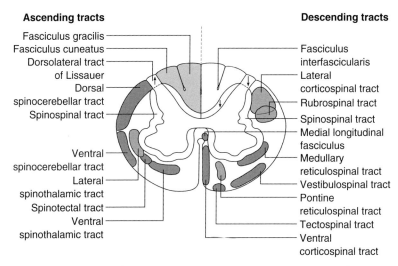

Ascending tracts

Fasciculus gracilis
Fasciculus cuneatus
Dorsolateral tract
of Lissauer
Dorsal
spinocerebellar tract
Spinospinal tract

Ventral
spinocerebellar tract
Lateral
spinothalamic tract
Spinotectal tract
Ventral
spinothalamic tract

Descending tracts

Fasciculus
interfascicularis
Lateral
corticospinal tract
Rubrospinal tract
Spinospinal tract
Medial longitudinal
fasciculus
Medullary
reticulospinal tract
Vestibulospinal tract
Pontine
reticulospinal tract
Tectospinal tract
Ventral
corticospinal tract

FIGURE 2–20. ■ The spinal cord showing ascending tracts on the *left* and descending tracts on the *right*. (Adapted with permission from Carpenter MB: *Core Text of Neuroanatomy,* 3rd ed. Baltimore, Williams and Wilkins, 1985, p 97.)

root, then veer off through the gray rami communicantes to enter the sympathetic chain ganglia.

The major ascending tracts are the posterior columns, the spinothalamic/anterolateral system, and the spinocerebellar tracts. Large myelinated fibers conveying light touch, position, and vibration enter via the posterior root, then turn upward in the fasciculi gracilis and cuneatus without synapsing. The dorsal columns are selectively affected in tabes dorsalis (tabes means "wasting away") and affected along with the pyramidal tracts in subacute combined degeneration of the spinal cord due to vitamin B_{12} deficiency.

Fibers originating from second-order neurons in the posterior horn cross the midline in the anterior white commissure and gather into the anterior and lateral spinothalamic tracts, or, in modern terminology, the anterolateral system. This tract ascends in an anterolateral position, just inside the anterior spinocerebellar tract. It is somatotopically organized. Because the sacral fibers lie most laterally, the phenomenon of sacral sparing suggests an intramedullary cord lesion. Fibers crossing in the anterior white commissure are affected early in syringomyelia. A syrinx classically produces the finding of "suspended" (only involving a certain segmental level with normal function above and below) or "dissociated" (only involving pain and temperature, because the touch fibers are safely tucked away in the posterior columns) sensory loss.

The spinocerebellar tracts contain axons arising from cells in Clarke column (nucleus dorsalis) and other nearby cells in the base of the posterior horn. Afferent fibers to these cells come primarily from muscle spindles. The anterior and posterior spinocerebellar tracts ascend along the far periphery of the cord and ultimately enter the cerebellum.

The major descending tracts are the corticospinal, rubrospinal, and vestibulospinal. Other tracts, such as the tectospinal and reticulospinal, are present as well, but have scant clinical significance. The lateral corticospinal tract is a massive bundle taking up most of the lateral funiculus of the cord. It contains descending pyramidal tract fibers from the giant pyramidal Betz cells in the motor cortex, but these comprise only 3% of the bundle; fibers making up the bulk of the tract come from other cortical areas. Lateral corticospinal axons drop off to innervate segmental motor neurons all along the cord, so the tract becomes progressively smaller as it descends. By the time it reaches sacral levels, there is almost nothing left.

The rubrospinal tract contains axons originating in the red nucleus, descends just anterior and adjacent to the lateral corticospinal tract, and influences segmental motor neurons to facilitate flexor muscle tone. The vestibulospinal tract descends in the anterior funiculus; its primary function is to facilitate extensor muscle tone.

Central Nervous System Blood Supply

CAROTID ARTERY

The carotid artery enters the skull through the carotid canal, courses through the petrous bone, and emerges intracranially within the cavernous sinus. The vessel has an S- shaped course in the sinus, referred to as the carotid siphon. Intracavernous carotid aneurysms can compress the neural contents of the sinus, and carotid-cavernous fistulas can markedly impair the venous drainage of the orbit and produce tremendous proptosis. Immediately after exiting the sinus, the ophthalmic artery arises, after which the posterior communicating artery arises. The carotid then divides into its major terminal branches, the anterior (ACA) and middle cerebral arteries (MCA).

The ACA runs forward and up, then gives off the anterior communicating branch to link with the ACA on the opposite side. The ACA then arches up and back in the interhemispheric fissure. Its main supply is to the leg area on the medial surface of the hemisphere.

After giving off the posterior communicating artery, the MCA turns laterally (its "M-1" segment in radiologic parlance), and along this segment gives off the lenticulostriate arteries. These pierce the anterior perforated substance and supply the basal ganglia and internal capsule. The lenticulostriates are the vessels most often involved in hypertension-induced fibrinoid necrosis, leading to either occlusion (lacunar stroke) or hemorrhage.

On entering the Sylvian fissure, the MCA turns up and back to course in the depths of the fissure, giving off branches that supply the lateral aspects of the frontal and temporal lobes (known to radiologists as the middle cerebral "candelabra"). The MCA breaks up into terminal cortical branches near the apex of the fissure, supplying the frontal, temporal, and parietal lobes.

VERTEBROBASILAR SYSTEM

The two vertebral arteries enter the skull through the foramen magnum and run upward along the clivus. The PICA, a very important branch supplying the lateral medulla, arises at approximately the midportion of the vertebral artery's course. The two vertebral arteries join to form the basilar artery, which is short (about 2 inches long) and thick.

From the basilar artery arise paramedian perforators, which supply the deep midline structures of the brainstem, much in the way the lenticulostriates supply the basal ganglia. Short and long circumferential arteries off the basilar artery run various distances around the brainstem. The major named arteries off the vertebrobasilar system are long circumferential vessels: PICA, anterior inferior cerebellar, and superior cerebellar.

Just before its termination, the basilar artery receives the posterior communicating arteries from the terminal carotid artery. A tuft of small vessels comes off the top of the basilar artery to supply the thalamus, after which it bifurcates into the two posterior cerebral arteries. The third nerve usually runs between the superior cerebellar and posterior cerebral arteries. The posterior cerebral artery proceeds back to the occipital lobe to perfuse the visual cortex.

The ACA, MCA, and PCA vessels communicate in their terminal ramifications via small collateral vessels, which are better developed in some individuals than others. The areas between the major vessels are a vascular no-man's land, marginally perfused and susceptible to ischemic injury when the perfusion pressure decreases (i.e., watershed stroke).

VENOUS DRAINAGE

Most superficial cortical venous drainage is into the superior sagittal sinus. Deeper regions drain into the inferior sagittal sinus in the inferior free margin of the falx or into the very deep internal cerebral venous system. The inferior sagittal sinus and deep cerebral veins converge at the vein of Galen, which is a short, squat structure that quickly dumps into the straight sinus. Infants sometimes develop an aneurysmal dilatation of the vein of Galen. The straight and superior sagittal sinuses converge at the torcula (confluence of sinuses), from which point transverse sinuses curve around the inner table of the posterior fossa to eventually join the jugular veins to exit through the jugular foramen (in company with the ninth, tenth, and eleventh cranial nerves).

Peripheral Nervous System

The anterior and posterior roots join to form the mixed spinal nerve (see Figure 2–2). As the spinal nerve exits the intervertebral foramen, it immediately divides into a large anterior primary ramus and a small posterior primary ramus. The posterior primary ramus arches backward to innervate the paravertebral or paraspinal muscles. The status of the paraspinal muscles is an important localizing feature in electromyography (Enrichment Box 2–18). The anterior primary rami continue to form the cervical, brachial, and lumbosacral plexi and the intercostal nerves.

BRACHIAL PLEXUS

The anatomy of the brachial plexus is intricate and hard to remember unless reviewed frequently. There is a dictum that only electromyographers and some surgeons understand the brachial plexus. If true, it is not because of intellectual gifts but because of daily use of the information. The details of the brachial plexus are available in any anatomy text; the following summarizes some of the clinically relevant information.

The brachial plexus is formed by the anterior primary rami of C5 through T1 (Enrichment Box 2–19). Figure 2–21 is a diagram that highlights most of the clinically important branches. Table 2–3 summarizes, from a clinical examination standpoint, the most important upper extremity muscles innervated by various structures.

The two terminal branches of the posterior cord are the axillary and radial nerves. The axillary nerve supplying the deltoid muscle veers off

---

ENRICHMENT BOX 2–18

A finding on needle electromyography of denervation in the paraspinal muscles is extremely helpful in distinguishing radiculopathy from other processes. If the lesion is proximal to the takeoff of the posterior primary ramus, as in radiculopathy or anterior horn cell disease, the paraspinals show abnormalities. If the lesion is distal to the posterior primary ramus, such as in plexopathy and other more peripheral processes, it involves only the structures that arise from the anterior primary rami; the paraspinals are normal.

ENRICHMENT BOX 2-19

The brachial plexus

The only important branch arising from root level is the nerve to the rhomboids, off C5. From the upper trunk, the suprascapular nerve comes off to supply the supraspinatus and infraspinatus muscles. The lateral cord divides into the musculocutaneous nerve and a large trunk that becomes part of the median. The medial cord also sends a large branch to the median before continuing as the ulnar nerve.

The radial nerve

The radial nerve is most often injured by external pressure at the level of the spiral groove (i.e., Saturday night palsy, bridegroom's palsy). Such patients have wrist and finger drop and brachioradialis weakness but no triceps weakness (its innervation occurs above the groove). Rarely, posterior interosseous lesions cause finger drop without wrist drop.

The median nerve

Carpal tunnel syndrome is caused by entrapment of the median nerve beneath the transverse carpal ligament. Carpal tunnel syndrome can cause hand pain and numbness, sensory loss, and weakness of the abductor pollicis brevis and opponens. Rarely, more proximal median lesions produce, in addition, weakness of finger flexion and pronation.

The ulnar nerve

Ulnar neuropathy at the elbow may occur from external pressure on the nerve in the groove, or from entrapment beneath the aponeurosis just distally. "Tardy ulnar palsy" is a classic neurologic condition in which patients develop ulnar neuropathy at the elbow many years after a fracture or dislocation of the elbow.

---

just before the posterior cord evolves into the radial nerve to supply the deltoid muscle and a small patch of skin on the shoulder. The axillary nerve is sometimes injured during shoulder injections, arthrograms, and arthroscopy. The radial nerve is a direct continuation of the posterior cord. In the upper arm it innervates the triceps muscle, then spirals around its humeral groove and gives off no further branches until the forearm. The main trunk of the radial nerve innervates the supinator, the brachioradialis, and the extensor muscles of the wrist. The purely motor posterior interosseous branch innervates the extensor muscles of the fingers. Sensory supply is to the radial aspect of the dorsum of the hand. The radial nerve commonly is the victim of compression injury (see Enrichment Box 2–19). The brachioradialis jerk is mediated by the radial nerve via the C6 root, and the triceps jerk is mediated by the radial nerve via the C7 and C8 roots.

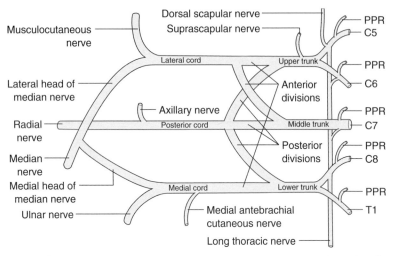

FIGURE 2–21. ■ A skeleton view of the brachial plexus showing only the major clinically important branches. (Adapted with permission from Campbell WW: *Essentials of Electrodiagnostic Medicine*. Baltimore, Williams and Wilkins, 1998, p 209.) PPR = posterior primary ramus.

The musculocutaneous nerve is a continuation of the lateral cord. It supplies the biceps and brachialis muscles and provides sensation to the radial aspect of the forearm. It seldom is injured in isolation. The bi-

---

TABLE 2–3. CLINICALLY IMPORTANT UPPER EXTREMITY MUSCLES INNERVATED BY VARIOUS STRUCTURES

Structure	Muscles
C5 root	Rhomboids
Brachial plexus upper trunk	Supraspinatus and infraspinatus
Axillary nerve	Deltoid
Musculocutaneous nerve	Biceps
Radial nerve	Triceps, brachioradialis, wrist and finger extensors
Median nerve	Forearm pronators, wrist flexors, FDS, FDP_{1-2}, APB, OP, FPL, lumbricals$_{1-2}$
Ulnar nerve	FCU, FDP_{3-4}, hypothenar muscles, interossei, lumbricals$_{3-4}$

APB = abductor pollicis brevis; FCU = flexor carpi ulnaris; FDP = flexor digitorum profundus; FDS = flexor digitorum sublimis; FPL = flexor pollicis longus; OP = opponens pollicis.

ceps jerk is mediated by the musculocutaneous nerve via the C5 and C6 nerve roots.

The median nerve is formed by a branch from the lateral cord of the plexus, which carries mostly C6 and C7 fibers, and a branch from the medial cord, which conveys primarily C8 and T1 fibers. All of the sensory fibers in the median nerve come from the lateral branch. The median nerve is almost like two separate nerves, with the lateral head supplying the pronator teres and flexor carpi radialis and providing sensation to the hand, and the purely motor medial head supplying the finger flexors and small hand muscles (e.g., abductor pollicis brevis and opponens pollicis). This distinction is useful conceptually, but all of these fibers are gathered into one nerve trunk. The most common disorder of the median nerve by far is carpal tunnel syndrome (see Enrichment Box 2–19).

The ulnar nerve is a direct continuation of the medial cord of the plexus. It descends through the upper arm in a common sheath with the median, then parts company to slant backward toward the ulnar groove. No branches exit in the upper arm. After passing through the ulnar groove, the nerve passes beneath an aponeurosis (the humeroulnar arcade, or cubital tunnel), which occasionally entraps it. It passes down the forearm, gives off a large sensory branch that curves around the ulna to supply the dorsum of the hand, and then enters the hand through Guyon's canal. The ulnar nerve supplies the hypothenar muscles, all of the interossei, and the third and fourth lumbricals. From a practical clinical standpoint, the "index muscle" for ulnar nerve lesions is the first dorsal interosseous, because weakness and wasting are usually evident there first, both to the patient and to the physician. The most common disorder of the ulnar nerve is ulnar neuropathy at the elbow (see Enrichment Box 2–19). Rarely, the nerve may be compressed at Guyon's canal.

LUMBOSACRAL PLEXUS

The lumbosacral plexus consists of two functionally different areas joined by a large communicating branch, the lumbosacral trunk. It is simpler to think of the lumbar plexus and the sacral plexus as separate structures, recalling that lesions can sometimes involve the lumbosacral plexus in its entirety. Figure 2–22 is a skeletonized diagram of the lumbosacral plexus, and Table 2–4 summarizes the major clinically important branches.

The lumbar plexus is composed of branches from L1 to L4. The major terminal branch is the femoral nerve, which innervates the iliopsoas and quadriceps muscles and supplies sensation to the thigh, the medial lower leg, and the medial aspect of the foot. The knee jerk is mediated by the femoral nerve and the L3 and L4 roots. The obturator nerve departs the lumbar plexus, exits through the obturator foramen, and innervates the adductors of the thigh. Several purely sensory nerves arise

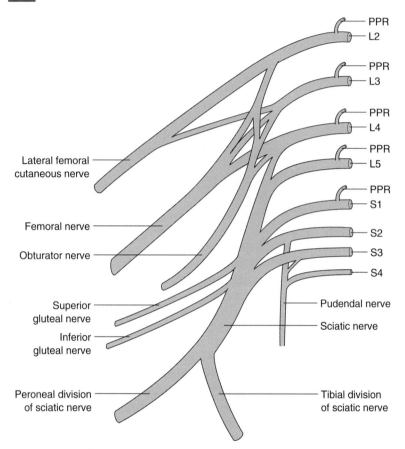

FIGURE 2–22. ▪ A skeleton view of the lumbosacral plexus showing only the major clinically important branches. (Adapted with permission from Campbell WW: *Essentials of Electrodiagnostic Medicine.* Baltimore, Williams and Wilkins, 1998, p 210.) PPR = posterior primary ramus.

from the lumbar plexus: ilioinguinal, iliohypogastric, genitofemoral, and lateral femoral cutaneous.

The sacral plexus is composed of branches from L5 to S2 with an L4 component from the lumbar plexus via the lumbosacral trunk. The major terminal sacral plexus branches are the sciatic nerve, inferior gluteal nerve, superior gluteal nerve, and posterior cutaneous nerve of the thigh.

The sciatic nerve has two divisions, the peroneal and the tibial. It exits the pelvis through the sciatic foramen and descends through the thigh, supplying the hamstrings. In the popliteal fossa, the sciatic nerve divides into its two terminal branches. The peroneal nerve winds

TABLE 2-4. CLINICALLY IMPORTANT LOWER EXTREMITY MUSCLES INNERVATED BY VARIOUS STRUCTURES

Structure	Muscles
Lumbosacral plexus	
Pudendal nerve	Anal sphincter
Superior gluteal nerve	Gluteus medius, TFL
Inferior gluteal nerve	Gluteus maximus
Femoral nerve	Iliopsoas, quadriceps
Obturator nerve	Adductor longus, adductor magnus
Sciatic nerve	
Peroneal division of sciatic	
Superficial peroneal nerve	Peroneus longus and brevis
Deep peroneal nerve	TA, EDL, EHL, EDB
Tibial division of sciatic	Hamstrings
Posterior tibial nerve	Gastrocnemius, soleus, TP, FDL, FHL

EDB = extensor digitorum brevis; EDL = extensor digitorum longus; EHL = extensor hallucis longus; FDL = flexor digitorum longus; FHL = flexor hallucis longus; TA = tibialis anterior; TFL = tensor fascia lata; TP = tibialis posterior.

around the fibular head and descends through the anterior compartment, supplying the foot and toe extensors and foot everters; it terminates by supplying the short toe extensors and sensation to the dorsum of the foot. The tibial nerve runs down the posterior compartment supplying the gastrosoleus, long toe flexors, and foot inverters; it terminates by supplying the small muscles of the foot in a manner very reminiscent of the ulnar nerve in the hand. The ankle jerk is mediated by the tibial branch of the sciatic nerve via the S1 root.

The lumbosacral plexus branches most commonly involved in injury or disease processes are the femoral, sciatic, and common peroneal (Enrichment Box 2–20).

Autonomic Nervous System

Descending autonomic influences arise in the hypothalamus, which is itself considerably influenced by the cerebral cortex via connections with the limbic system. This hypothalamic autonomic control is mediated by sympathetic and parasympathetic effector systems in the brainstem and spinal cord.

ENRICHMENT BOX 2-20

In its proximal course, the femoral nerve lies near the psoas muscle and can be severely damaged by hemorrhage into the psoas mass, usually due to anticoagulant medications. The sciatic nerve can be injured by misplaced injections into the hip, by stretch during total hip replacement, and sometimes through other mechanisms. The peroneal nerve is most often injured by external pressure at the fibular head, such as from habitual leg crossing ("crossed leg palsy"). Lesions limited to the tibial branch are rare.

The parasympathetic system consists of cranial and sacral parts. The cranial part consists of the Edinger-Westphal nucleus in the midbrain, which innervates the iris and ciliary body via the third nerve; the brainstem nuclei, which innervate the lacrimal and salivary glands; and the dorsal motor nucleus of the vagus. The sacral portion consists of neurons in segments S2–S4, which innervate the bladder, rectum, and sexual organs via the pelvic splanchnic nerves. The parasympathetic system is characterized by long preganglionic fibers, ganglia located in or near the organ innervated, and short postganglionic fibers. Acetylcholine is the transmitter.

Sympathetic neurons occupy the intermediolateral gray column in the thoracic and upper lumbar spinal cord. Axons exit through the anterior root. White rami communicantes exit the spinal nerve just beyond the foramen, and the axons enter the sympathetic paravertebral chain. Postganglionic gray rami leave the chain to provide sympathetic fibers to each spinal nerve in its course to the periphery. There are thus 31 pairs of gray rami, one for each spinal nerve, but only 17 or so white rami, one for each level T1–L2 plus the three cervical ganglia. Some preganglionic fibers pass through the chain to eventually synapse in the prevertebral ganglia located in the celiac, mesenteric, and other plexuses, from which long postganglionic fibers travel to innervate blood vessels, glands, and viscera. In the cervical region, the superior, middle, and inferior (stellate) ganglia provide sympathetic innervation to the head, neck, upper extremities, and heart. Horner syndrome (i.e., ptosis, miosis, and anhydrosis) results from a lesion involving the cervical sympathetic chain. From the upper lumbar cord, sympathetic fibers travel along the lumbar and pelvic splanchnic nerves to innervate the bladder, rectum, sexual organs, blood vessels, and glands. Preganglionic sympathetic fibers synapse directly on the adrenal medulla, which is in effect a sympathetic ganglion. All sympathetic transmission is adrenergic except for sweat glands, which are cholinergic.

TABLE 2-1. OVERVIEW OF NEUROANATOMY

Brain Region or Structure	Primary Function	Clinical Manifestation of Damage
Frontal lobe		
General	Thinking, judgment, reasoning, modulation of emotions	Dementia, abulia (lack of initiative and motivation), social disinhibition, poor judgment
Precentral gyrus	Cortical motor control	Weakness (usually hemiparesis/hemiplegia)
Broca area	Cortical motor control of speech	Nonfluent aphasia
Frontal eye fields	Contralateral conjugate horizontal gaze	Impairment of gaze to the opposite side, often accompanied by gaze deviation to the ipsilateral side due to the unopposed action of the opposite frontal eye fields (destructive lesion); forced horizontal conjugate gaze to the opposite side (irritative lesion)
Parietal lobe		
General	Sensory association cortex, visuospatial integration	Cortical sensory loss (astereognosis, agraphesthesia, impaired two-point discrimination), apraxia (ideational, ideomotor, constructional, dressing)
Wernicke area	Auditory reception and speech processing	Fluent aphasia
Temporal lobe	Memory, emotion (limbic lobe connections), lower retinal fibers of the optic radiations	Partial complex seizures (irritative), memory loss (with bilateral damage), contralateral upper quadrantanopia ("pie-in-the-sky")
Occipital lobe	Vision and visual processing	Hemianopia
Limbic lobe	Emotions, sexual function (rich connections with hypothalamus, temporal lobe, and olfactory regions)	Changes in emotionality and sexuality

(continued)

TABLE 2–1. OVERVIEW OF NEUROANATOMY (*Continued*)

Brain Region or Structure	Primary Function	Clinical Manifestation of Damage
Hypothalamus	Control of appetite, thirst, osmolality, temperature, and sexual function	Diabetes insipidus, syndrome of inappropriate anti-diuretic hormone, hyper-phagia, anorexia with wasting, hypersexuality, hyposexuality, hyper-thermia, hypothermia
Thalamus	Sensory relay station between cerebral cortex and lower centers, arousal and alert-ness (interlaminar nuclei), integration and modulation of cortical activity (rich reciprocal connections with all cortical regions), motor integration between cortex, cerebellum, and basal ganglia	Contralateral sensory loss, contralateral pain (thalamic pain syndrome), memory loss (if involvement of dorsomedial nucleus)
Basal ganglia	Contralateral extrapyramidal motor control	Extrapyramidal motor signs and/or abnormal involun-tary movements (rigidity, cogwheeling, bradykinesia, dystonia, chorea, athetosis)
Internal capsule	Contains descending cortico-fugal motor fibers (cortico-spinal and corticobulbar tracts) and thalamic radiations (posterior limb); reciprocal connections between frontal lobe and lower centers (anterior limb); optic radiations (retrolentic-ular, i.e., posterior to the posterior limb)	Contralateral hemiparesis/ hemiplegia affecting arm, leg, and face equally
Pretectum	Control of pupillary reactivity	Light near dissociation of pupils
Brainstem		
Midbrain		
Tectum	Vertical gaze, ocular reflexes	Impairment of upward gaze (Parinaud syndrome)

(continued)

TABLE 2-1. OVERVIEW OF NEUROANATOMY (*Continued*)

Brain Region or Structure	Primary Function	Clinical Manifestation of Damage
Tegmentum	Oculomotor control (CN III and CN IV cranial nerve nuclei)	CN III nerve palsy, CN IV nerve palsy
Base	Descending corticospinal and corticobulbar tract, substantia nigra	Contralateral hemiparesis, Parkinson disease
Pons		
Tectum		
Tegmentum	CN VI nerve nuclei, CN VII nerve nuclei, PPRF, relay nuclei between the cerebral cortex and cerebellum giving rise to the middle cerebellar peduncle, long ascending sensory pathways	Ipsilateral CN VI nerve palsy, ipsilateral CN VII nerve palsy, impairment of horizontal conjugate gaze to the ipsilateral side (PPRF), contralateral hemisensory loss
Base	Descending corticospinal and corticobulbar fibers	Contralateral hemiparesis/ hemiplegia
Medulla		
Tectum		
Tegmentum	Hypoglossal nuclei, nucleus ambiguus, spinal tract of CN V, vestibular nuclei, cochlear nuclei, and connections of spinal cord and vestibular system with cerebellum (inferior cerebellar peduncle), long ascending sensory tracts	Hypoglossal nerve palsy; ipsilateral face, contralateral face, and contralateral body loss of pain and temperature; vertigo; dysphagia; ipsilateral cerebellar ataxia; Horner syndrome (lateral medullary syndrome)
Base	Descending corticospinal tract (medullary pyramid)	Hemiparesis/hemiplegia, contralateral or ipsilateral depending on the relationship of the lesion to the decussation
General	Long sensory and motor tracts, control of arousal and alertness (reticular formation), coordination of binocular horizontal conjugate gaze (MLF), descending sympathetic fibers	Contralateral weakness or sensory loss, alterations in level of consciousness, internuclear ophthalmoplegia, ipsilateral Horner syndrome

(*continued*)

TABLE 2-1. **OVERVIEW OF NEUROANATOMY** (*Continued*)

Brain Region or Structure	Primary Function	Clinical Manifestation of Damage
Cerebellum		
Flocculonodular lobe	Vestibular function, eye movement control	Nystagmus
Vermis	Control of midline coordination, especially walking	Gait ataxia
Hemisphere	Control of extremity (appendicular) coordination	Ipsilateral appendicular ataxia
Spinal cord		
Posterior root	Ipsilateral sensory function	Ipsilateral dermatomal sensory loss
Anterior root	Ipsilateral motor and autonomic function	Ipsilateral myotomal weakness and possibly wasting
Posterior gray horn	Sensory relay mechanism into the ipsilateral posterior columns and contralateral spinothalamic tracts	Ipsilateral variable sensory loss (extremely rare)
Anterior gray horn	Ipsilateral lower motor neurons	Ipsilateral weakness and wasting (seldom, if ever, limited to a single myotome)
Posterior columns	Ipsilateral touch, pressure, position sense, and vibration (destined to decussate in the medulla and ascend in the medial lemniscus to the thalamus)	Ipsilateral loss of touch, pressure, position sense, and vibration
Lateral column	Ipsilateral descending motor control (corticospinal tract) and contralateral ascending pain and temperature perception (lateral spinothalamic tract)	Ipsilateral hemiparesis/hemiplegia or monoparesis/monoplegia, depending on the level of involvement; contralateral loss of pain and temperature
Anterior columns	Anterior corticospinal tract (descending motor responses) and anterior spinothalamic tract (ascending crude touch)	None significant
Cranial nerves		
Olfactory (I)	Olfaction	Anosmia

(*continued*)

TABLE 2–1.   OVERVIEW OF NEUROANATOMY (*Continued*)

Brain Region or Structure	Primary Function	Clinical Manifestation of Damage
Optic (II)	Vision	Impaired vision, visual field defects, pupillary abnormalities
Oculomotor (III)		
Motor component	Innervation of ipsilateral inferior oblique and medial, superior and inferior recti; innervation of eyelid	Paresis of ipsilateral ocular adduction, elevation, and depression; ptosis
Autonomic component	Pupillary control	Impaired constriction of pupil
Trochlear (IV)	Innervation of superior obliques	Impaired depression of adducted eye
Trigeminal (V)		
Motor component	Innervation of muscles of mastication	Weakness and possibly wasting of masseter and temporalis, jaw deviation to the side of the weakness
Main sensory nucleus	Light touch and pressure innervation of the ipsilateral face	Impaired light touch and pressure over the ipsilateral face
Spinal tract	Pain and temperature innervation to the ipsilateral face	Impaired pain and temperature sensation over the ipsilateral face
Abducens (VI)	Innervation of the ipsilateral lateral rectus	Impaired abduction of the ipsilateral eye
Facial (VII)	Innervation of muscles of facial expression	Facial paralysis
Vestibulocochlear (VIII)		
Vestibular portion	Vestibular function	Vertigo, nausea and vomiting, imbalance, nystagmus
Cochlear portion	Hearing	Deafness
Glossopharyngeal (IX)	Innervation of pharynx and larynx	Difficulty with speech and swallowing
Vagus (X)	Innervation of pharynx and larynx; parasympathetic function	Difficulty with speech and swallowing; parasympathetic dysfunction

(*continued*)

TABLE 2–1. **OVERVIEW OF NEUROANATOMY** (*Continued*)

Brain Region or Structure	Primary Function	Clinical Manifestation of Damage
Spinal accessory (XI)	Innervation of trapezius and sternomastoid	Weakness and possibly wasting of trapezius and SCM, scapular winging
Hypoglossal (XII)	Innervation of tongue	Weakness and possibly wasting of the tongue

CN = cranial nerve; MLF = medial longitudinal fasciculus; PPRF = pontine paramedian reticular formation; SCM = sternocleidomastoid.

3

An Overview of Neurophysiology

This chapter provides a broad overview of some of the clinically relevant concepts of basic neurophysiology, with the expectation that the material has been studied in depth previously. More advanced material for elective reading is included in the Enrichment Boxes.

Cells in the Nervous System

Most neurons have four distinct morphologic regions: the cell body or soma, the dendrites, the axon, and the axon terminals. The cell body is chiefly responsible for the metabolic integrity of the neurons. Cytoskeletal proteins, neurotransmitters, and other substances necessary for function of the axon are moved from the cell body through the axon by the process of axonal transport (Enrichment Box 3–1).

A neuron's dendritic tree has a large surface area and serves as the major mechanism for receiving input from other neurons. The axon is a single process arising from the axon hillock and is the neuron's output mechanism. The axon terminals are tiny ramifications at the end of the axon that make synaptic contact with the dendrites or the cell bodies of other neurons, muscles, glands, and other structures. The axon terminals release neurotransmitters, providing a basis for interneuronal communication.

There are two basic types of neurons: interneurons and projection neurons. *Interneurons* are cells with short axons that function within a circumscribed area; they have no projections outside the central nervous system (CNS), and they play an important role in communication between other neurons. Interneurons are the most common type of neurons. *Projection neurons* have long axons. They convey impulses to and from the periphery and between brain regions.

Renshaw cells are inhibitory interneurons found in the spinal cord. They are excited by recurrent collateral fibers off the motor neuron

---

ENRICHMENT BOX 3–1 Axonal Transport

The axoplasm is in constant flux, containing cytoskeletal elements, neurofilaments, neurotubules, and other substances that flow to and fro along the length of the axon between the cell body and the periphery. There are three types of axoplasmic flow: fast antegrade, slow antegrade, and retrograde.

Abnormalities of axonal transport are likely important in the mechanism of dying back or length-dependent neuropathies. Several substances produce neuropathy by disrupting the cytoskeletal elements: vinca alkaloids, taxols, and hexacarbons, for example (see Chapter 11). Retrograde flow moves materials from the periphery back to the cell body, and is the mechanism through which some neurotrophic viruses (e.g., rabies) reach the central nervous system.

---

axon and function to inhibit the motor neuron that gave rise to the impulse, or other nearby motor neurons. This serves to restrict the firing rate of motor neurons and may help to limit activity to the motor neurons that are firing most strongly. In "stiff man syndrome," patients develop rigidity because of dysfunctioning inhibitory interneurons in the spinal cord.

Glial cells are much more numerous than neurons and serve many vital functions. *Oligodendrocytes* and *Schwann cells* synthesize myelin. *Astrocytes* are involved in forming the blood–brain barrier and in the buffering of extracellular potassium ion (K^+) concentration. *Microglia* are a type of macrophage and function as scavengers.

Synaptic Transmission

In response to nerve impulses in the terminal axon, neurotransmitters are released and diffuse across the *synaptic cleft*. There, transmitter molecules interact with receptors to produce a change in the ionic permeability of the postsynaptic membrane. This process requires some finite time to occur, producing a synaptic delay.

Chemical synaptic transmission produces postsynaptic electrical potentials. The postsynaptic potentials result from slight depolarization or hyperpolarization of the postsynaptic membrane (Table 3–1). Postsynaptic potentials play an important role in epilepsy. Inhibitory postsynaptic potentials (IPSPs) produce an increase in K^+ conductance, causing an outward leak of K^+, which increases the internal net negativity of the cell, hyperpolarizing the membrane and making it more difficult to depolarize. Excitatory postsynaptic potentials (EPSPs) cause an increase

TABLE 3-1. POSTSYNAPTIC POTENTIALS*

Ion	Direction of Change in Permeability	Effect on Membrane Voltage
K^+	Increase	Hyperpolarize (IPSP)
Na^+	Increase	Depolarize (EPSP)
K^+	Decrease	Depolarize (EPSP)
Na^+	Decrease	Hyperpolarize (IPSP)

Modified and reprinted with permission from Haines DE: *Fundamental Neuroscience.* New York, Churchill Livingstone, 1997.
   EPSP = excitatory postsynaptic potential; IPSP = inhibitory postsynaptic potential; K^+ = potassium ion; Na^+ = sodium ion.
   *Voltage fluctuations that can result from changes in the permeability of ions to produce excitatory and inhibitory postsynaptic potentials.

in sodium ion (Na^+) conductance, partially depolarizing the membrane and making it easier to excite.

THE RESTING MEMBRANE POTENTIAL

The cell membrane is a *lipid-protein bilayer* sparsely studded with specialized pores or channels. The membrane is relatively permeable to lipid-soluble substances but impermeable to water and water-soluble substances. It separates two electrolytic solutions of different ionic composition and concentrations: the extracellular fluid and the intracellular fluid. The channels control the passage of ions through the membrane. Under certain circumstances, channels may be open to a particular ion, and under other circumstances may be closed. An essential feature of excitable membranes is selective ionic permeability, mediated by the action of ion channels.

Ion channels are complex protein macromolecules that are embedded in and span the membrane, connecting the intracellular and extracellular compartments. The channel has a central pore selective for one or more ions. When the pore is open, ions can traverse the channel. Channels may alternate between the open and closed configuration, depending on chemical or electrical events in the microenvironment. Channels may be voltage gated or ligand gated. Abnormalities in the behavior of these channels produce a wide variety of clinical syndromes, referred to as *channelopathies*. Selected conditions and agents affecting channel function are listed in Table 3–2.

Electrolytes on either side of the semipermeable membrane are distributed in different concentrations related to the electrochemical forces

---

TABLE 3–2. SOME CLINICAL CONDITIONS AND AGENTS THAT AFFECT CHANNEL FUNCTION

Myasthenia gravis

Lambert-Eaton myasthenic syndrome

Hyperkalemic periodic paralysis

Normokalemic periodic paralysis

Hypokalemic periodic paralysis

Continuous muscle-fiber activity syndromes

Myotonia congenita

Local anesthetics

Cardiac antiarrhythmics

Some anticonvulsants (e.g., phenytoin, carbamazepine)

Cocaine

Calcium-channel blocking agents

---

acting on them. Electrical equilibrium requires electrical neutrality of the intracellular space, as well as neutrality of the extracellular space. However, the intracellular and extracellular spaces are at different electrical equilibrium levels. The intracellular space is approximately -90 to -70 mV, as compared with the extracellular space. Along the boundary between these compartments, a charge differential exists. This creates an electrical potential across the membrane, which favors the movement of each ion species in a particular direction depending on its charge. Positively charged ions tend to diffuse into the cell, and negatively charged ions diffuse out of the cell. There also is an impetus for ions to diffuse from an area of higher concentration to an area of lower concentration, which is the chemical potential. These two forces create a *net electrochemical potential gradient* for each ion. In some cases, both the concentration and the electrical gradient favor movement in a given direction; in other instances, the forces counterbalance. The Na^+ concentration outside the cell is approximately 140 mEq/L, K^+ is approximately 4 mEq/L, and Cl^- is approximately 125 mEq/L (i.e., the levels of normal serum electrolytes). The concentration of different electrolytes inside the cell varies from cell to cell; as an approximation, the concentration of K^+ is nearly 30 times greater inside than out, and the concentration of Na^+ is approximately 12 times greater outside than in (Figure 3–1).

Whether an ion moves across the membrane along its electrochemical gradient depends on the permeability (k) or the conductance (g) of

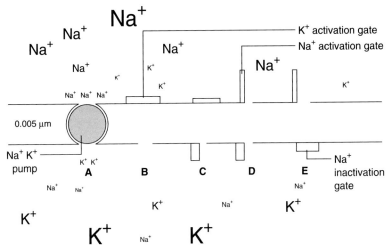

FIGURE 3–1. ■ A representation of the excitable cell membrane, which is 0.005 μm thick, with the relative concentrations of sodium ions (Na$^+$) and potassium ions (K$^+$) on the extracellular (*top*) and intracellular (*bottom*) sides. The gaps in the membrane indicate the position of channels. (*A*) The *Na$^+$/K$^+$ pump,* which has exchanged 3 Na$^+$ molecules for 2 K$^+$ molecules. (*B*) The *K$^+$ channel* in its inactivated (closed) state. (*C*) The *Na$^+$ activation gate* (*top*) is closed and the inactivation gate (*bottom*) is open; the Na$^+$ channel is at rest and ready for activation. (*D*) The Na$^+$ channel's activation and inactivation gates are both open, and the channel is conducting. (*E*) The *inactivation gate has closed,* the channel is no longer conducting, and it cannot again conduct until the channel returns to a resting configuration. (Adapted with permission from Campbell WW: *Essentials of Electrodiagnostic Medicine.* Baltimore, Williams and Wilkins, 1998, p 45.)

the membrane, which, for ions using voltage-gated channels, depends on the transmembrane potential (TMP). The TMP in turn depends on the electrochemical equilibrium potential of the membrane-permeable ions. It is a complex, reciprocal relationship. In the resting state, essentially all the voltage-gated Na$^+$ channels (VGNCs) are closed and permeability is very low, but enough voltage-gated K$^+$ channels (VGKCs) are open that the membrane at rest is more permeable to K$^+$ than to Na$^+$ (by a factor of 50–100), and the equilibrium potential for K$^+$ therefore largely determines the level of the resting potential. Enrichment Box 3–2 contains further discussion of the membrane potential, including the equations.

Considering the delicate balance required for normal function, the profound clinical effects of hypokalemia/hyperkalemia and hyponatremia/hypernatremia are not surprising. These include lethargy, confusion, seizures, muscle paralysis, cramps and fasciculations, cardiac arrhythmias, and more.

ENRICHMENT BOX 3–2 The Membrane Potential

When the membrane is permeable to an ion, its electrochemical equilibrium potential (E), at which there is no net flow across the membrane, is described by the *Nernst equation*. At physiologic temperature, the Nernst equation can be reduced to:

$$E_{ion} = 58 \log \frac{[ion]_{outside}}{[ion] \, inside}$$

Where [ion] = the concentration of a particular ion.

The *Goldman constant field equation* is a refinement of the Nernst equation that takes into account the conductance of the membrane to each individual ion, as well as its intracellular and extracellular concentration, to yield a value for the membrane potential, E_M. Because the membrane potential depends primarily on sodium ions (Na^+) and potassium ions (K^+), the Goldman equation can be simplified to:

$$E_M = 58 \log \frac{g_K [K+]_{outside} + g_{Na} [Na+]_{outside}}{g_K [K+]_{outside} + g_{Na} [Na+]_{inside}}$$

Where g_K = the conductance of K^+ and g_{Na} = the conductance of Na^+. The level of the transmembrane potential depends on the ratio of g_{Na+} to g_{K+}. Because the membrane at rest is 50–100 times more permeable to K^+ than to Na^+, g_{K+} is the primary determinant of E_M. Additionally, because $[K^+]_{inside}$ is much greater than $[K^+]_{outside}$, E_M at rest is a large negative number. The value of E_M at rest is approximately -70 mV for a nerve cell and -90 mV for a muscle cell. Therefore, when g_{K+} is much higher, the membrane potential approximates E_{K+}, which is the normal resting membrane potential (RMP). When g_{Na+} is much higher, the membrane potential approaches E_{Na+}, as during the rise of the action potential. Conductances are equal just at threshold and at the peak of the action potential.

In summary, the membrane at rest is much more permeable to K^+ than to Na^+. It is in dynamic equilibrium, a steady state with no net ionic fluxes across it. The concentration of K^+ is high on the interior; K^+ tends to move outward down its concentration gradient but is held in check by the strong intracellular negativity. The E_K is at -90 to -70 mV, and the voltage-dependent channels are largely closed. Na^+ is at a high concentration outside, and both the electrical and chemical gradients favor movement inside, but the VGNCs are closed. The few Na^+ ions entering the cell are extruded by the Na^+/K^+/adenosine triphosphatase (ATPase) pump (Enrichment Box 3–3). With the membrane more permeable to K^+ than Na^+, the resting TMP is near the E_K of

---

ENRICHMENT BOX 3-3 The NA$^+$/K$^+$ Pump

The sodium ions (Na$^+$)/potassium ion (K$^+$) pump helps maintain the membrane potential. Energy derived from adenosine triphosphate (ATP) is expended in maintaining the potential by reinforcing the exclusion of Na$^+$. The voltage-gated sodium channels, although mostly closed, permit a slight inward leak. The Na$^+$/K$^+$ pump simultaneously moves 3 Na$^+$ ions from inside to outside and 2 K$^+$ ions from outside to inside. The 3:2 ratio causes a continuous net loss of positive charge and contributes a small additional internal negativity of approximately -4 mV beyond that because of ionic diffusion alone.

-90 mV, and far from the E_{Na} of $+60$ mV. The membrane is poised for action.

THE ACTION POTENTIAL

The membrane potential can change in two ways. If it moves toward zero, becoming less negative, it is depolarized. If it moves away from zero, becoming more negative, it is hyperpolarized. There are two basic types of changes in the membrane potential: propagated and nonpropagated. Generator potentials and end-plate potentials are nonpropagated, local, or graded responses. The action potential is a propagated potential conducted in an all-or-none fashion down the nerve or muscle membrane because of the sequential activation and deactivation of the voltage-gated Na$^+$ and K$^+$ channels. Whether a propagated potential develops depends on whether a membrane depolarization reaches threshold (Enrichment Box 3–4).

Once initiated, the action potential runs through a fixed cycle of events determined by the inherent kinetics of the different channels. The refractory period (RP) is an interval during the action potential cycle when a second action potential can be produced with difficulty (the relative RP) or not at all (the absolute RP).

Conduction Along Nerve and Muscle Fibers

Knowledge of the physiology of conduction is important, especially for understanding demyelinating disorders, appreciating some of the clinical manifestations of peripheral nerve and muscle disease, and understanding the concepts of clinical neurophysiology.

An action potential tends to crawl along the membrane of an unmyelinated nerve fiber or a muscle cell by *continuous conduction* (Figure 3–2). As any finite point is depolarized, the positive charges now

ENRICHMENT BOX 3-4 Membrane Depolarization

In the course of the action potential, three different events occur, each with its own kinetics. Of these, the voltage-gated sodium channel (VGNC) activation is quickest; both VGNC inactivation and voltage-gated potassium channel (VGKC) activation/deactivation are approximately 10 times slower than VGNC activation. Once triggered, changes in the VGNC cycle according to a fixed-time course, but the VGKCs remain open as long as the membrane is depolarized. Each channel alteration produces a corresponding change in membrane permeability. Threshold is defined as the voltage level at which an action potential will be generated half of the time. With depolarizations greater than the threshold, the sodium ion (Na^+) gates open *en masse,* and the process becomes overwhelming, generating a self-perpetuating all-or-none action potential.

The action potential can be conceptualized as two separate events: a depolarization cycle and a repolarization cycle. Once the threshold is exceeded, the opening of VGNCs becomes self-perpetuating, and the membrane becomes freely permeable to Na^+, with a conductance approximately 5000-fold higher than at baseline. As the most permeable ion, Na^+ determines the level of the membrane potential, which very rapidly approaches the equilibrium potential (E_{Na+}) of approximately +60 mV. This is the main spike of the action potential. After the action potential, there is transient membrane hyperpolarization, or overshoot, as potassium ions ($K+$) continue to flow out of the cell along its concentration gradient, increasing the internal negativity by a further 10–20 mV. As all the ion permeabilities normalize, the membrane potential returns to its baseline resting level.

on the membrane interior tend to attract and neutralize the negative charges on the immediately contiguous inner membrane. This makes the neighboring segment of membrane less interior-negative, depolarizing it to threshold and spawning another action potential. The depolarization cycle in the active sector must bring the abutting inactive membrane to threshold, which is a laboriously slow process.

All other things being equal, the impulse conduction velocity (CV) of a nerve or muscle fiber is directly related to its size. However, increasing fiber size is not a feasible way to increase CV in the mammalian nervous system. To achieve nerve CVs in the range seen in mammals, an individual axon might have to be as big around as the median nerve, and the nerve would have to be as large as the patient's arm! CV can be increased much more efficiently and dramatically by myelination. By insulating the membrane, the myelin sheath increases the transverse mem-

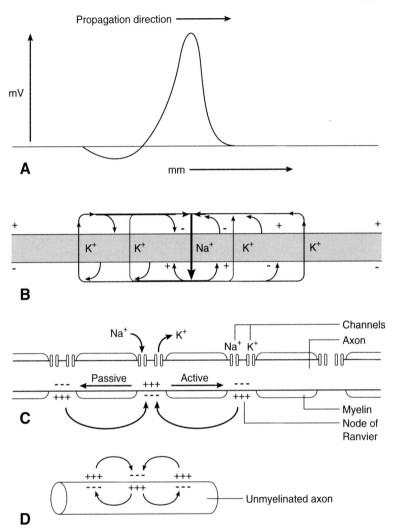

FIGURE 3–2. ■ Current paths during (*A*) the propagation of the action potential are shown in (*B*) an electrical circuit of a membrane and in (*C*) a myelinated and (*D*) an unmyelinated axon. (Reprinted with permission from Haines DE: *Fundamental Neuroscience.* New York, Churchill Livingstone, 1997, p 50.) Na$^+$ = sodium ions; K$^+$ = potassium ions.

brane resistance and lessens transverse current leakage across the membrane, enhancing current flow down the axon. In addition, conduction in myelinated fibers is saltatory (from the Latin *salio,* to leap), jumping from one node of Ranvier to the next (see Figure 3–2).

Saltatory conduction is very efficient. A 20-μm myelinated fiber has a CV 10 times faster than an unmyelinated fiber of the same diameter. Large myelinated human nerve fibers studied clinically in the electromyography (EMG) laboratory are in the 6- to 12-μm-diameter range and conduct at up to approximately 70 m/s, which is more than 150 miles/hour.

Axons are divided into three major size groups: large myelinated, small myelinated, and unmyelinated. Small myelinated fibers are approximately three times more numerous than large myelinated axons. The compound nerve action potential (NAP), recorded in vitro from mixed peripheral nerve, separates fibers into groups based on their CV. Peripheral nerve fibers are then classified by CV according to either of two schemes, the ABC and the I/II/III/IV systems, both ranging from largest (A, I) to smallest (C, IV) (Enrichment Box 3–5).

Most diseases involving peripheral nerves affect all types of fibers, but some have a special predilection for large fibers or for small fibers. When working with such patients, it is important to understand the differences between large-fiber functions and small-fiber functions.

THE MOTOR UNIT

The motor unit consists of an anterior horn motoneuron, its axon, and all its subject muscle fibers; it is the final common pathway for all motor activity, both voluntary and involuntary (Figure 3–3). Clinical dis-

---

ENRICHMENT BOX 3–5 Nerve Fiber Classification

The conduction velocity (CV) of a fiber depends on its diameter and degree of myelination; it ranges from < 1 m/sec for small, unmyelinated fibers to > 100 m/sec for large, myelinated fibers. The A group of nerve fibers is further divided into four Greek-letter–designated subgroups. A-alpha and A-gamma fibers are efferent fibers from alpha and gamma motoneurons respectively. A-beta and A-delta fibers are primarily cutaneous afferent nerves. Group-B fibers are preganglionic autonomic fibers. Group-C fibers are postganglionic autonomics, visceral afferent fibers, and pain and temperature fibers.

The Roman numeral system applies only to afferent fibers. Ia fibers arise from nuclear bag muscle spindle fibers and joint receptors, Ib fibers from Golgi tendon organs, and II fibers from nuclear chain muscle spindle fibers. Class III fibers are cutaneous axons, which correspond more or less to A-delta pain fibers; class IV fibers correspond to C fibers. The familiar classification of nerve fibers into general versus special, and somatic versus visceral has little if any clinical utility.

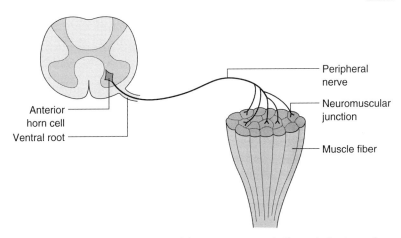

FIGURE 3–3. ■ The motor unit. An alpha motor neuron in the anterior horn gives rise to an axon, which branches and arborizes in the periphery to innervate scattered muscle fibers within a muscle fascicle.

orders may affect any portion of the motor unit (e.g., cell body, nerve root, plexus, peripheral nerve, neuromuscular junction, or muscle), and diseases at different sites have different clinical features. Abnormal, spontaneous involuntary activity can occur in all or part of the motor unit, and produces such clinical phenomena as fasciculations, cramps, and myokymia.

The anterior horn of the spinal cord and the brainstem motor nuclei contain alpha and gamma motoneurons. The alpha motoneurons innervate common, extrafusal muscle fibers, whereas the gamma motoneurons innervate intrafusal, muscle spindle fibers (*fusus* is the Latin word for spindle). The peripheral nerve enters the muscle at the motor point and divides into intramuscular branches. These arborize within a muscle fascicle and terminate as fine twigs, which end as axon boutons. Terminal boutons abut the motor end plates of individual muscle fibers across a synaptic cleft, forming neuromuscular junctions. Each muscle fiber has only a single end plate.

Terminal axonal twigs ramify in the muscle and innervate widely dispersed muscle fibers. A motor unit may have anywhere from a handful of muscle fibers to more than 1000, depending on the precision of control required. To produce a smoothly graded muscle contraction, motor units are recruited, more or less, in order of increasing size. Small motoneurons are first recruited, and increasing force of contraction calls forth activity from increasingly larger motoneurons. This is referred to as the *size principle*.

Motor units are classified histochemically as type 1 or type 2 (Enrichment Box 3–6). This classification is instrumental in the clinical and pathologic evaluation of patients with neuromuscular disease.

ENRICHMENT BOX 3–6 Classification of Motor Units

Muscles were broadly divided into red muscle and white muscle (dark meat and light meat) long before the basis for the difference was understood. The red or dark color is now known to result from the presence of the instruments for oxidative metabolism: myoglobin, mitochondria, and a vascular network for delivery of oxygen to the metabolizing muscle cells. When examining a muscle biopsy, pathologists apply histochemical stains, which help to separate the different types of muscle fibers and often allow the appreciation of structural detail and abnormalities not seen with routine hematoxylin and eosin (H&E) stains. The myosin adenosine triphosphatase (ATPase) histochemical stain identifies two distinct populations of muscle fibers, referred to as type 1 and type 2. An average muscle contains approximately 40% type 1 fibers and 60% type 2 fibers, but this ratio varies with the anatomic location and function of the muscle, and similar muscles may vary among individuals. The fiber type mix in the leg muscles of runners may have some rough correlation with their athletic talents for sprinting as opposed to distance running. All fibers in a particular motor unit are of the same type, and the fiber type mix of a muscle is determined by its innervation and ultimately by its function.

Type-1 fibers are rich in oxidative enzymes and mitochondria but sparse in glycogen, and are designed for sustained, long-duration contraction under aerobic conditions. Red meat is high in type-1 fibers (e.g., the leg meat of a bird that mostly walks but the wing meat of a bird that flies long distances). *Type-2 fibers* are rich in glycogen and glycolytic enzymes; are sparse in oxidative enzymes, mitochondria, and lipids; and are designed for brief, intense bursts of activity under anaerobic conditions. The mnemonic *"one, slow, red ox"* helps recall the essentials: type-1 fibers, slow muscle, red meat, oxidative metabolism.

In another functional and physiologic scheme, motor units are classified into three different types: fast twitch, fatigue sensitive (FF); slow twitch, fatigue resistant (S); and intermediate (FR). Type FF units are fast twitch, fatigue sensitive; type 2B histochemically; rich in glycogen but poor in oxidative enzymes; and designed for brief, phasic activity. Type S units are slow twitch, fatigue resistant; type 1 histochemically; low in glycolytic but high in oxidative enzymes; and designed for sustained, tonic activity. Type FR is intermediate, fast twitch but is more fatigue resistant than type FF.

All muscle fibers of a motor unit are of the same type, and there is good correlation between the mechanical properties and other attributes of a motor unit and the histochemical reactions of its muscle fibers.

Anatomy And Physiology Of The Neuromuscular Junction

Neuromuscular transmission is complex, and defects may develop at a number of points in the process, causing conditions such as myasthenia gravis and the Lambert-Eaton syndrome. Knowledge of the physiology of the neuromuscular junction is helpful in dealing with these patients, and especially for understanding some of the electrodiagnostic features of neuromuscular transmission disorders.

As the motor nerve approaches its termination point, it divides into fine terminal arborizations. Each "twig" ends by forming a bulbous swelling, the *terminal bouton*. The primary synaptic cleft separates the terminal bouton from the postsynaptic muscle membrane, which is in turn divided into a number of secondary synaptic clefts. The postsynaptic muscle membrane is blanketed by a dense array of nicotinic acetylcholine receptor (AChR) molecules. Acetylcholine esterase (AChE) molecules lurk on both presynaptic and postsynaptic membranes (Figure 3–4).

The terminal bouton is a beehive of metabolic activity. It is packed with cytoskeletal proteins, mitochondria, and numerous chemicals. Most importantly, it contains vesicles that are membrane-bound collections of

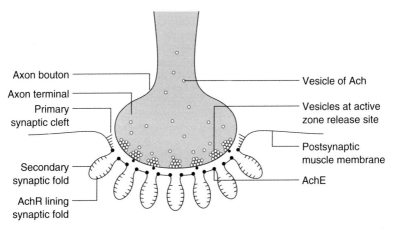

FIGURE 3–4. ■ The neuromuscular junction. An axon bouton abuts a postsynaptic muscle membrane across the primary synaptic cleft. Acetylcholine (ACh) is released and diffuses across the cleft to interact with receptors on the postsynaptic membrane. (Modified with permission from Campbell WW: *Essentials of Electrodiagnostic Medicine.* Baltimore, Williams and Wilkins, 1998, p 280.)

acetylcholine (ACh). In the cytoplasm of the terminal bouton, ACh is packaged into vesicles, which then migrate to and collect at primary release sites, or *active zones*. The active zones of the presynaptic membrane tend to line up opposite the secondary synaptic clefts of the postsynaptic membrane. The presynaptic membrane contains voltage-gated calcium channels. In response to nerve depolarization, these channels permit the influx of calcium into the presynaptic terminal, which greatly facilitates the release of neurotransmitter with the next nerve impulse.

Vesicles of ACh are released sporadically and irregularly while the membrane is at rest, and they are released in flurries when the terminal bouton undergoes depolarization. Upon activation, the vesicles fuse with the presynaptic membrane and pour their ACh contents out into the primary synaptic cleft. The molecules of ACh diffuse rapidly across the primary synaptic cleft and into the secondary synaptic clefts. Anywhere two molecules of ACh encounter an AChR, a chemical interaction takes place that opens sodium channels in the postsynaptic membrane, producing a brief nonpropagated, localized depolarization. The 5000–10,000 molecules of ACh contained within a single vesicle are also referred to as a *quantum*. The release of 1 quantum of ACh results in the opening of approximately 1500 channels in the postsynaptic membrane and produces a miniature end-plate potential. The summation of many miniature end-plate potentials produces a localized, nonpropagated depolarization in the region of the end plate, referred to as an *end-plate potential*. These can summate, and if above threshold, they spawn a propagated, all-or-none muscle fiber action potential.

Anatomy And Physiology Of Muscle

A muscle is composed of hundreds to thousands of individual muscle fibers (Figure 3–5). Each fiber is a multinucleated syncytium, roughly cylindrical in shape and encased in a connective tissue covering of endomysium, which extends over a long distance within a muscle fascicle. A muscle fascicle is a group of fibers lying together within a sheath of perimysium. Intramuscular nerve twigs, capillaries, and muscle spindles also occupy the perimysium.

Epimysium separates groups of fascicles and also provides a covering for the entire muscle. The surface epimysium, which encases the muscle proper, is continuous with the fascia, which covers the muscle, and in turn with the tendons, which anchor it at the origin and insertion points. The nuclei supporting a muscle fiber lie peripherally just under the sarcolemmal membrane. Just external to the sarcolemma is the dense basement membrane.

Each muscle fiber is composed of thousands of myofibrils, which are in turn made up of myriad myofilaments, the contractile elements. The

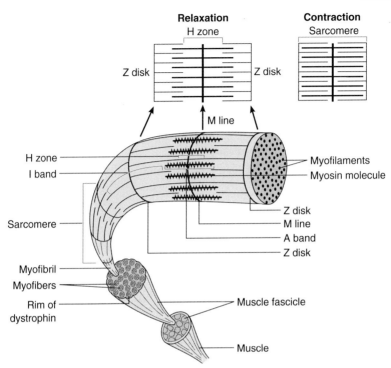

FIGURE 3-5. ■ Myofibrils are composed of repeating sarcomeres. The sarcomere extends from *Z line* to *Z line* and consists of the *I band* (actin filaments only), the *A band* (actin and myosin filaments overlapping), the *H zone* (myosin filaments only), and the *M line* (a central condensation of the myosin filaments). The myosin molecules have cross-bridges that interact with the actin molecules. When the muscle shortens, the overlapping of the myosin and actin molecules increases as the filaments slide, drawing the Z lines together and obliterating the I band. Dystrophin lies beneath the sarcolemma and helps reinforce it against the stretching and buckling. (Adapted with permission from Campbell WW: *Essentials of Electrodiagnostic Medicine.* Baltimore, Williams and Wilkins, 1998, p 301.)

myofibril is composed of repeating identical segments called *sarcomeres*. Components of the sarcomere include the A band, I band, Z disk, and H zone (Enrichment Box 3–7).

Actin. There are twice as many actin filaments as myosin filaments. During muscle contraction, the filaments slide past each other as side arms on the myosin molecule ratchet the actin molecule and draw it past. At maximal shortening, the Z disks are drawn together, and the I bands are obliterated as the overall length of the sarcomere decreases (see Figure 3–5).

ENRICHMENT BOX 3-7 Sarcomeres

A sarcomere is anchored at each end by a condensation of protein referred to as a Z disk. From each Z disk arise thin filaments of actin, which project toward the center of the sarcomere. At the center of the sarcomere, the M line anchors the thick filaments of myosin, which project outward toward the Z lines. Where the myosin and actin filaments overlap, the sarcomere appears more dense and transmits less light (i.e., the anisotropic or A band). At the ends of the sarcomeres, where thin actin filaments exist alone, the appearance is lighter (i.e., the isotropic or I band). In the paramedian zone, where myosin filaments exist alone, the appearance is intermediate (i.e., the H zone).

Myosin. Myosin is composed of two fragments: heavy meromyosin, which has ATPase activity, and light meromyosin, which does not. Actin is composed of three fragments: actin, troponin, and tropomyosin. Troponin can reversibly bind with calcium. A troponin–tropomyosin complex inhibits the interaction of myosin and actin while the muscle is at rest. The binding of calcium to troponin disinhibits the interaction and allows reactions to occur between the cross-bridges on the myosin molecule and active sites on the actin molecule.

At the junction of the A and I bands, the transverse (T) tubular systems arise as invaginations of the plasmalemma and ramify as an intricate network within the sarcomere. The T tubules allow communication between the muscle interior and the extracellular space, and are the conduits along which the action potential is transmitted to the depths of the sarcomere.

The *sarcoplasmic reticulum (SR)* is a closed internal labyrinth of vesicles that surrounds the myofibrils. The SR ends as focal dilatations, the terminal cisterns, which contain calcium. The action potential conducted into the fiber along the T tubule causes calcium release from the terminal cisterns, which in turn activates myosin ATPase and initiates sliding of the filaments. This sequence is referred to as *excitation contraction coupling*. After contraction, calcium ions are sequestered back into the terminal cisterns of the SR. Failure of normal resequestration of calcium causes at least two important clinical conditions: malignant hyperthermia and neuroleptic malignant syndrome. Both are associated with high fever, muscular rigidity, and rhabdomyolysis because of failure of skeletal muscle to relax normally.

In addition to the contractile elements, skeletal muscle contains important *cytoskeletal proteins,* which help provide structure. Elastic elements are essential, and allow for contraction and relaxation. One of the key cytoskeletal proteins is *dystrophin,* a large molecule that forms a reinforcing meshwork just beneath the sarcolemma and links the sarcomere to the sarcolemma and the extracellular matrix. Dystrophin appears to lend mechanical support to the sarcolemma to help stabilize and brace it against the forces of muscle contraction. Genetic derangements of these cytoskeletal proteins underlie some of the muscular dystrophies. Duchenne muscular dystrophy is caused by a derangement on the X chromosome, which causes a near total absence of membrane dystrophin.

Cellular organelles, glycogen granules, and lipids lie interspersed between the myofibrils and near the sarcolemmal nuclei. The relative abundance of different components varies with the function of a particular muscle (see Enrichment Box 3–6).

SPINAL REFLEXES

In addition to the motor unit, the next level of nervous system integration is at the spinal cord level. The simplest example of spinal cord segmental modulation of motor unit activity is the *monosynaptic stretch reflex.*

The motor unit consists of an alpha motor neuron and all its subject muscle fibers. A parallel system of innervation arises from gamma motor neurons. These are smaller motor neurons, which are also located in the anterior horn of the spinal cord. The gamma motor neurons innervate muscle spindles. These are compact, specialized units that lie widely interspersed among the extrafusal muscle fibers. The extrafusal fibers provide the force for muscle contraction. The muscle spindles provide modulation and control of that force. They also help regulate the underlying tone in the muscle. Muscle contraction always occurs against some setting of background tone. When the underlying, background level of muscle tone is either too high or too low, voluntary activity cannot occur with normal effectiveness. Thus, the gamma efferent system is a critical component of motor control.

The tiny muscle spindles are composed of specialized muscle fibers, which are affixed with connective tissue to the larger, extrafusal muscle fibers. The gamma motor neurons are also known as fusimotor neurons, as opposed to the alpha motor neurons, which are also known as skeletomotor neurons. Tonic firing of the gamma motor neuron produces slight contraction of the intrafusal fibers, leaving them under tension. The spindles send information regarding the level of tension to the spinal cord via large, heavily myelinated, rapidly conducting, primary spindle afferent nerve fibers. Centrally, these primary spindle afferent fibers connect monosynaptically to alpha motor neurons. They also send collaterals to the gamma motor neurons innervating the same muscle, as well as inhibitory collaterals to alpha motor neurons innervating antagonist muscles.

Given this arrangement, imagine the chain of events if a muscle were suddenly stretched, as if by percussion of its tendon with a reflex hammer. The passive stretch of the tendon stretches the muscle belly, which in turn leads to passive stretch of the muscle spindle. This lengthening of the intrafusal fibers triggers a volley of impulses in the primary spindle afferent nerve fibers. These synapse with alpha motor neurons innervating the muscle, causing them to fire, producing a contraction of the muscle, which then unloads or takes the stretch off of the muscle spindles. The muscle then returns to a state of relaxation. This sequence of percussion, contraction, then relaxation is a *deep tendon reflex* or *muscle stretch reflex*.

If the resting tone of the muscle spindles is increased, and the tension of the intrafusal fibers is at a higher-than-normal level, then the additional passive stretch due to percussion of the tendon produces a markedly exaggerated response. This is *hyperreflexia*, and it is seen with upper motor neuron lesions.

The activity of the motor neurons in the spinal cord is regulated and modulated by descending motor pathways that originate from the pyramidal cells in the motor cortex (pyramidal pathways) and elsewhere (extrapyramidal pathways). These descending motor pathways are generally inhibitory to spinal cord motor neurons, and act to suppress any excess activity. When the influence of the descending motor pathways is removed, as in a spinal cord injury, the result is a disinhibition of the segmental motor neuron pools below the level of the lesion, resulting in a higher level of gamma efferent resting traffic. This increases the gain on the muscle spindles, leaving them under an increased level of resting tone, which leads to spasticity and hyperreflexia.

In addition to this "simple" monosynaptic reflex arc, there are complex polysynaptic spinal reflexes that involve excitation or inhibition of agonists, synergists, and antagonist muscles. These segmental spinal cord reflexes can be responsible for fairly complex motor phenomena, such as the withdrawal reflex. Brain-dead patients can display impressive local reflex movements, including the so-called Lazarus effect, in which they virtually sit up in bed. These all are ostensibly caused by local spinal cord reflexes that have become autonomous and are under no suprasegmental control.

The major descending motor pathways that modulate segmental spinal cord activity include the corticospinal, rubrospinal, and vestibulospinal tracts (see Figure 2–12). There are several other minor tracts involved as well. The corticospinal tract preferentially innervates certain muscle groups. These include the extensors, supinators, and external rotators in the upper extremity, and the hip flexors, knee flexors, and foot dorsiflexors in the lower extremity. The pyramidal tract also preferentially innervates distal muscles and is responsible for fine motor control. Corticospinal tract functions are discussed further in Chapter 5.

The rubrospinal tract originates from the red nucleus and acts to generally enhance flexor muscle tone, primarily in the upper extremities. The vestibulospinal tract arises from the vestibular nuclei and acts to facilitate extensor tone. The functional significance of the rubrospinal and vestibulospinal tracts can be best appreciated by observing a patient progress from decorticate rigidity to decerebrate rigidity to the flaccidity of brain death. After rostrocaudal deterioration to a certain level, the patient lies with arms flexed and legs extended (i.e., *decorticate rigidity*). This is attributable to the fact that the rubrospinal pathways are still intact and are enhancing flexor tone to the upper extremities, producing a flexed arm posture with an extended leg posture. With further rostrocaudal deterioration, the rubrospinal tracts cease to function, but the vestibulospinal tracts remain intact, facilitating extensor tone to all four extremities and resulting in an extension posture of both arms and legs. This is *decerebrate rigidity*. With further rostrocaudal deterioration, the vestibulospinal tracts cease to function, and the patient become flaccid in all four extremities, an agonal condition.

The extrapyramidal pathways include all of those descending motor fibers that are not contained in the corticospinal tract. Many of these arise from the basal ganglia. Abnormalities in the extrapyramidal pathways can produce striking alterations in muscle tone as well as spontaneous motor activity (e.g., tremor). A classic example of an extrapyramidal disorder is Parkinson disease.

The final important link in motor control is the cerebellum. Its effects are mediated primarily by projections to the thalamus, red nucleus, and vestibular nuclei, and by reciprocal connections with the basal ganglia and motor cortex. At a cortical level, the primary motor cortex in the precentral gyrus is chiefly responsible for executing movement. The premotor and supplementary motor areas, which lie anterior to the motor strip in the frontal lobe, probably are involved in planning and preparation for movement.

Enrichment Box 3–8 provides an overview of motor physiology as applied to a movement (see also Enrichment Box 2–6). In the absence of disease, the movement is smooth and precise. Lesions involving any of the descending motor pathways can interfere with the normal execution of the movement. Learning how lesions of the corticospinal tract, the extrapyramidal pathways, and the cerebellum interfere with normal movement is one of the foundations of clinical neurology.

ENRICHMENT BOX 3-8 Motor Physiology

The premotor or supplementary motor area decides that a certain body part should move. It sends messages to that effect to the primary motor cortex. Impulses begin to descend through the corticospinal system toward the spinal cord. En route, collateral impulses are sent to the pontine nuclei, which then project to the cerebellum. Other portions of the cortex are co-activated and also send signals to the pontine nuclei. The pontine nuclei project to the cerebellum via the middle cerebellar peduncle. Cerebellar outflow then travels via the dentatorubrothalamic tract in the superior cerebellar peduncle to the red nucleus and to the thalamus. Impulse traffic in the rubrospinal tract interacts with the impulse traffic in the corticospinal tract to influence the stage of background muscle tone on which the muscle movement may be carried out. Additional cerebellar outflow via the vestibulospinal tract accomplishes the same function.

Impulse traffic to the thalamus is projected back to the motor cortex as well as to the basal ganglia. The descending traffic from the basal ganglia further interacts with the descending corticospinal impulses to regulate and coordinate the movement. The projections from the basal ganglia to the cortex via the thalamus act as a feedback loop in regard to the specifics of performance. All of the descending impulse traffic (i.e., corticospinal, extrapyramidal, rubrospinal, and vestibulospinal) converge on the spinal cord motor neuron pool responsible for the final execution of the intended movement.

The resting background excitability level of the segmental motor neuron pool is determined by all the noncorticospinal impulse traffic. The corticospinal tract impulses ultimately converge on the anterior horn cells innervating the muscle that needs to move; collateral impulses are sent to antagonist and synergist muscles for further coordination. The anterior horn cells comprising the appropriate motor units are then activated, and the movement is executed.

Further modulation at the local segmental level is provided by the muscle spindle afferent nerves, which help regulate tone in the gamma system. Also, afferent fibers coming from skin and joints help to convey additional information regarding the position of the limb in space to fine-tune the movement. Another important component in this system is the Golgi tendon organ (GTO). The GTO, from its position in the tendon, further helps to regulate muscle tone. It is a mechanism for force feedback to the contracting muscle. It also may serve as a protective mechanism against overstretch of the muscle tendon, either from active contraction of the muscle or from passive stretch. When tension in the tendon increases beyond a certain level, afferent traffic travels centrally via type Ib fibers from the GTO to inhibit contraction of the agonist and to cause contraction of the antagonist. At least for tension generated by active muscle contraction, this helps to unload the tension on the tendon by causing the muscle to relax. The GTO may be involved in two interesting clinical manifestations of spasticity: the clasp-knife reflex and clonus (Enrichment Box 3–9).

CEREBELLUM

The cerebellum is necessary for normal control of muscle contraction. Without it, movements are gross, uncoordinated, and tremulous. Precise movements, such as placing the finger on a target (as in the finger-to-nose/finger-nose-finger test), become impossible. Other manifestations of cerebellar disease include nystagmus, difficulty walking, and difficulty with sitting balance (titubation).

From a physiologic standpoint, the cerebellum can be viewed as having three components: the flocculonodular lobe, the vermis, and the hemispheres (Figure 3–6). The flocculonodular lobe is phylogenetically

---

ENRICHMENT BOX 3–9 Spasticity and Clonus

When a spastic muscle (e.g., the biceps) is stretched, there may be sudden loss of resistance near the end of the range of motion. This may be caused by Golgi tendon organ (GTO) impulses inhibiting contraction in the spastic muscle to prevent excessive tension from building up in the tendon. *Clonus* refers to a series of rhythmic contractions that can occur in a spastic muscle subjected to sudden, rapid, passive stretch. It is seen most often at the ankle (ankle clonus), occasionally at the patella (knee clonus), and in the forearm pronators (pronator clonus). To elicit ankle clonus, the examiner passively dorsiflexes the patient's foot using a rapid motion and holding the foot in a dorsiflexed position. This sudden stretch of the gastrosoleus muscle elicits a contraction essentially analogous to a deep tendon reflex. This causes a contraction with resultant plantar flexion of the foot. The foot goes down. This contraction increases tension in the gastrosoleus tendon GTOs, which then inhibits the contraction of the gastrocnemius muscle and facilitates contraction of its antagonist, the tibialis anterior muscle. The foot goes up. This in turn passively stretches the gastrosoleus, and the cycle is repeated. Plantar flexion of the foot also may initiate a stretch reflex in the dorsiflexors, and vice versa. These alternating stretch reflexes also may play a role in the production of clonus. The result is a rhythmic oscillation due to alternating contraction and relaxation of agonist and antagonist. Sustained clonus can persist indefinitely.

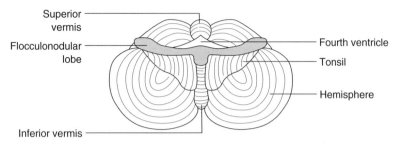

FIGURE 3–6. ■ The cerebellum depicting major functional divisions. The flocculonodular lobe is the archicerebellum and consists primarily of vestibular connections. The vermis is the paleocerebellum and is concerned with gait and locomotion. The hemispheres are the neocerebellum and are responsible for extremity coordination. The tonsils are the most inferior part of the hemispheres and are the part that may herniate through the foramen magnum in patients with increased intracranial pressure.

the oldest and is referred to as the archicerebellum. It has extensive connections with the vestibular nuclei and is concerned primarily with eye movement and gross balance. The archicerebellum can be viewed as "man the fish," the only concerns being eye movement control and gross orientation in space. The next area of the cerebellum to evolve was the vermis. There are extensive connections between the vermis and spinal cord pathways. The vermis is the paleocerebellum or spinocerebellum. It is concerned primarily with gait and locomotion. The paleocerebellum can be viewed as "man the snake." Snakes must attend to locomotion, but they do not have to worry about extremity control. The most phylogenetically recent part of the cerebellum is the neocerebellum, or the cerebellar hemispheres. These are concerned with precise movements of the extremities. The neocerebellum can be viewed as "man the monkey." The clinical signs of dysfunction in these three parts of the cerebellum are different. The clinical manifestations of cerebellar disease are discussed in more detail in Part II (Approach to the Patient) and Part III (Neurologic Disorders). The cerebellar anatomic connections are discussed in more detail in Chapter 2.

Sensory Physiology

The sensory system can be categorized in several different ways. There is the division between exteroceptive and interoceptive sensation. Exteroceptive sensation provides information about the external environment, including somatosensory functions and special senses. The interoceptive system conveys information about things internal, such as the orientation of the limbs and body in space, blood pressure, or the concentration of chemical constituents in bodily fluids. Sensory systems may function on a conscious or unconscious level. The monitoring of limb position has both a conscious component (i.e., the posterior column pathways) and an unconscious component (i.e., the spinocerebellar pathways). On routine clinical examination, sensory testing usually is restricted to exteroceptive, conscious sensation, but information may be gathered about other sensory functions using special techniques.

RECEPTORS

The interface between the sensory nervous system and the environment is the receptor. There are many different types of receptors to subserve the transduction of various types of information into nerve impulses. Receptors may respond to more than one type of stimulus, but have specificity because they have the lowest threshold for a particular type of stimulus.

When a stimulus is applied to a receptor, there is some change in the permeability of the membrane, which gives rise to a receptor or generator potential. These are local, nonpropagated potentials whose intensity is proportional to the intensity of the stimulus. Receptors may adapt to a stimulus to varying degrees. Some receptors are rapidly adapting and most sensitive to on-and-off stimuli. Others adapt slowly and function to constantly monitor a stimulus. Receptors are the terminal part of (and are continuous with) a sensory nerve. Receptor potentials induce action potentials in the nerve, with the frequency of the action potential discharge usually in proportion to the amplitude of the receptor potential, which is in turn proportional to the intensity of the applied stimulus. Each neuron has a specific receptive field, which consists of all the receptors it can respond to. The receptive fields form more or less discrete maps in the nervous system, in which specific regions of the body are represented in specific regions of the brain. Some systems have a highly organized map, for instance the somatosensory *homunculus* in the postcentral gyrus. In other systems, the maps are crude. In the cortex, neurons subserving the same modality and with similar receptive fields are organized into vertical rows that extend from the cortical surface to the white matter, referred to as cortical columns.

The impulses generated by the receptors are conveyed by afferent nerve fibers to the spinal cord or brainstem, then to the brain. The somatosensory system subserves external somatic sensation and can be divided into two primary components: the fine discriminative touch, position, vibration system and the pain, temperature, crude touch system. The latter also conveys other sensations, such as itch and tickle. These afferent inputs terminate in the ventral posterior complex of the thalamus. The information is then relayed from the thalamus via the thalamic radiations to the somatosensory cortex (see Figure 2–8).

The spinocerebellar tracts subserve unconscious proprioception. They are not relayed through the thalamus. Input from muscle spindles, GTOs, and receptors in muscles, skin, and joints is conveyed to the spinal cord and then via the anterior and posterior spinocerebellar tracts to the ipsilateral cerebellum (Enrichment Box 3–10). This information helps the cerebellum coordinate and control movement.

Throughout this system, at every level, there is constant processing and refinement of sensory impulses to produce meaningful and useful information. At the receptor level, there is the phenomenon of the *inhibitory surround,* in which stimuli not in a neuron's receptive field suppress its activity to more sharply focus applied stimuli. Each sensory relay neuron receives impulses from more than one input source, *convergence,* then sends impulses to more than one relay up the chain, *divergence.* Stimuli applied repetitively over a short time produce temporal summation. Stimuli applied repetitively to the same site produce spatial summation. Collaterals activated by incoming sensory volleys may produce local feedback inhibition of surrounding neurons in the posterior gray horn to help focus the signal and decrease divergence. All this complex activity serves to convert a given stimulus into a pattern of neural activity that is recognizable by the nervous system.

Pain Physiology

Pain physiology has become a complex topic. The *gate control theory* describes an inhibitory function of large myelinated fiber traffic on ac-

---

ENRICHMENT BOX 3–10 Unconscious Proprioception

In the spinal cord, the nucleus dorsalis of Clarke for the lower extremities and the nucleus cuneatus for the upper extremities give rise to the posterior spinocerebellar and cuneocerebellar tracts, respectively. These tracts enter the ipsilateral cerebellum through the inferior peduncle. Other cells in the intermedioposterior gray matter of the spinal cord give rise to the anterior spinocerebellar tract, which crosses the midline, enters the cerebellum via the superior peduncle, then crosses back to wind up ipsilateral to the cells of origin (see also Chapter 2). Impulse traffic in these tracts keeps the cerebellum appraised of the positions of the limb in space, and of the rate of movement. The cerebellar outflow tracts then communicate with other elements of the motor system to improve the precision of movements.

tivity in the neurons in the dorsal horn, which mediates pain impulses. Stimulation of large myelinated fibers can decrease simultaneous activity in pain fibers. At one time or another, everyone has experienced the attenuation of an acutely painful stimulus (e.g., cracking one's shin on a sharp edge) by vigorously rubbing the injured area. Rubbing stimulates large myelinated touch fibers and "closes the gate" for the incoming pain fibers. A transcutaneous electrical nerve stimulator (TENS) produces a constant stimulation of large myelinated fibers and is sometimes useful for the treatment of chronic pain.

Analgesia also can be produced by *electrical stimulation of the midbrain periaqueductal gray matter*. The midline raphe nuclei in the brainstem project downward in the dorsolateral funiculus of the spinal cord to synapse on neurons in the dorsal gray matter. These projections inhibit spinothalamic tract neurons and can attenuate pain, perhaps also by affecting the "gate" in the region of the first synapse of the pain pathways. Electrical stimulation of the dorsal columns can activate these projections below the level of the stimulator and affect pain perception. Clinically, both dorsal column stimulators and midbrain stimulators have been used in an attempt to manage chronic pain. These effects are likely mediated through the activity of endorphins and other opioid peptides. Neither has lived up to their initial promise based on the physiology.

Special Senses
The physiology of vision and eye movements is discussed in the chapter on NEUROOPHTHALMOLOGY (Chapter 7). Most diseases that cause hearing loss are not neurologic, and the reader is referred to other sources for a discussion of auditory physiology. However, disorders of the vestibular system are very common, and some understanding of the physiology is necessary for dealing with neurologic patients.

The Vestibular System
There are five components: the utricle, the saccule, and the three semicircular canals. The utricle and saccule respond to linear acceleration, the semicircular canals to angular acceleration. These responses are mediated by hair cells and transmitted to the vestibular ganglion and subsequently to the vestibular nuclei. Under normal circumstances, the neural activity in the labyrinths is equal on both sides, and the vestibular system is in balance. It is convenient to visualize the action of each vestibular system as pushing toward the opposite side (Figure 3–7). When the two labyrinths push equally, the system is in balance, and function is normal. When one labyrinth is underactive, the opposite labyrinth pushes the eyes, extremities, and body toward the side of un-

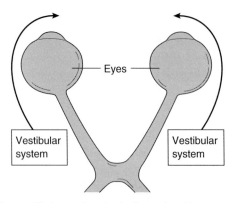

FIGURE 3–7. ■ The vestibular system tonically pushes the eyes, limbs, and body in the opposite direction. When the vestibular systems are equally active bilaterally, function is normal. When one vestibular system is more active, the eyes, limbs, and body tend to deviate to the opposite side.

deractivity. The clinical manifestations of vestibular dysfunction include vertigo, nausea, vomiting, nystagmus, past pointing, and lateropulsion.

Nystagmus results from a corrective saccade initiated by the frontal eye fields in response to the deviation of gaze toward the side of the less active labyrinth. The fast component of the nystagmus is therefore in the opposite direction from the hypoactive labyrinth. Without visual information to correct for errors (i.e., with eyes closed), patients with an acutely hypoactive labyrinth will have deviation of their extremities toward the underactive side on finger-to-nose testing. When attempting to walk with eyes closed, they will drift toward the side of the hypoactive labyrinth.

Caloric responses frequently are used clinically to check for brainstem integrity in patients with possible brain death. Ice water instilled into one ear canal will abruptly decrease the tonic activity from the labyrinth on the irrigated side. The normal labyrinth will then push the eyes tonically toward the irrigated side. This is the normal response in a comatose patient. In an awake subject, cold calorics produce nystagmus because of the cortically initiated corrective saccade in the opposite direction (hence the familiar mnemonic COWS: cold opposite, warm same). This refers to the fast, saccadic component of the nystagmus, not to the tonic gaze deviation. Nystagmus is seen only when the cortex is functioning normally.

When both labyrinths are diseased or malfunctioning, as might occur with ototoxic drug effects, there is no vestibular imbalance and therefore no nystagmus, vertigo, past pointing, or the like. However, patients with bilateral labyrinthine disease may nonetheless have great difficulty with balance and equilibrium.

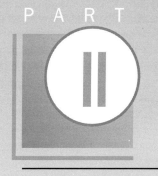

P A R T

II

Approach To The Patient

4

The Neurologic History

"Never believe what a patient tells you his doctor said."
—Sir William Jenner

INTRODUCTION

Introductory textbooks of physical diagnosis cover the basic aspects of medical history taking. This chapter is designed to point out some aspects of history taking that are of particular relevance to neurologic patients. Space does not permit an exhaustive treatment. Important historical points to be explored in some common neurologic conditions are summarized in the tables.

HISTORY TAKING

The history is the cornerstone of medical diagnosis, and neurologic diagnosis is no exception. More often than not, the diagnosis is in the history, and specifically in the details of the present illness. Many students and house officers seem to get so caught up in obtaining a complete database that they give short shrift to the details of the present illness. They may learn the cause of death of the patient's paternal grandmother and the year of the patient's old herniorrhaphy, while treating the symptoms of the present illness superficially. The majority of the time spent with a new patient should be devoted to the history, and the majority of the history-taking time should be devoted to the details of the presenting problem. It should go without saying that the most important aspect of history taking is attentive listening. Physicians should always ask open-ended questions and avoid suggesting possible responses. Although patients are frequently accused of being "poor historians," there are, in fact, as many poor history takers as there are poor history givers.

THE INTERVIEW

At the beginning of the interview, it is worthwhile to attempt to put the patient at ease. If possible, the physician should try to appear unhurried and engage in some small talk with the patient. Asking where the patient is from and what they do for a living not only helps to make the encounter less rigid and formal, but also helps physicians to discover very interesting things about their patients. Knowing patients as people is one of the greatest sources of pleasure in clinical practice.

Many physicians find it useful to take notes during the interview. A useful approach is simply to "take dictation" as the patient talks, particularly in the early stages of the encounter. Osler advised using the patient's own words, and a note sprinkled with patient quotations often is very illuminating. However, the physician must not be fixated on note taking. The trick is to interact with the patient while taking notes unobtrusively. The patient must not be left with the impression that the physician is paying attention to the note taking and not to them. Such notes typically are used for later transcription into some final format.

Deciding whether the physician or the patient should control the pace and content of the interview is a frequent problem. Patients do not practice history giving. Some are naturally much better at relating the pertinent information than others. Many patients digress frequently into extraneous detail. The physician adopting an overly passive role under such circumstances often prolongs the interview unnecessarily. When possible, the patient should give the initial part of the history without interruption. It is appropriate to keep the patient on track with focused questions, but the patient should not be interrogated. If the patient pauses to remember some irrelevancy, he or she should gently be encouraged not to dwell on it. A reasonable method is to let the patient run as long as they are giving a decent history, then take more control to clarify necessary details. Some patients may need to relinquish more control than others. Patients should be discouraged from grousing about their past medical care.

PAST HISTORY

Introduction to clinical medicine courses and internal medicine clerkships usually teach a traditional approach to history taking in which the clinician begins with the chief complaint and present illness. In fact, many experienced clinicians begin with the *pertinent* past history. This does not mean going into detail about unrelated past surgical procedures and the like. It does mean identifying major comorbidities that might have a direct or indirect bearing on the present illness. This technique helps to put the present illness in context and to prompt early consideration about whether the neurologic problem is a complication of some underlying condition or an independent process. It is inefficient to go through taking a long and laborious history from a patient with peripheral neuropathy, only to subsequently find out in the past history that the patient has known, long-standing diabetes. Therefore, major underlying past or chronic medical illnesses should be identified at the outset.

PRESENT ILLNESS

Gather information on the present illness by beginning with an open-ended question, such as, "What sort of problems are you having?" Asking "What brought you here today?" generates responses regarding a mode of transportation. And, asking patients, "What is wrong with you?" only invites wisecracks.

The preferred technique for taking the history of the present illness is to have the patient start at the beginning of the story and go through developments chronologically. However, many patients will not do this without direction. The patient should be encouraged to talk about symptoms, not about what previous physicians have thought.

HYPOTHESIZING THE DIAGNOSIS

Chapter 8 discusses the process of diagnostic reasoning. For now, suffice it to say that experienced clinicians generally make a diagnosis through a process of hypothesis testing. At some point in the interview, the physician must assume greater control to ask the patient about specific details of their symptomatology in order to test hypotheses and help to rule in or rule out diagnostic possibilities.

It is important to clarify important elements of the history that the patient is unlikely to spontaneously describe. Symptoms must be analyzed systematically, which is done by asking the patient a series of questions to clear up any ambiguities. The physician should determine exactly when the symptoms began; whether they are present constantly or intermittently; and, if intermittently, what are the character, duration, frequency, severity, and any relationship to external factors. Any specific precipitating or relieving factors should be identified. However, the physician should clarify what the patient means by a term (e.g., numbness or dizziness) that is used in different ways by different patients.

Some patients have difficulty describing the character of pain. Although spontaneous descriptions have more value, and leading questions should be avoided, it is perfectly permissible when necessary to offer possible choices, such as "dull like a toothache" or "sharp like a knife."

INFORMATION GLEANED FROM NEW PATIENTS

Several different types of information may be obtained during the initial encounter. There is direct information from the patient describing their symptoms, information from the patient regarding what previous physicians may have thought about their problem, and information that might be obtained from medical records or from previous caregivers. All of this information potentially is important. Usually, the most essential information is the patient's own description of his or her symptoms. Therefore, physicians should work from information obtained firsthand from the patient when possible. The patient should be steered away from a description of what previous physicians have thought, at least initially. Many patients tend to jump quickly to describing encounters with caregivers, glossing over any description of the details of the illness. The patient should be encouraged to focus on the symptoms instead.

INFORMATION FROM PAST CAREGIVERS

Usually, it is best to see the patient de novo with minimal prior review of the medical records. Too much information in advance of the patient encounter may bias the physician's opinion. If it later turns out that previous caregivers reached similar conclusions based on primary information, then the likelihood of a correct diagnosis is increased. The patient should be seen first; old records should be reviewed later. If medical records are not available, it is certainly useful and appropriate for the patient to relate what they have been told by previous caregivers. Bear in mind, however, that patient recollections may be flawed because of faulty memory, misunderstanding, or other factors.

There are three approaches to utilizing information from past caregivers, whether from medical records or as relayed by the patient. In the first instance, the physician takes too much at face value and assumes that previous diagnoses must be correct. An opposite approach, actually used by some, is to assume that all previous diagnoses are incorrect. However, this forces the extreme skeptic into a position of having to make some other diagnosis, even when the preponderance of the evidence indicates that previous physicians were correct. The logical middle ground is to make no assumptions regarding the opinions of previous caregivers. Information should be used appropriately, matching it against what the patient relates and whatever other information is available. The physician should not automatically believe it all, but also not automatically disbelieve it.

REVIEWING PAST MEDICAL RECORDS

One efficient way to work is to combine reviewing past notes with talking directly with the patient. If the records contain a reasonably complete history, review it with the patient for accuracy. For instance, read from the records and say to the patient, "Dr. Payne says here that you have been having pain in the left leg for the past 6 months. Is that correct?" The patient might verify that information or may say, "No, it's the right leg, and it's more like 6 years." Such an approach can save considerable time when dealing with a patient who carries extensive previous records. A very useful method for summarizing a past work-up is to make a table with two vertical columns, listing all tests that were done, placing those with normal results in one column and those with abnormal results in the other column.

RE-TAKING THE HISTORY

The history may need to be taken more than once. A good general working rule is that whenever the diagnosis is in doubt, take the history again. The *attending effect* occurs when an attending physician takes the history from a patient after the history has been taken by one or more trainees. History taking improves with experience because the clinician is able to generate more hypotheses to explain the patient's complaint, and has more questions available to verify or exclude candidate conditions. It is not uncommon for a great deal of relevant information to suddenly come out under the attending physician's questioning, sometimes to the chagrin of students and house staff. Although the attending effect may be attributable to the more highly evolved history-taking skills of an experienced clinician, there are other potential explanations. Patients sometimes forget important details of their history during the initial encounter. They also may be sick, in pain, or inattentive. Many initial histories are taken by trainees at a very late hour. By the time of attending rounds, after the patient has had some sleep, a little breakfast, and some time to ponder, the history has evolved because the patient has recalled information prompted by the earlier questioning. The previous history serves as a warm-up. When working alone, take advantage of the attending effect by simply repeating and verifying the key portions of the history after some time has elapsed.

TAKING THE HISTORY OF NEUROLOGIC PATIENTS

In neurologic patients, pay particular attention to the time course of the illness because this is often instrumental in determining the etiology. An illness might evolve hyperacutely, as in stroke; subacutely over a period of days to weeks, as in Guillain-Barré syndrome; chronically over a period of many months to several years, as in Alzheimer disease; or very chronically over many years, as in hereditary spinocerebellar degeneration. Some illnesses are characterized by recurrent attacks, between which there is partial or complete recovery. Such a relapsing-remitting course is typical of multiple sclerosis.

In patients presenting with neurologic symptoms, a *neurologic re-*

view of systems is useful after exploring the present illness. Some question areas worth probing into are summarized in Table 4–1. Symptoms of depression often are particularly relevant and are summarized separately in Table 4–2.

The family history is occasionally quite important in neurologic patients. Many neurologic disorders that are generally considered pediatric (e.g., congenital malformations, some hereditary conditions) occasionally present in adulthood. But there are traps, and a negative family history is not always really negative. Some diseases may be rampant in a family without the affected individuals being aware of it. With Charcot-Marie-Tooth disease, for example, so many family members bear the stigmata that it is not recognized as abnormal. Chronic, disabling neurologic conditions in a family member may be attributed to another cause, such as arthritis.

Sometimes, family members deliberately withhold information about a known familial condition. This seems to happen most often in cases of Huntington chorea. Patients themselves may also occasionally conceal important information. In some cases, they may not realize the information is important. In other cases, they may be too embarrassed to reveal certain details.

Family members sometimes accompany the patient during the inter-

---

TABLE 4–1. A NEUROLOGIC SYSTEM REVIEW

Any history of seizures or unexplained loss of consciousness

Headache

Vertigo

Loss of vision

Diplopia

Difficulty hearing

Tinnitus

Difficult with speech or swallowing

Weakness

Numbness or tingling

Problems with gait, balance, or coordination

Difficulty with sphincter control or sexual function

Difficulty with thinking or memory

Depressive symptoms

TABLE 4–2. SOME SYMPTOMS SUGGESTING DEPRESSION

Unexplained weight gain or loss

Increased or decreased appetite

Sleep disturbance

Lack of energy, tiredness, or fatigue

Anhedonia

Depressed mood or sadness

Feelings of guilt or worthlessness

Suicidal ideation

Psychomotor agitation or retardation

Sexual dysfunction

Difficulty concentrating or making decisions

Difficulty with memory

view. Often they provide important supplementary information; however, family members must not be permitted to dominate the patient's account of their illness unless the patient is incapable of giving a history.

It is useful at some point to ask the patient what is worrying them. Occasionally it turns out that the patient is very concerned about the possibility of some disorder that the physician had not even thought to consider. Patients with neurologic complaints often are apprehensive about having some dreadful disease, such as a brain tumor, amyotrophic lateral sclerosis, multiple sclerosis, or muscular dystrophy. All of these conditions are well known to the lay public, and patients or family members occasionally jump to outlandish conclusions about the cause of some symptom. Simple reassurance is usually all that is necessary.

Some of the important historical features to explore in patients with certain neurologic complaints are summarized in Tables 4–3 to 4–11. There are too many potential neurologic presenting complaints to cover them all, so these tables should be regarded only as a starting point and an illustration of the process.

Space does not permit an explanation of the differential diagnostic relevance of each of these elements of the history. These details regarding all the possible presenting complaints, or even just the common ones, would comprise a textbook of neurology. Suffice it to say that each of these elements in the history has significance in ruling in or ruling out

TABLE 4–3. IMPORTANT HISTORICAL POINTS IN THE PATIENT WITH CHRONIC HEADACHE

Location of the pain (e.g., hemicranial, holocranial, occipitonuchal, bandlike)

Pain intensity

Pain quality (e.g., steady, throbbing, stabbing)

Average daily caffeine intake

Average daily analgesic intake (including over-the-counter medications)

Precipitating factors (e.g., alcohol, sleep deprivation, oversleeping, foods, bright light)

Relieving factors (e.g., rest/quiet, dark room, activity, medications)

Neurologic accompaniments (e.g., numbness, paresthesias, weakness, speech disturbance)

Visual accompaniments (e.g., scintillating scotoma, transient blindness)

Gastrointestinal accompaniments (e.g., nausea, vomiting, anorexia)

Associated symptoms (e.g., photophobia, phonophobia/sonophobia, tearing, nasal stuffiness)

Any history of head trauma

TABLE 4–4. IMPORTANT HISTORICAL POINTS IN THE PATIENT WITH NECK AND ARM PAIN

Onset and duration (acute, subacute, chronic)

Pain intensity

Any history of injury

Any history of preceding viral infection or immunization

Any past history of disc herniation, disc surgery, or previous episodes of neck or arm pain

Location of the worst pain (e.g., neck, arm, shoulder)

Pain radiation pattern, if any (e.g., to shoulder, arm, pectoral region, periscapular region)

Relation of pain to neck movement

Relation of pain to arm and shoulder movement

Relieving factors

Any exacerbation with coughing, sneezing, straining at stool

Any weakness of the arm or hand

Any numbness, paresthesias, or dysesthesias of the arm or hand

Any associated leg weakness or bowel, bladder, or sexual dysfunction suggesting spinal cord compression

TABLE 4–5. IMPORTANT HISTORICAL POINTS IN THE PATIENT WITH BACK AND LEG PAIN

Onset and duration (acute, subacute, chronic)

Pain intensity

Any history of injury

Any past history of disc herniation, disc surgery, or previous episodes of back or leg pain

Location of the worst pain (e.g., back, buttock, hip, leg)

Pain radiation pattern, if any (e.g., to buttock, thigh, leg, or foot)

Relation of pain to body position (e.g., standing, sitting, lying down)

Relation of pain to activity and movement (e.g., bending, stooping, leg motion)

Any exacerbation with coughing, sneezing, straining at stool

Any weakness of the leg, foot, or toes

Any numbness, paresthesias, or dysesthesias of the leg or foot

Relieving factors

Any associated bowel, bladder, or sexual dysfunction suggesting cauda equina compression

Any associated fever, weight loss, or morning stiffness

TABLE 4–6. IMPORTANT HISTORICAL POINTS IN THE DIZZY PATIENT

Patient's precise definition of dizziness

Presence or absence of an illusion of motion

Whether symptoms are constant or intermittent

If intermittent, the duration and timing of attacks

Relation of dizziness to body position (e.g., standing, sitting, lying)

Any precipitation of dizziness by head movement

Associated symptoms (e.g., nausea, vomiting, tinnitus, hearing loss, weakness, numbness, diplopia, dysarthria, dysphagia, difficulty with gait or balance, palpitations, shortness of breath, dry mouth*, chest pain)

Medications, especially antihypertensives or ototoxic drugs

*Dry mouth may suggest hyperventilation.

TABLE 4–7. IMPORTANT HISTORICAL POINTS IN THE PATIENT WITH HAND NUMBNESS*

Whether symptoms are constant or intermittent

If intermittent, the timing of symptoms, especially any relationship to time of day or tendency for nocturnal symptoms

Relationship to activities (e.g., driving)

Part of hand that is most involved

Any involvement of arm, face, or leg

Any problems with speech or vision associated with the hand numbness

Neck pain

Hand or arm pain

Hand or arm weakness

Any history of injury, especially to the wrist

Any involvement of the opposite hand

*The primary considerations in the differential diagnosis are carpal tunnel syndrome and cervical radiculopathy.

TABLE 4–8. IMPORTANT HISTORICAL POINTS IN THE PATIENT WITH SUSPECTED TIA*

Date of first spell

Frequency of attacks

Duration of attacks

Specific body parts and functions involved

Any associated difficulty with speech, vision, or swallowing

Other associated symptoms (e.g., chest pain, shortness of breath, nausea and vomiting, headache)

Any history of hypertension, diabetes mellitus, hypercholesterolemia, coronary artery disease, peripheral vascular disease, or drug abuse

Any past episodes suggestive of retinal, hemispheric, or vertebrobasilar TIA

Current medications, especially aspirin, oral contraceptives, antihypertensive agents

TIA = transient ischemic attack.
  *TIA is suspected in patients who have had one or more spells of weakness or numbness involving one side of the body, transient loss of vision, symptoms of vertebrobasilar insufficiency, and similar problems.

TABLE 4–9. IMPORTANT HISTORICAL POINTS IN THE PATIENT WITH EPISODIC LOSS OF CONSCIOUSNESS (SYNCOPE VERSUS SEIZURE)

Timing of attack (e.g., frequency, duration)

Patient's recollection of events

Circumstances of attack (e.g., in church, in the shower)

Events just prior to attack

Body position just prior to attack (e.g., supine, sitting, standing)

Presence of prodrome or aura

Any tonic or clonic activity

Any suggestion of focal onset

Symptoms following the spell (e.g., sleeping, focal neurologic deficits, incontinence, tongue biting)

Time until complete recovery

Family history

Witness description of attacks

TABLE 4–10. IMPORTANT HISTORICAL POINTS IN THE PATIENT WITH NUMBNESS OF THE FEET*

Whether symptoms are constant or intermittent

If intermittent, any relation to posture, activity, or movement

Any associated pain in the back, legs, or feet

Any weakness of the legs or feet

Any history of back injury, disc herniation, or back surgery

Symmetry of symptoms

Any bowel, bladder, or sexual dysfunction

Any history of underlying systemic disease (e.g., diabetes mellitus, thyroid disease, anemia, low vitamin B_{12} level)

Any weight loss

Drinking habits

Smoking history

Any history to suggest toxin exposure, either vocational or recreational

Dietary history

Medication history, including vitamins

Family history of similar symptoms

Family history of diabetes, pernicious anemia, or peripheral neuropathy

*The differential diagnosis is usually between peripheral neuropathy and lumbosacral radiculopathy. There is a further extensive differential diagnosis of the causes of peripheral neuropathy.

TABLE 4–11. IMPORTANT HISTORICAL POINTS IN THE PATIENT COMPLAINING OF MEMORY LOSS*

Duration of the problem

Getting worse, getting better, or staying the same

Examples of what is forgotten (e.g., minor things, such as dates and anniversaries, compared with major things)

Does the patient still control the checkbook

Any tendency to get lost

Medication history, including over-the-counter drugs

Drinking habits

Any headache

Any difficulty with the senses of smell or taste

Any difficulty with balance, walking, or bladder control

Any depressive symptoms (see Table 4–2)

Any recent head trauma

Past history of stroke or other vascular disease

Past history of thyroid disease, anemia, low vitamin B_{12} level, or any sexually transmitted diseases

Any risk factors for HIV

Family history of dementia or Alzheimer disease

*The primary consideration here is to distinguish Alzheimer disease from conditions (especially treatable ones) that may mimic it.

some diagnostic possibility. Such a list exists for every complaint in every patient. Learning and refining these lists is the challenge of medicine.

For example, Table 4–3 lists some of the specific important historical points helpful in evaluating a patient with chronic headache. The following features are general rules and guidelines, not absolutes. Patients with migraine headaches tend to have unilateral hemicranial or orbitofrontal throbbing pain associated with gastrointestinal upset. Those patients suffering from migraine with aura, or classic migraine, have visual or neurologic accompaniments. Patients usually seek relief by lying quietly in a dark, quiet environment. Patients with cluster headache tend to have unilateral nonpulsatile orbitofrontal pain with no visual, gastrointestinal, or neurologic accompaniments and tend to get some relief by moving around. Patients with tension or muscle contraction headaches tend to have nonpulsatile pain that is bandlike or occipitonuchal in distribution, and is unaccompanied by visual, neurologic, or gastrointestinal upset.

Table 4–4 lists some of the important elements in the history in patients with neck and arm pain. The primary differential diagnosis is usually between cervical radiculopathy and musculoskeletal conditions, such as bursitis, tendonitis, impingement syndrome, and myofascial pain. Patients with a herniated cervical disc usually have pain primarily in the neck, trapezius ridge, and upper shoulder region. Patients with cervical myofascial pain have pain in the same general distribution. Patients with radiculopathy may have pain referred to the pectoral or periscapular regions, which is unusual in those with myofascial pain. Patients with radiculopathy may have pain radiating in a radicular distribution down the arm. Pain radiating below the elbow usually means radiculopathy. Patients with radiculopathy have pain on movement of the neck; those with shoulder pathology have pain on movement of the shoulder. Patients with radiculopathy may have weakness or sensory symptoms in the involved extremity.

5

A Screening Neurologic Examination

"Life is short, the art long, opportunity fleeting,
experience treacherous, judgement difficult."
—*Hippocrates*

INTRODUCTION

There is no more important task during a neurology rotation than learn-ing to do a competent neurologic examination. Identifying the abnormal findings is a vital step toward an accurate formulation of the problem and the formation of a differential diagnosis. The neurologic examination can be a complex and arduous undertaking. The arcane techniques and em-phasis on completeness can make an encounter with a neurologic patient an intimidating task. Although some neurologists think that anything short of a complete neurologic examination is inadequate, it is better to do some neurologic examination than none at all. The interpretation of abnormalities found on the examination is discussed in Chapter 6.

Neurologists have generally concluded that the commonly seen no-tation "neuro grossly intact" means that little if any examination was done. In fact, few neurologists do a truly complete examination on every patient. As with the general physical examination, the history fo-cuses the neurologic examination so that certain aspects are empha-sized in a given clinical situation. The examination done on a typical patient with headache is not the same as that done on a patient with low back pain, or dementia, or cerebrovascular disease. With co-matose, combative, or uncooperative patients, a complete examination is impossible. However, in each of these situations, at least some ma-neuvers are used to screen for neurologic dysfunction that is not nec-essarily suggested by the history. A primary care physician nearly always listens to the heart and lungs, no matter what the presenting complaint. But she will not auscultate the heart while having the patient perform a Valsalva maneuver or squat unless there is a specific need to characterize or bring out a murmur driven by some detail of the history or a finding on the routine screening cardiac examination. So it is with the neurologic examination. Every patient does not require every conceivable test, but all require a screening examination.

INCORPORATING THE GENERAL PHYSICAL EXAMINATION INTO THE NEUROLOGIC EXAMINATION

Rather than thinking about how to incorporate the neurologic examination into the general physical examination, think about incorporating the general physical into the neurologic examination. Any neurologic examination, even a cursory one, provides an opportunity to accomplish much of the general examination. A head-eyes-ears-nose-throat (HEENT) examination is a natural byproduct of an evaluation of the cranial nerves. After listening for carotid bruits, it requires very little additional effort to palpate the neck for masses and thyromegaly. A good motor and reflex examination and an evaluation of gait and station provide a great deal of information about the patient's orthopedic condition. It is difficult to miss a bad knee, shoulder, or hip during the process. Testing sensation and plantar responses provides an opportunity to coincidentally look at the skin and nails and feel the peripheral pulses. At the end of a good neurologic examination, one only has to listen to the heart and lungs and palpate the abdomen to have also done a fairly complete general physical examination.

THE "NAVY NEUROLOGIC"

A crusty Air Force neurosurgeon once described what he referred to as a "Navy neurologic." The concept is that of a screening examination that requires the nervous system to perform at a high level. If the nervous system can execute a complex task flawlessly, it is very unlikely there is significant pathology present, and going through a more extensive evaluation is not likely to be productive.

Try doing a Navy neurologic on yourself. Stand with feet together and arms outstretched to the sides. Now touch your nose alternately with the right and left index fingers. Keeping up this motion, close your eyes, get a rhythm going, then hop on one foot. Now switch to the other foot. You probably found this maneuver difficult but doable. If a patient successfully performs this complex maneuver, all that is then necessary is to look at the fundi and test the plantar responses. If these are normal, the chance of significant neurologic pathology is remote.

The "Navy neurologic" is too brief to be appropriate for ordinary medical practice, but the concept of a screening examination is valid. A neurologic examination that addresses complex functions and seeks signs that are sensitive indicators of pathology is efficient and not overly time consuming. It can also serve as a core around which a general physical examination can be built. The examination techniques that follow use these concepts. Common errors and areas that cause particular technical problems are highlighted.

For those who would like to explore a more complete traditional examination, visit the Internet site *www.neuroland.com,* click on the brain, and follow the links to "Best Neuro Sites" then to "Best Neuro Exam," which will take you to the University of Florida medical information site. Here there is an excellent description of a full neurologic examination in outline format compiled by Dr. Richard Rathe. There are several textbooks of varying lengths devoted to the neurologic examination for those who are interested in further detail.

A SCREENING NEUROLOGIC EXAMINATION

There are two basic approaches to a traditional neurologic examination: regional and systemic. A systemic approach evaluates the motor system in its entirety, the sensory system, and so on. A regional approach evaluates all the systems in a given region, such as the upper extremities, then the lower extremities. Regardless of the approach, the results are recorded in the same way (Table 5–1). The rapid screening examination is an amalgam of the regional and systemic approaches geared for speed and efficiency (Table 5–2) . The following sections describe the mechanics of performing a screening neurologic examination that relies heavily on sensitive signs, especially the flawless execution of complex functions.

TABLE 5–1. SCHEME FOR RECORDING THE RESULTS OF THE NEUROLOGIC EXAMINATION

Mental status

Cranial nerves

Motor system

Sensory system

Reflexes

Cerebellar function and coordination

Gait and station

TABLE 5–2. STEPS IN A RAPID SCREENING NEUROLOGIC EXAMINATION

Mental status examination (during history taking or dispersed during the rest of the examination)

Penlight examination

　Pupils (at distance)

　Extraocular movements

　Pharynx, oral cavity, and tongue (watch the jaw open to be sure it drops vertically to screen for trigeminal motor dysfunction)

Facial motor functions (e.g., grimacing, closing eyes tightly)

Visual fields

Fundi

Upper extremity strength examination (i.e., deltoid, triceps, wrist extensors, and hand intrinsics)

Examination for pronator drift (eyes closed)

Examination of upper extremity stereognosis and upper and lower extremity double simultaneous stimulation, While waiting for drift, with the patient's eyes closed. (Evaluate fine motor control during the patient's manipulation of the stereognosis test objects.)

Examination of finger-to-nose coordination (eyes closed)

Examination of arm and finger roll

Examination of lower extremity strength (hip flexors, hamstrings, foot dorsiflexors)

Examination of deep tendon reflexes in upper and lower extremities

Elicitation of plantar responses

Examination of station and gait, heel and toe walking, hopping on each foot, tandem gait, Romberg test, or eyes closed tandem

MENTAL STATUS EXAMINATION

This screening examination begins with taking the medical history, which serves as a fair barometer of the mental status. Patients who can relate a logical, coherent, pertinent, and sensible narrative of their problem will seldom be found deficient on more formal bedside mental status testing. Conversely, a rambling, disjointed, incomplete history may be a clue to the presence of some cognitive impairment, although there may be no direct complaint of thinking or memory problems from the patient or the family. Similarly, psychiatric disease is sometimes betrayed by the patient's demeanor and style of history giving.

If there is any suggestion of abnormality from the interaction with the patient during the history-taking phase of the encounter, then a more detailed mental status examination should be performed. This usually begins with assessing orientation. Other commonly used questions include the current president, past presidents, inquiries about current events, serial 7s, and spelling the word "world" backward. The Katzmann Orientation-Memory-Concentration questionnaire is a very useful, brief instrument that has been standardized (Table 5–3). The Folstein mini-mental questionnaire also is commonly used for a quick, quantitative assessment of cognitive abilities (Table 5–4).

EXAMINATION OF THE CRANIAL NERVES

The screening examination continues with checking the lids and pupils and proceeds to finish everything that requires use of a penlight. Begin by noting the position of the eyelids and the width of the palpebral fissures bilaterally. The upper eyelid should cross the iris just below the superior limbus; there should be no sclera showing above the iris. Any asymmetry of lid position should be noted, such as ptosis or lid retraction. The width of the palpebral fissures should be equal on both sides. Check the pupils for light reaction with the patient fixing at a distance (see Common Errors). If the pupillary light reaction is normal and equal in both eyes, there is little to be gained by routine testing for the pupillary near reaction that is part of the accommodation reflex. Continue the examination by assessing extraocular movements in the six cardinal positions of gaze, having the patient follow the penlight. Six positions are used rather than four because the oblique muscles insert at an angle, and the globe must be in a moderately adducted position for the

---

TABLE 5–3. THE SHORT ORIENTATION-MEMORY-CONCENTRATION TEST FOR COGNITIVE IMPAIRMENT

Ask the patient to:

1. Name the month

2. Name the year

3. State the time of day

4. Remember the following memory phase: "John Brown, 42 Market Street, Chicago"

5. Count backward from 20 to 1

6. Name the months of the year in reverse

7. Recall the memory phrase

Reprinted with permission from Katzman R, Brown T, Fuld P, et al: Validation of a short orientation-memory-concentration test of cognitive impairment. *Am J Psychiatr* 140:734, 1983.

TABLE 5–4. MINI MENTAL STATE EXAMINATION

Maximum Score	Item Tested
	Orientation
5	What is the day, date, month, season and year?
5	Where are we? Country, state, city, hospital, floor?
	Registration
3	Name three objects: 1 second to say each. Then ask patient to repeat all three. Give 1 point for each correct answer. Then repeat until all three are registered.
	Attention and calculation
5	Serial sevens. 1 point for each correct. Stop after 5 answers. Alternatively, spell "world" backward.
	Recall
3	Ask for the three objects repeated above. Give 1 point for each correct.
	Language
9	Name a pencil and watch (2 points)
	Repeat the following: "No ifs, ands, or buts." (1 point)
	Follow a three-stage command: "Take a piece of paper in your right hand, fold it in half, and put it on the floor." (3 points)
	Read and obey the following: "Close your eyes." (1 point)
	Write a sentence. (1 point)
	Copy design. (1 point)

Reprinted with permission from Folstein MF, Folstein S, McHugh P: "Mini-mental state": A practical method for grading the cognitive state of patients for the clinician. *J Psychiatr Res* 12:189–198, 1975.

oblique muscles to exert their pull. With the eye adducted, the superior oblique depresses the globe; with the eye in primary position, the superior oblique acts only to intort it. Be sure the patient has no diplopia or limitation of movement with the eyes fully right, fully left, right and up, right and down, left and up, and left and down. Ocular movements in pursuit of a target should be smooth and fluid; degeneration into coarse, ratchety movements (referred to as saccadic pursuit) is abnormal. With the eyes in primary and eccentric positions, look for any nystagmus. Abnormalities of eye movement are discussed in detail in Chapter 7. For an excellent simulation of normal and abnormal eye movements visit the Web site *cim.ucdavis.edu/eyes*. A program in beta testing also simulates normal and abnormal pupillary reactions.

For purposes of the general physical examination, take the opportunity during this phase to note any abnormalities of the eyes, lids, and ocular adnexa (e.g., conjunctivitis, exophthalmos, lid lag, ectropion, xanthelasma, arcus senilis).

With the light still in hand, the pharynx and oral cavity should be examined. Examination of the motor branch of the trigeminal nerve is accomplished by watching the patient's jaw drop open. When the pterygoids are unilaterally weak, the jaw invariably deviates toward the weak side on opening. This deviation, although subtle, is a more sensitive indicator of trigeminal motor root pathology than the traditional palpation of the masseter and temporalis muscles. For general examination purposes, note any prognathism, micrognathia, trismus, and the like.

Observe the tongue for atrophy or fasciculations. Note any glossitis or other abnormality. Have the patient phonate and be sure the median raphe of the palate elevates in the midline. There is little to be gained by checking the gag reflex if the patient has no complaints of dysphagia or dysarthria and if there is no reason from the history to suspect a brainstem or cranial nerve lesion. Routine elicitation of the gag reflex is rarely informative and is unpleasant for the patient. As an extension to the general physical examination, the physician can search for any intraoral lesions, leukoplakia, or other abnormality.

When the penlight examination is completed, observe the nasolabial folds for depth and symmetry, and note whether there is any asymmetry in forehead wrinkling or in the width of the palpebral fissures to suggest facial nerve dysfunction. Ask the patient to grimace, vigorously baring his teeth, while closing his eyes tightly. Note the symmetry of the grimace, the number of teeth seen on each side, the relative amplitude and velocity of the lower facial contraction, and the symmetry of the upper facial contraction. How completely the patient buries the eyelashes on the two sides is a sensitive indicator of orbicularis oculi strength.

If the patient has no complaints of hearing loss, tinnitus, vertigo, facial numbness, or weakness, and there is no specific reason suggested by the history to do so, routine examination of hearing is seldom productive. If there is a need to examine hearing, a quick comparison of the patient's ability to hear a soft whisper in each ear is very effective. Most neurologically significant hearing loss involves frequencies in the range of the spoken voice. Attempts to pick up high-frequency sensorineural hearing loss of the type associated with noise exposure or presbycusis is not usually necessary in a screening neurologic examination. The Weber and Rinne maneuvers are seldom of significant help.

At this point, the cranial nerve examination is nearly complete, and only the visual fields and fundi must be checked. The confrontation visual field examination can be tailored to the circumstances. Fairly sophisticated techniques can be used to explore the visual fields in detail if circumstances warrant. If the patient has no specific visual complaint, and if other aspects of the history and examination do not suggest that a field defect is likely, then a screening examination is appropriate. This can be accomplished rapidly and with great sensitivity by using small-amplitude finger movements in the far periphery of the visual field. The normal visual field extends 60° nasally and superiorly, 70° inferiorly, and 90°+ temporally. All visual field testing is based on the patient's fixating on a central point and not deviating from it.

Extending elbows and index fingers, the examiner should position the fingers nearly directly lateral to the lateral canthus at a distance of approximately 24 inches (Figure 5–1). Superficially, this appears to be a binocular examination, but, properly placed, the finger targets actually are in the unpaired monocular temporal crescent part of the visual field. With the targets positioned, a small-amplitude flexion movement should be made with the tip of one index finger, perhaps 2 cm in amplitude. Ask the patient to "point to the finger that moves." This language is much more efficient than getting into a right-left verbal description situation in which the patient's and examiner's rights and lefts are reversed. Stimuli should be delivered in each upper quadrant individually, then both together, then similarly for the lower quadrants. Including bilateral simultaneous stimuli is necessary to detect mild, subtle defects that may be manifested only by extinction of one stimulus on double simultaneous stimulation. Always bear in mind that primary ophthalmologic disorders such as glaucoma, diabetic retinopathy, and retinal detachment also can alter the visual fields.

With the visual field examination completed, the cranial nerve examination is finished by examination of the fundi. For neurologic purposes, the structure of primary concern is the disc, and the two chief abnormalities that might be encountered are disc swelling and disc atrophy. For purposes of the general physical examination, note any evidence of diabetic or hypertensive retinopathy. Discussion of the fundus examination is beyond the scope of this chapter; see Chapter 7 for further details. Enrichment Box 5–1 describes how to construct a simulator for practicing fundus examination.

MOTOR EXAMINATION

Screening examination of motor function, sensory function, and coordination in the upper extremities can be completed as one compound, multifaceted maneuver. However, for purposes of clarity, these will be considered separately.

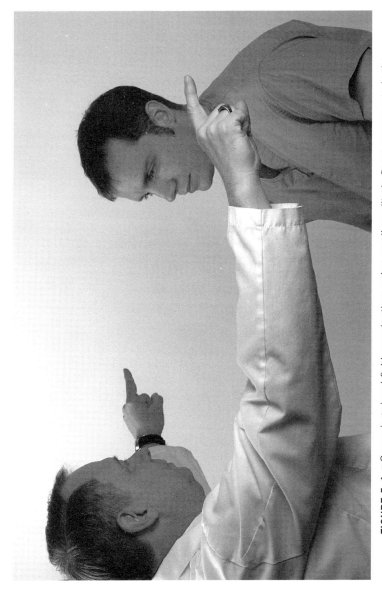

FIGURE 5–1. ■ Screening visual field examination; using small-amplitude finger movements in the far periphery of the visual field, instruct the patient to point to the finger that moves.

ENRICHMENT BOX 5–1 CRAFTS FOR CLERKS—MAKING A FUNDUS SIMULATOR

To practice holding and focusing an ophthalmoscope, roll a printed piece of paper into a tube approximately 1 inch in diameter with the print on the inside, and punch a small hole approximately 5 mm in diameter through the paper. Look through the hole (the pupil) and try to read the print on the "fundus."

A quick fundus simulator can be made simply by placing a piece of paper with an aperture over a small single-slide viewer, the sort used to preview slides (e.g., the Photoco 3 Model #PH3 works well). Cut the paper (e.g., a sticky note) so that it slightly overlaps the edges, and tape it in place over the front of the viewer. Make a hole in the middle of the paper, using an initial opening that is 6–8 mm in diameter. This aperture is the "pupil." Obtain some 2 × 2–inch color slides of normal and abnormal fundi. Visit the eye clinic and request extra copies of interesting fundus photographs, or have slides made from textbooks or other sources. Using an ophthalmoscope and with the slide illuminated, look through the "pupil" at the slide that simulates the fundus. Practice focusing and navigating. This is a reasonably close simulation of the clinical examination of the fundus. By changing the slides, one can get a realistic look at different sorts of abnormalities. One can make the pupil smaller or larger, depending on the skill level of the examiner.

A homemade fundus simulator can be constructed as follows. Using heavy cardboard, cut a strip 2 inches wide and 8 inches long. Score the strip at 2-inch intervals, then fold at the scores to form a cube open at front and back. About 0.5 inch inside the "back" of the cube, tape an empty slide carrier or similarly cut piece of cardboard. Insert a fundus slide into the back of the cube so that it rests against and is held in place by the empty slide carrier. For ease of insertion and removal of the fundus slides, it helps if the cube is ever-so-slightly larger than the slide.

With the fundus slide in place, the simulator should be enclosed on all sides; the sides being simply the cardboard, the front being the index card with the "pupil" aperture, and the back being the "fundus" to be examined. Hold the cube up toward a diffuse, moderately bright but not intense light source, such as a window in daylight or an overhead fluorescent light. Depending on the light source, the ophthalmoscope light may or may not need to be on.

Before discussing the motor examination, it is necessary to briefly review some neurophysiology. In most clinical situations in which a screening examination is appropriate, the primary concern is to detect a lesion involving the corticospinal tract (CST). The CST preferentially innervates certain muscle groups. An effective way to remember the

CST's preferential innervation is to visualize the posture of a patient with a spastic hemiparesis, in which the involved muscles (i.e., the CST-innervated muscles) have been overpowered by the uninvolved, non–CST-innervated muscles. The arm is held tightly adducted and internally rotated at the shoulder, flexed at the elbow, and flexed at the wrist. The forearm is pronated, even hyperpronated, and the hand is fisted. The CST-innervated muscles are the ones that have been defeated and can be deduced: finger extensors, wrist extensors, forearm supinators, external rotators of the shoulder, triceps, and deltoid. In addition, the CST preferentially innervates distal muscles, and one of its most important functions is to provide fine motor control to these groups in both the upper and lower extremity. Fine motor control, including rapid alternating movements (RAMs), would furthermore be impossible without normal cerebellar input to provide further coordination.

The patient with a spastic hemiparesis often can stand by using the leg as a passive support and usually has a foot drop. The non-CST muscles lock the hip and knee into extension and provide antigravity power. The leg is held in an adducted position with the knee and hip in a tightly extended position. The leg becomes a pillar on which the patient can bear weight and ambulate despite poor coordination and control. The patient circumducts the leg during the stride phase, dragging it along, then vaults on it during the stance phase. The cardinal CST muscles in the lower extremity therefore are the muscles that have been overcome to produce this posture: the hip flexors, the hamstrings, and the dorsiflexors of the foot and toes.

Bearing in mind the neurophysiology, the screening examination therefore focuses on detecting weakness in the CST distribution. In the upper extremity, the best muscles for strength testing are the deltoid, triceps, wrist and finger extensors, and intrinsic hand muscles, especially the interossei. In the lower extremity, the best muscles to test are the hip flexors, hamstrings, and foot dorsiflexors.

Strength Testing

Although strength is the primary focus of the motor examination, it is important to note any changes in muscle bulk (e.g., atrophy, hypertrophy, or pseudohypertrophy) or muscle tone (e.g., rigidity, spasticity, or hypotonia), and to note any abnormal involuntary movements (e.g., tremor, fasciculations, or chorea). Assessment of fine motor control and screening for pronator drift are other important parts of the motor examination.

The MRC scale. Strength is most commonly graded using the five-level MRC (Medical Research Council) scale (Table 5–5), which was

TABLE 5–5. THE MRC SCALE FOR MUSCLE STRENGTH GRADING

Grade	Functional Strength
5	Normal power
4	Able to contract the muscle against gravity and resistance
3	Able to contract against gravity but not against resistance
2	Able to contract only with gravity eliminated
1	A flicker
0	No contraction

MRC = Medical Research Council.

developed in Britain during World War II to evaluate patients with peripheral nerve injuries. The MRC scale has been widely applied to the evaluation of strength in general. However, the scale is heavily weighted toward the evaluation of very weak muscles. In a peripheral nerve injury, improvement from grade 0 (no contraction) to grade 1 (a flicker) is highly significant because it signals the beginning of reinnervation. A patient with a nerve injury who eventually recovers to grade 4 has had an excellent outcome. In contrast, a patient with polymyositis who is diffusely grade 4 has severe involvement and is doing poorly. So, the most commonly used strength-grading scale has significant limitations when dealing with most patients.

The levels of the MRC scale are precisely defined and are not linear. It is a common error to believe the MRC grades are evenly spaced and that grade 5 is normal, grade 4 is mild weakness, grade 3 is moderate weakness, and so forth. In fact, anything less than grade 5 denotes significant weakness. Grade 4 is moderate weakness, and anything less is severe weakness. A physician or medical student who does not understand the scale may attempt to describe a patient with Guillain-Barré syndrome, for example, as having grade 4 strength, intending to convey that there is mild weakness. To someone who understands the scale, this description indicates high-grade involvement. One must not confuse poor effort with weakness.

The different levels of the MRC scale are so precisely defined that there is good interexaminer consistency once the fine points of proper positioning and so forth are mastered. In clinical practice, the MRC scale often is expanded to include subgrades (e.g., 5−, 4+). The subgrades are not as precisely defined, and there is much less interexaminer and even intraexaminer consistency. Approximate guidelines are all that is possible.

Strength mismatch and reliable testing. Before attempting to describe these guidelines, the problem of examiner/examinee mismatch should be recognized. Physicians come large and small, young and old, male and female, physically strong and relatively weak. So do patients. A large, young, powerful, male resident examining a small, old, sick, female patient may tend to think she is weak, when she is, in fact, normal for her age, gender, and circumstances. Conversely, a small, relatively weak female physician examining a large, powerful man may miss significant weakness because of strength mismatch.

As a general principle, reliable strength testing should attempt to break a given muscle. Muscles are most powerful when maximally shortened, as anyone who has attempted to do heavy biceps curls in the weight room is well aware. Another consideration is the lever effect. Attempting to overpower a muscle (e.g., deltoid) using a very short lever (e.g., examiner's hand at the mid-upper arm) is much less likely to meet with success than using a long lever (e.g., patient's elbow extended and examiner's hand pressing down on the wrist). A small, weak examiner can overcome the deltoid of the most powerful man by keeping the examinee's elbow extended and using both hands to pull down the wrist. Technique matters.

By varying the length of lever and the shortening of the muscle permitted, the examiner may give or take mechanical advantage as necessary to compensate for strength mismatch. Many patients of different ages, sizes, and strength levels must be examined in this fashion to develop an appreciation of the expected strength of a muscle for a given set of circumstances.

Therefore, for an examiner of average size and strength examining a patient of average size and presumed normal strength, the following is a useful guideline for assessing power in the major muscle groups. Using the extremity positions and pressure points described in Table 5–6 and in Figures 5–2 through 5–8 as an approximation, if it requires the whole hand and a firm push to break the muscle, the power is grade 4+. If the muscle can be broken using three fingers, it is grade 4. If it can be broken using one finger, it is grade 4−. The subgrades of muscles weaker than grade 4 are beyond the scope of this discussion.

Some muscles are special cases. The small hand muscles are best examined by matching them precisely against the examiners like muscle (e.g., abductor pollicis brevis to abductor pollicis brevis). This method is beautifully described and illustrated in *Segmental Neurology* by John K. Wolf (University Park Press, Baltimore, 1981). The gastrocnemius muscles normally are so powerful that it is virtually useless to examine them using hand and arm strength, unless they are very weak. Having the patient walk on tiptoe, hop, support the entire body

TABLE 5–6. TECHNIQUES FOR MUSCLE STRENGTH TESTING

Muscle	Limb Position	Pressure Point	Muscle Action
Deltoid	Elbow fully flexed, arms horizontal	Elbow	Shoulder abduction
Biceps	Elbows at sides, flexed 90°, fore-arms horizontal	Wrist	Elbow flexion
Triceps	Same as for biceps	Wrist	Elbow extension
Wrist extensors	Wrist extended	Dorsum of hand	Wrist extension
Hip flexors	Patient sitting, hip flexed 30°–45°	Knee	Hip flexion
Quadriceps	Patient sitting, knee flexed 90°, lower leg perpen-dicular to floor	Ankle	Knee extension
Hamstring	Same as for quadriceps	Ankle	Knee flexion
Tibialis anterior	Foot dorsiflexed	Distal dorsum of the foot	Ankle dorsiflexion

weight on one tiptoe, or do one-legged toe raises usually are better methods.

Although commonly done, it is very poor technique to use grip power to assess strength. The finger and wrist flexors are not inner-vated through the CST and are not likely to be weak with a mild CST lesion. So insensitive is grip strength to corticospinal pathology that many patients with a severe, spastic hemiparesis have a tightly fisted hand, so much so that palmar hygiene may become a major problem. In addition, grip is a complex function and involves many different muscles, so it is insensitive to peripheral pathology as well.

Ancillary Maneuvers

The motor examination is not concluded only with the strength as-sessment. Patients with mild CST lesions may have normal strength, but the neurologic deficit may be brought out using ancillary maneu-vers. The most important of these maneuvers is the examination for pronator drift. With the patient's upper extremities outstretched to the front, palms up, and with the eyes closed, observe the position of each

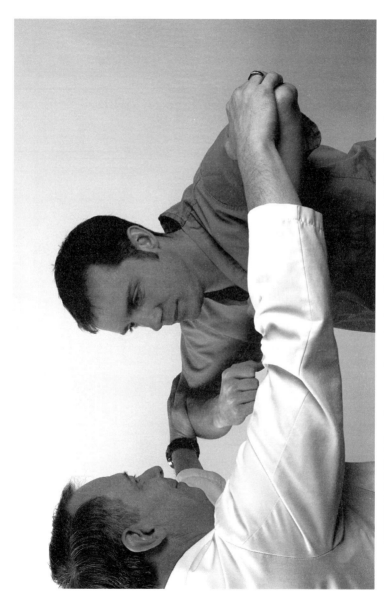

FIGURE 5–2. ■ Technique for manual muscle strength testing of the deltoid, with examiner and examinee of approximately equal strength.

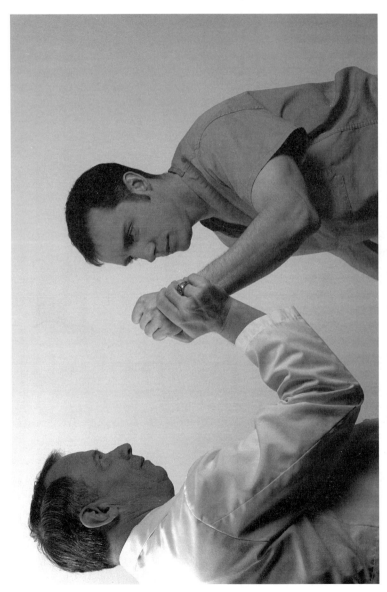

FIGURE 5–3. ■ Technique for manual muscle strength testing of the triceps.

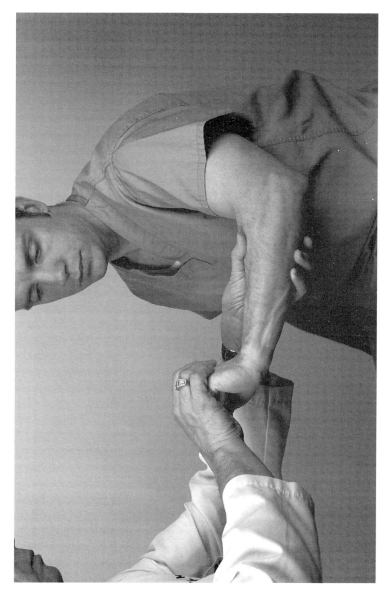

FIGURE 5–4. ■ Technique for manual muscle strength testing of the wrist extensors.

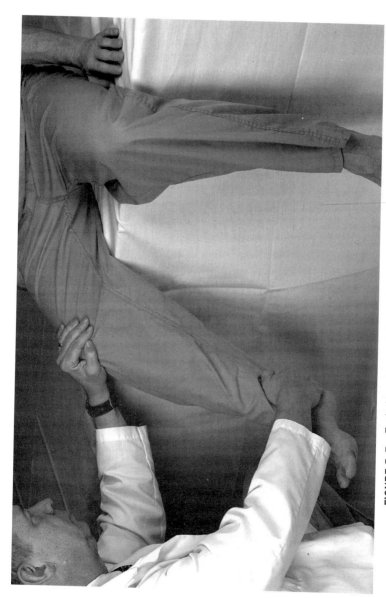

FIGURE 5–7. ■ Technique for manual muscle strength testing of the hamstrings.

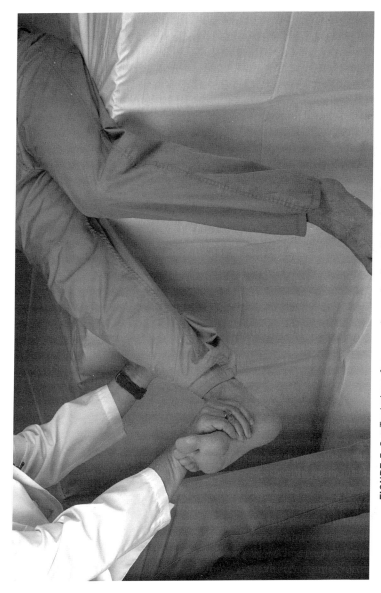

FIGURE 5–8. ■ Technique for manual muscle strength testing of the tibialis anterior.

extremity (Figure 5–9). In normal patients, the palms will remain flat, the elbows straight, and the limbs horizontal. Any deviation from this position will be similar on the two sides. One exception to the usual symmetry is that the dominant hand occasionally may pronate slightly because the nondominant extremities tend to be more flexible than the dominant extremities, and it is slightly more difficult to stretch the dominant hand to a horizontal position. Except for this, and for coincidental orthopedic or musculoskeletal problems, there should be no difference between the positions of the two limbs.

The patient with a mild CST deficit may demonstrate pronator drift to varying degrees. With mild drift there is simply pronation on the abnormal side; with more severe drift, there is also flexion of the elbow, and there may be downward drift of the entire arm (Figure 5–10). Drift can be understood by remembering the innervation pattern of the CST and by understanding that the minimally weak CST-innervated muscles are overcome by the non-CST muscles. With a mild CST lesion, the strong muscles are the pronators: the biceps and the internal rotators of the shoulder. As these overcome the slightly weakened CST-innervated muscles, the hand pronates, the elbow flexes, and the arm drifts downward. Imagine what would occur if this motion continued to the extreme: the hand would become hyperpronated, the elbow fully flexed, and the shoulder internally rotated, that is, the position of spastic hemiparesis (Figure 5–11). The abnormal upper limb positions in minimal pronator drift and in severe spastic hemiparesis are caused by the same underlying phenomenon: strong non-CST muscles overcome variably weak CST muscles involved by the disease process.

The examination for pronator drift is a very important part of the screening neurologic examination. If only one motor test could be done on a patient, the best single test to use would be examining for drift. While waiting for drift to occur, since it is not instantaneous, the examiner may simply wait or may hasten the development of drift by tapping on the palms or having the patient turn their head back and forth. Alternatively, the examiner may use the short period of time waiting for drift to occur by examining upper extremity sensory functions.

SENSORY EXAMINATION

The quick sensory examination screens for sensory dysfunction by having the nervous system perform a complex and difficult task. If this function is executed flawlessly, the likelihood of finding clinically significant sensory loss through a more detailed examination is low. Testing for stereognosis and performing double simultaneous stimulation are efficient and sensitive tools for screening for sensory deficits.

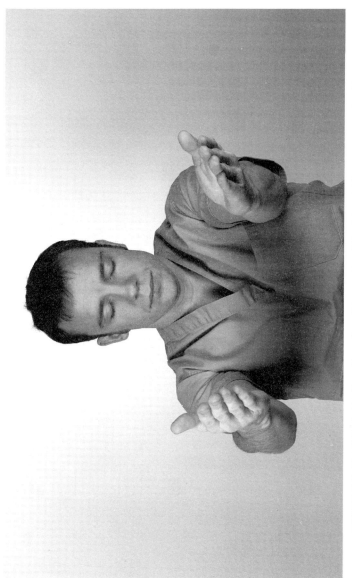

FIGURE 5-9. ■ In this illustration, there is *mild pronator drift* of the right upper extremity. The selectively weakened muscles (shoulder abductors, supinators, and elbow extensors) are overcome by their antagonists to cause pronation, elbow flexion, and downward drift.

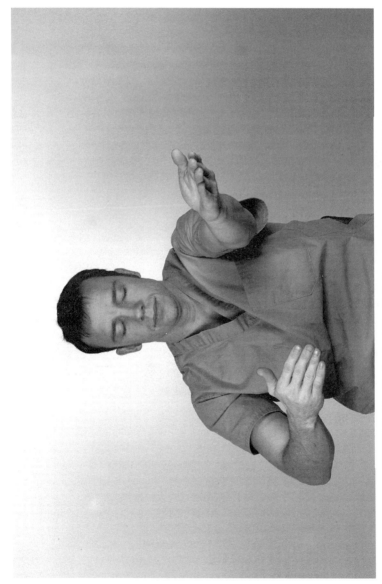

FIGURE 5–10. ■ Moderate drift with further development of the posture.

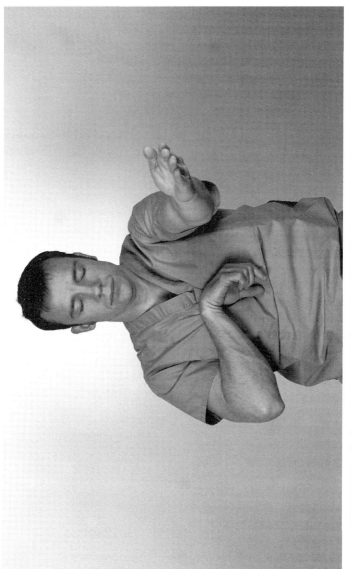

FIGURE 5-11. ▇ Further development of pronator drift, with the evolution of severe drift to show how marked weakness of the muscles innervated by the corticospinal tract produces the posture of spastic hemiparesis.

Double Simultaneous Stimulation

At the conclusion of the initial screening motor examination, the patient is still in "drift position;" that is, arms outstretched in front, palms up, and eyes closed. Instruct the patient to indicate which side is touched, then very lightly touch the patient on first one hand, then the other, then both. Convenient stimuli might be minimal finger pressure, a cotton wisp, or a tissue. A set of stimuli to the lower extremities also is convenient at this point. If all the responses are correct, proceed with testing for stereognosis.

Stereognosis

Stereognosis is the ability to recognize and identify an object by touch and feel. The inability to do so is referred to as astereognosis. For purposes of a screening examination, stereognosis is an excellent modality. Stereognosis can only be normal when all of the peripheral sensory pathways and the parietal lobe association areas are normal. If it is executed flawlessly, then all of the sensory pathways must be functioning normally and a detailed examination is not likely to be productive. However, if there is astereognosis on this preliminary assessment, a detailed examination of sensory function will be necessary to localize the site of the abnormality.

An efficient technique is to test stereognosis by placing objects (e.g., coin, key, safety pin, paper clip) into the patient's upgoing palms while the patient has his arms outstretched and his eyes closed during observation for pronator drift. If the patient cannot identify the object, place it in the other hand. If the object is then identified correctly, the patient has unilateral astereognosis, the most common type of abnormality.

Additional useful information can be gained by dropping the small object more or less in the center of the palm. A patient with normal fine motor control, which is a CST function, will adroitly manipulate the object, move it to the fingertips, rub it between the thumb and opposed fingers, and announce the result. A patient with a mild CST lesion that produces relatively subtle clinical signs without major weakness may be clumsy in manipulating the object and will occasionally drop it.

Only when the primary sensory modalities (i.e., touch, pressure, pain, and temperature) are normal can the unilateral failure to identify an object be termed astereognosis, and be attributed to a parietal lobe lesion. A patient with severe carpal tunnel syndrome and numb fingers may not be able to identify a small object by feel; this finding is *not* astereognosis.

CEREBELLAR EXAMINATION
Finger-To-Nose Test

After completing the assessment of double simultaneous stimulation and stereognosis, with eyes still closed, the patient is instructed to spread the fingers, then touch first one index finger and then the other to the tip of his nose. This is the finger-to-nose (FTN) test, which is used primarily to examine cerebellar function.

Ordinarily, the FTN test is carried out with the patient's eyes open, and several trips are made between the nose and finger looking for intention tremor and incoordination. It is useful to then have the patient continue the alternate finger and nose touching with eyes closed. In the presence of either cerebellar disease or vestibular disease, the FTN test may reveal so-called past pointing, in which the patient misses the target with eyes closed but is accurate with eyes open. The pattern of abnormal past pointing may vary. In patients with vestibular disease, the patient will past point to the same side of the target with either upper extremity. With unilateral cerebellar hemispheric disease, the patient will past point to either side of the target randomly, but only with the upper extremity ipsilateral to the lesion. The opposite side will be normal, with no past pointing to either side.

For purposes of the screening examination, the more difficult maneuver of eyes-closed FTN is performed first. If it is executed flawlessly, then neither cerebellar nor vestibular disease is likely.

The examination of upper extremity motor, sensory, and cerebellar function is nearing completion. If time does not permit, the examination could be terminated at this point, and the likelihood of missing significant intracranial pathology would be remote if all assessments were normal.

Additional Maneuvers

A few quick additional maneuvers can provide extra information at little cost of time. These are examination of *arm roll, finger roll,* and rapid alternating movements (*RAMs*).

Arm and finger roll. *Arm roll* is a sensitive indicator of neurologic pathology. The patient is instructed to make fists, then to hold the forearms horizontally so that the fists and distal forearms overlap with the palms pointed more or less toward the umbilicus, then to rotate the fists around each other, first in one direction then the other (Figure 5–12). Normal patients will have an approximately equal excursion of both forearms, so that the fists and forearms roll about each other symmetrically. With a unilateral CST lesion, the involved side does not move as much as the normal side, so the patient will appear to hold one forearm still and to rotate the opposite forearm around it.

Finger roll is an even more sensitive version of the same test. The patient is asked to extend the forefingers from the clenched fists and to rotate just the fingers around each other (Figure 5–13) . Again, the fin-

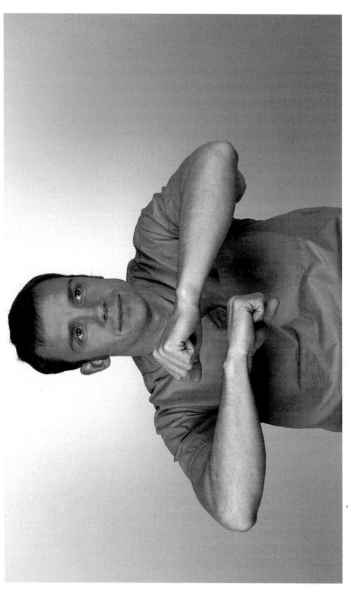

FIGURE 5–12. ■ Testing for a corticospinal tract lesion using *arm roll*. The involved extremity tends to have a lesser excursion as the forearms roll about each other, so that the normal extremity tends to rotate around the abnormal extremity, which tends to remain relatively fixed. Patients with mild corticospinal tract lesions may have an abnormal arm roll test result in the absence of clinically detectable weakness to formal strength testing.

ger on the abnormal side will move less than its fellow. Occasionally, patients with a unilateral CST lesion will have an abnormal finger roll as the only abnormal test.

Rapid alternating movements. Testing for RAMs requires the patient to quickly start and stop or reverse simple movements. Some of the usual tests include patting the palm of one hand alternately with the palm and dorsum of the other hand, repetitively touching the interphalangeal joint of the thumb with the ipsilateral index finger, touching the thumb to each fingertip in rapid succession, tapping out a complex rhythm, or tapping the foot in steady beat. Dysfunction of any of the motor pathways (corticospinal, extrapyramidal, or cerebellar) may impair the ability to perform RAMs. The specific characteristics of the impairment in RAMs vary with the cause. When the patient is able to perform these maneuvers with speed and dexterity, it is good evidence that all of these motor pathways are functioning normally.

In the course of performing all of these testing maneuvers in the upper extremities, one has had ample opportunity to observe for the presence of clubbing, cyanosis, other nail changes, hand deformity, arthropathy, and so forth to complete the upper extremity examination portion of the general physical examination. In stroke patients, it is wise to palpate both radial pulses simultaneously to screen for brachiocephalic vascular occlusive disease.

Lower Extremity Examination

After completing examination of motor, sensory, and cerebellar function in the upper extremities, attention is turned to strength assessment of the lower extremities. Recall that the primary corticospinal innervated muscles in the lower extremity are the hip flexors, knee flexors, and the dorsiflexors of the foot. The power of these muscle groups should be assessed. For purposes of a screening examination, there is no corollary to the upper extremity quick examination of cerebellar function or stereognosis. A few double simultaneous stimuli to the legs should be included during examination of the upper extremities. Certainly, if there is any clinical reason to do so, there are many ways to assess sensory and cerebellar function in the lower extremities, but then this is going beyond a screening examination.

REFLEX EXAMINATION

At this point, it is convenient to examine the deep tendon reflexes (DTRs), also referred to as muscle stretch reflexes, in both upper and lower extremities. During the reflex examination, the patient should be instructed to keep his or her head straight, because looking to one side,

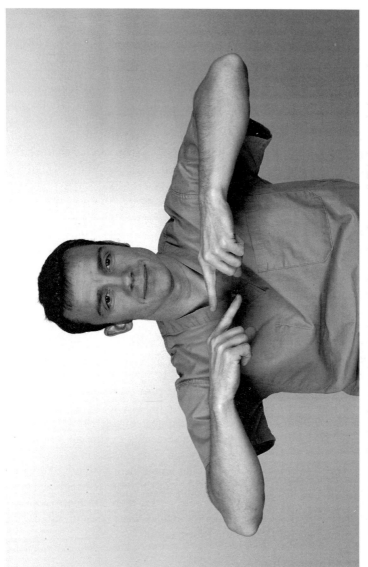

FIGURE 5–13. ■ Testing for a corticospinal tract lesion using *finger roll*. This is a variation on the arm roll test for reciprocating motion, and is even more sensitive.

as is the temptation, can alter reflex tone, especially in the arms. The DTRs usually examined include the biceps, triceps, brachioradialis, knee (quadriceps), and ankle (Achilles tendon) reflexes (Table 5–7) .

After examining the DTRs, the plantar responses should be assessed. Make sure the knee is straightened for the plantar examination because a bent knee can, for some unclear reason, cause a positive Babinski reflex to become negative. Plantar stimulation must be carried out far laterally, in the S1 root/sural nerve sensory distribution. More medial plantar stimulation may fail to elicit a positive response. Far medial stimulation may actually elicit a plantar grasp response causing the toes to flex strongly. The stimulus should begin far posteriorly near the heel and be carried slowly up the side of the foot and, if necessary, across the base of the toes. The only movements of significance are those of the great toe. Fanning of the lateral toes without an abnormal movement of the great toe is seldom of any clinical significance.

The plantar stimulus should be firm enough to elicit a consistent response. It need not necessarily be truly and deliberately noxious, although most patients find it at least somewhat uncomfortable even if the examiner is trying to be considerate. Babinski first observed the extensor plantar response when the wind blew the curtains across the feet of patients with spinal cord injuries at the Salpetriere in Paris, hardly a noxious stimulus. Every physician should undergo plantar stimulation to appreciate the discomfort usually associated with elicitation of plantar responses. Some patients are very sensitive to plantar stimulation, and only a slight stimulus suffices to elicit a consistent response; stronger stimuli may produce confusing withdrawal. Other patients require a very firm stimulus. Sometimes a response cannot be elicited from a patient, in which case the plantar reflexes are said to be mute or silent. Occasionally, there is so much withdrawal that one cannot be certain whether the toe was truly extensor or not; these are equivocal plantar responses.

TABLE 5–7. THE DEEP TENDON (MUSCLE STRETCH) REFLEXES

Deep Tendon Reflex	Segmental Level	Peripheral Nerve
Biceps	C5–6	Musculocutaneous
Triceps	C7–8	Radial
Brachioradialis	C5–6	Radial
Quadriceps	L3–4	Femoral
Achilles	S1	Sciatic

With a true extensor plantar response, the upward movement of the great toe is often a quick, flicking motion mistaken for withdrawal by inexperienced physicians. Asymmetry of the plantar responses may be significant, even if the toe does not frankly go up.

In the course of examining the legs and feet for strength and reflexes, the pattern of hair growth and any dystrophic changes in the nails should be noted. In addition, the pulses should be felt in the feet. The patient should be checked for pretibial edema, leg length discrepancy, swollen or deformed knee or ankle joints, the odd missing toe, or any other abnormalities.

Reflex Grading

DTRs are most commonly graded on a scale of 0–4. Other scales are in use, but not widely. Some add a grade 5 for the patient with extreme spasticity and clonus. The Mayo Clinic uses a scale in which 0 is normal, and reflexes are either increased (1+ to 4+) or decreased (1− to 4−). A similar scale exists for grading muscle strength.

The common 0–4 scale works as follows: Level 2+ DTRs are completely and unequivocally normal. Level 1+ DTRs are still normal but somewhat sluggish and difficult to elicit; hypoactive, but in the examiner's opinion, not pathologic. Level 3+ reflexes are "fast normal," quicker than 2+, sometimes very quick, but not accompanied by any other signs of CST pathology (e.g., increased tone, upgoing toes, or sustained clonus). In the presence of CST pathology, the DTRs are increased, but the superficial reflexes (i.e., abdominal and cremasteric reflexes) are decreased or absent (see Chapter 6). Normality of the superficial reflexes, normal lower extremity tone, and downgoing toes are reassuring evidence of fast normal rather than pathologically quick reflexes. Level 4+ reflexes are unequivocally pathologically increased. The speed of the response is very fast, and there are accompanying signs of CST dysfunction. Level 0 reflexes are absent.

Another level, trace, is frequently used to refer to a reflex (most often an ankle reflex) that appears absent to routine testing but can be elicited with reinforcement. A reflex can be reinforced or brought out using several methods. In the Jendrassik maneuver, the patient attempts to pull the hands apart with the fingers flexed and locked, palms facing. A simple and effective method to reinforce a knee or ankle reflex is to have the patient exert a slight, steady contraction of the muscle whose tendon is being tested (e.g., slight plantar flexion to reinforce the ankle jerk). Using a driving analogy and advising the patient to imagine pressing on an accelerator enough to go "17 mph" communicates the need for a low level but precisely graded contraction, which is then easy to adjust up or down to the proper level.

The DTRs are normally symmetric, and reflexes that are otherwise normal may be abnormal if they are different from expected. For example, a 1+ biceps jerk in a patient with suspected cervical radiculopathy, although normal, may be judged abnormal if the opposite biceps jerk is 2+. Ankle jerks of 1+ when all the other reflexes are 2+ and symmetric may signal mild peripheral neuropathy. When asymmetry is the main finding, it may sometimes be difficult to tell whether one side is abnormally increased or the other side is decreased.

GAIT EXAMINATION

It is likely possible to learn more about neurologic status from watching a patient walk than from any other single maneuver. Observation of gait should therefore always be part of a neurologic examination.

The first step in analyzing gait is to check the width of the base. Widening of the base is the first compensatory effort in most gait disorders. Just as the novice skier is most comfortable in the very wide "snowplow" position, a patient with a gait disorder first seeks stability by widening the base. Under normal circumstances, the medial malleoli pass within approximately 2 inches of each other during the stride phase of a narrow and well-compensated gait. A spread larger than this may signal some problem with gait or balance. While observing the distance between the medial malleoli, the physician should assess whether the forefoot on each side clears the ground to approximately the same degree. Asymmetry here may be the earliest evidence of foot drop. A shortened stride length may be early evidence of bifrontal or extrapyramidal disease. Excessive movement of the hips may occur with any process causing proximal muscle weakness. Note the reciprocal arm swing; a decreased swing on one side is sometimes an early indicator of hemiparesis. Watch the hands for tremor or chorea.

Tandem walking stresses the gait and balance mechanisms even further. Elderly patients may have difficulty with tandem gait because of obesity or deconditioning. The Romberg test assesses proprioceptive functions by having the patient stand with eyes closed. However, the Romberg test often is misunderstood and misinterpreted. The essential finding is a difference between standing balance with eyes open and with eyes closed. To test this, the patient must have a stable stance with eyes open and then demonstrate decreased balance with eyes closed, when the patient must rely on proprioception to maintain balance. Patients with cerebellar disease, or those with severe weakness and similar problems, may not have a stable base with their eyes open. It may help to have the patient widen her stance to the point where she is stable with eyes open, then close the eyes and check for any difference. A patient who cannot maintain balance with feet together and eyes open does not have a Romberg sign! Minimal amounts of sway with eyes closed, especially in elderly patients, are seldom significant.

In relatively young patients with a low likelihood of neurologic disease, a quick and effective substitute for the Romberg test is simply to have the patient close his eyes while doing tandem gait. This is a difficult maneuver and has high value as a screening test. Another excellent screening test is to have the patient hop on either foot. This simultaneously assesses lower extremity strength, especially of the gastrosoleus, plus balance functions. Individuals who can hop adroitly on either foot are unlikely to have significant neurologic disease. (Recall that hopping is an integral part of the "Navy neurologic.")

Although the gait examination portion of the general physical examination is largely for neurologic purposes, the physician should note whether the patient has any obvious orthopedic limitations, such as a varus deformity of the knee, genu recurvatum, pelvic tilt, or any other abnormalities.

The gait examination concludes the screening neurologic examination. At this point, if not already done, the examiner may find it convenient to complete the examination of the heart, lungs, and abdomen. While using the stethoscope, it is a convenient time to listen for carotid bruits, which provides an expedient opportunity to do the general physical neck examination, palpating for nodes and masses.

COMMON ERRORS

In the course of watching many students and residents examine patients, and of having students and residents examine one of the authors in the role of simulated patient, certain common errors and omissions have become apparent.

CRANIAL NERVE EXAMINATION

The most common error in the cranial nerve examination is to fail to test the visual fields. This is a major mistake because 80% of the afferent information entering the brain is visual. The visual system is a very important system. Visual field defects are fairly common and of major localizing significance when present. The screening examination is rapid and sensitive and should not be omitted.

When visual fields are checked, the most common problem is getting into verbal confusion with lefts and rights. With double simultaneous stimulation, the patient says left. Did they mean their left or the examiner's left? The instruction "point to the finger that moves" eliminates any ambiguity.

PUPIL EXAMINATION

The most common error with pupil examination is to have the patient fixing at near, by instructing him to look at the examiner's nose. Pupils will constrict to light or to near, and this technique provides both a light stimulus and a near stimulus simultaneously. The pupil constriction to near is more powerful than to light, so the pupils may well constrict to the near target of the examiner's nose even when the reaction to light is impaired or absent. Using this technique, the examiner would always miss light-near dissociation of the pupils, which is an important clinical sign. The patient should always fix at a distance when one is checking the pupillary light reaction.

EXTRAOCULAR MOVEMENT EXAMINATION

The most common error in examining extraocular movements is to use four movements rather than six, checking vertical gaze in primary position rather than eccentric position to each side, potentially missing any limitation of oblique muscle function.

FACIAL NERVE EXAMINATION

The most common error in facial nerve examination is to rely solely on the "purse your lips" or "puff out your cheeks" technique, which detects only fairly marked facial weakness. This technique is not sensitive to mild or subtle facial weakness, is a poor screen for central nervous system disease, would never detect a dissociated facial palsy, and fails to examine upper facial movements. Facial weakness is discussed further in Chapter 6.

TONGUE EXAMINATION

The most common error made when examining the tongue is to be duped by "pseudodeviation." Many patients, especially stroke patients, have facial weakness producing a droopiness and lack of mobility of the side of the mouth on the involved side. When protruding the tongue, there may appear to be a deviation of the tongue toward the side of the facial weakness. The tongue is closer to the corner of the mouth on that side, but this is because the corner of the mouth has not moved out of the way, not because the tongue is deviating. Manually pulling up the weak side of the face eliminates the "deviation." It may also be helpful to gauge tongue position in relation to the tip of the nose or the upper incisors.

MOTOR EXAMINATION

There are several common errors in the motor examination. Failure to exert sufficient force to truly test a muscle's strength is typical. A cursory push will only detect very gross weakness. Using too short a lever, as in pushing down on the middle of the upper arm to test deltoid strength, is a frequent mistake. Other perennial problems include failure to understand the nonlinearity of the MRC scale and failure to adjust for examiner/examinee strength mismatch. The worst possible upper extremity strength examination, unfortunately not rare, is a cursory push on the mid-upper arm of the abducted shoulder to test the deltoid muscle, followed by testing grip strength. Very significant pathology can be missed using such a technique.

SENSORY EXAMINATION

The most common error in sensory testing is to fail to perform double simultaneous stimulation, potentially completely missing a major parietal lobe lesion. Although not included as part of the rapid screening examination, there is frequently a need to check vibratory sensation. A frequent problem is failure to adequately instruct the patient in the desired response. The novice examiner strikes the tuning fork, touches it to the patient's great toe, and says "Do you feel that?" A deceptive problem lies in the definition of "that." A patient with absent vibratory sensation may feel the touch of the handle of the tuning fork, misinterpret it as the "that" inquired about, and respond affirmatively. Therefore, very gross defects in vibratory sensibility are completely missed. The physician should always set the fork in motion, touch it to some presumably normal body part, and tell the patient "this is vibrating or buzzing," then dampen the tines, reapply the stimulus, and tell the patient "this is just touching," or something similar that clearly differentiates the nature of the two stimuli, then proceed with the testing.

ELICITING DEEP TENDON REFLEXES

The primary problem areas in eliciting DTRs are poor tools and poor technique. To properly obtain a reflex, a crisp blow must be delivered to quickly stretch the tendon. A heavy, high-quality reflex hammer is immensely helpful for this task, but most students use the cheapest hammer they can find, usually poor, pitiable, and inferior instruments. The worst possible hammers are pharmaceutical company giveaways; they have no heft, and are worth just what was paid for them. A genuine, high-quality, purchased tomahawk is the lowest level of acceptable hammer, and these often are inadequate in the hands of novices. A variety of passably decent hammers are available in the $15–$20 range.

Proper technique is much more difficult to describe than to demonstrate. The best blow is delivered quickly with a flick of the wrist, holding the handle of the hammer near its end, and letting it spin through loosely held fingertips. Putting the index finger on top of the handle and using primarily elbow motion, both of which are common faults, make it much harder to achieve adequate velocity at the hammer head. Another common mistake is "pecking": striking the tendon with a timid, decelerating blow, pulling back at the last instant, perhaps in fear of hurting the patient.

In eliciting DTRs, unique problems arise with each reflex. With the biceps jerk, the most common error is too much pressure exerted with the thumb or finger against the tendon. To elicit this reflex, the usual technique (for a right-handed examiner) is to gently place the palmar surface of the extended interphalangeal joint of the left thumb on the biceps tendon, then strike the extensor surface of the interphalangeal joint smartly with the reflex hammer. Squeezing down too firmly makes the reflex much harder to obtain. The most common error in eliciting the triceps jerk is simply too timorous a blow. For the brachioradialis, the most common mistake is hitting the muscle belly rather than the tendon. The muscle becomes tendinous approximately at the middle of the forearm. A contraction can be elicited from any muscle by directly striking the belly of the muscle. The point in eliciting a DTR is to stretch the muscle by lengthening its tendon. Some physicians try to obtain the brachioradialis reflex by striking the muscle belly in the proximal third of the forearm; this is not a DTR. The blow should be struck at about the junction of the middle and distal third of the forearm.

By far the most difficult reflex to master is the ankle jerk. There are two critical variables: proper stretch on the tendon and efficient striking. Of the two, proper stretch is the more difficult to learn. The ankle should be passively dorsiflexed by the examiner to about a right angle. Too little dorsiflexion leaves the tendon slack and able to absorb the blow without stretching the muscle. Too much passive dorsiflexion makes the tendon too taut and unable to be stretched. Learning the proper tension requires instruction and practice. When the ankle reflexes prove difficult to elicit, reinforcement (e.g., Jendrassik or "17 mph") may be helpful.

In attempting to obtain the plantar responses, or Babinski signs, the most common mistakes made are insufficiently firm stimulation, placement of the stimulus too medially, and moving the stimulus too quickly so that the response does not have time to develop. Many novices use a motion resembling striking a match on the sole of the foot, a stimulus that is both too light and too quick. Imagine striking a large, heavy, wooden kitchen or fireplace match, starting near the heel and trying to ignite it before passing the midsole. That is about the right pressure and speed.

6

Interpretation of Neurologic Examination Abnormalities

Chapters 4 and 5 discussed the techniques of history taking and neurologic examination. The following sections elaborate on the meaning and significance of increased or decreased reflexes, weakness, gait abnormalities, and similar abnormal findings.

The most common abnormalities likely to be found on a patient's neurologic examination include altered mental status (AMS), impaired cognition, deficits in higher cortical function, weakness, sensory loss, abnormal reflexes, and incoordination.

Altered Mental Status

The term "AMS" is often used in a haphazard and imprecise fashion to describe a variety of abnormalities of cerebral function. It is variably used to describe patients who have impaired alertness, impaired cognition, or a deficit of higher cortical function. Strictly speaking, AMS should only be used to describe patients who have impaired alertness, confusion, or delirium.

The term AMS implies a change in the level of consciousness, somewhere on a continuum between confusion and coma. AMS should not be used to describe patients who have impaired cognition with a clear sensorium; those patients have dementia, which is an abnormality in the content of consciousness. AMS should not be used to describe patients who have focal deficits of higher cortical function, such as aphasia, nor should AMS be used to describe patients who have psychiatric disorders such as psychosis or mania. Neurologically naive clinicians may lump all of these conditions together under the rubric AMS. These conditions are, in fact, distinctly different, with different etiologies and treatments, and especially with different prognostic implications.

True AMS most often results from a metabolic derangement, such as electrolyte imbalance, renal or hepatic failure, substance intoxication, and substance withdrawal. Occasionally, patients with cerebral mass lesions, such as subdural hematoma, may present with AMS. Even more rarely, patients may exhibit AMS as a result of such things as a central nervous system (CNS) infection, head trauma, and subclinical status epilepticus. If the condition causing AMS and a clouded sensorium is not corrected, it may progress to coma and even death. This is the essential and critical difference between AMS and conditions such as aphasia, dementia, and psychosis. Diseases causing AMS pose an acute threat to life and health, whereas the other conditions do not progress to coma or worse, at least not in the short term.

Some patients may be alert but confused and disoriented. This is an acute confusional state. Patients with delirium are confused, disoriented, and often agitated. The best example is delirium tremens.

Patients with aphasia are alert but suffer from a disorder of language function. They are aphasic, not confused. They may speak fluently or nonfluently. Those who speak fluently make little sense (jargon aphasia). Sometimes the language content of a patient with Wernicke aphasia is so bizarre that he is thought to have AMS or an acute confusional state. The aphasias and related disorders of higher cortical function are discussed later in this chapter.

Patients with dementia are awake and alert, but suffer from defects in memory, judgment, reasoning, and other intellectual functions. Demented patients are susceptible to superimposed systemic processes, such as infection or drug intoxication. They may then develop acute AMS superimposed on the underlying dementia, a so-called beclouded dementia.

Dementia

Dementia refers to loss of mental capacity and can occur either as a primary degenerative condition (e.g., Alzheimer disease) or as a secondary complication of another disease (e.g., hypothyroidism). The thrust of a dementia workup is exclusion of a treatable dementia, wherein an underlying condition has produced dementia as a complication.

Demented patients may exhibit a variety of other clinical signs that provide a clue as to cause, such as a prominent gait disturbance in normal pressure hydrocephalus, Argyll Robertson pupils in neurosyphilis, focal deficits in multi-infarct dementia, or myoclonus in Creutzfeldt-Jakob disease. The core features consistent with a dementing illness are progressive loss of memory, of cognitive function, of judgment, and of social skills. Aberrant behavior often becomes a major management problem. Sundowning refers to the common tendency of demented patients to become more confused and restless at night.

The most commonly used instrument for the office or bedside assessment of cognitive functioning is the Folstein Mini-Mental State Examination (see Chapter 4). The patient is asked a series of questions and the responses are graded. The grades are summed to produce a mini-mental score. A normal score is 27 or more. Scores of less than 25 suggest cognitive impairment. The Mini-Mental State Examination is only a screening examination, and there are problems with both false positives and false negatives.

Abnormalities of Speech and other Higher Cortical Functions

Focal brain disease produces several types of neurologic dysfunction. When a stroke, tumor, or other condition affects the primary cortex, the resulting dysfunction reflects the affected area; for example, hemiparesis occurs with conditions affecting the posterior frontal lobe, or visual field defects occur with conditions affecting the occipital lobe. When disease affects the association cortex or areas of the brain that subserve high-level integrative function, a variety of interesting abnormalities of higher cortical function may result. The most common of these is a disturbance of language, referred to as aphasia. Other disturbances of higher cortical function include apraxias, agnosias, and various disconnection syndromes, in which the communications between cortical areas are disrupted.

The left cerebral hemisphere is dominant in 99% of right-handers (dextrals), and about 60% of left-handers. Anomalous dextrals are naturally left-handed individuals forced by parents or teachers early in life to function right-handed. This approach to dealing with left-handedness has largely died out, but anomalous dextrals are still encountered. The physician can therefore encounter right-handed patients who are left-hemisphere dominant (normal), left-handed patients who are left-hemisphere dominant (common), right-handed patients who are right-hemisphere dominant (anomalous dextrals), and left-handed patients who are right-hemisphere dominant (true sinistrals). Since clinical abnormalities of higher cortical function, especially language, are heavily influenced by dominance, determination of the patient's handedness and dominance status is of paramount importance.

ABNORMAL SPEECH

Many diseases can cause abnormal speech, which ranges from conditions as common as a lisp or stutter to those as esoteric as spasmodic dysphonia. In neurologic patients, the speech abnormalities most often encountered are dysarthria and aphasia. The essential difference is that aphasia is a disorder of language and usually affects other language functions such as reading and writing. Dysarthria is a disorder of speech, it leaves other language functions intact, and it is often accompanied by other abnormalities such as dysphagia. Dysarthria is a problem with articulation of speech, whereas aphasia is a problem with language function. The implications of these two conditions are different. A good general rule is that no matter how garbled the patient's speech, if he is speaking in correct sentences and using proper grammar and syntax, he has dysarthria and not aphasia.

THE APHASIAS

Aphasia refers to a disorder of language, including various combinations of impairment in the ability to spontaneously produce, understand, and repeat speech, as well as defects in the ability to read and write. In the patient with aphasia, if speech output is high, the aphasia is referred to as fluent; if speech output is sparse and effortful, the aphasia is classed as nonfluent. Nonfluent aphasias are expressive. Fluent aphasias with poor comprehension are receptive. One major problem with the expressive versus receptive classification of aphasia is that every aphasic patient has trouble expressing himself. Hence, there is a tendency among many to classify almost all aphasias as expressive, even when they are flagrantly receptive. The Broca/Wernicke and fluent/nonfluent classification schemes have no such built-in terminological bias. The systematic assessment of language function should include testing of spontaneous speech (fluency), auditory comprehension, naming, repeating, reading, and writing. The changes in some of these functions with the major aphasic disorders are summarized in Table 6–1.

Broca Aphasia (Nonfluent or Expressive Aphasia)

Broca aphasia is a nonfluent aphasia caused by a lesion in the inferior frontal convolution just anterior to the motor speech area serving the face and lips. Patients with Broca aphasia have nonfluent speech with a low word output and a tendency to leave out filler words such as "a," "an," "the," and various adjectives. Such speech is sometimes referred to as telegraphic, because it resembles the parsimonious language of a telegram. Ability to comprehend speech is unimpaired. Because of the severe nonfluency, patients are unable to name objects or to repeat spoken phrases. Patients with Broca aphasia usually have a contralateral

TABLE 6-1. CLASSIFICATION OF THE APHASIAS

Aphasia	Relative Severities			
	Fluency	Auditory Comprehension	Repetition	Naming
Broca	−	+	−	−
Global	−	−	−	−
Wernicke	+	−	−	−
Conduction	+	+	−	±
Anomic	+	+	+	−
Isolation of the speech area	−	−	+	−

− = abnormal function; + = relatively intact function; ± = mild or equivocal involvement.

hemiparesis, but no field cut. Writing is always abnormal, even with the nonparetic hand.

Wernicke Aphasia (Fluent Aphasia)

Not to be confused with Wernicke encephalopathy, Wernicke aphasia is due to a lesion in the posterior temporal region that involves the speech reception area (auditory association cortex). Patients with Wernicke aphasia are fluent. They typically have a high word output (logorrhea), but language is virtually meaningless, often filled with paraphasias (word substitutions), and neologisms (made up, nonsensical words). Although speech is abundant, it is devoid of meaningful content (sometimes referred to as word salad or jargon aphasia). Naming and repetition deficits arise from poor comprehension. Often the patient lacks awareness of the deficit and may actually appear euphoric. Patients with Wernicke aphasia classically have a visual field deficit but no hemiparesis.

Global Aphasia

In global aphasia, a large lesion, such as a middle cerebral artery occlusion, has destroyed both the Wernicke area and the Broca area. Grossly nonfluent speech is combined with a severe comprehension deficit and inability to name or repeat. Typically there is both a hemiplegia and a field cut.

Anomic Aphasia

Patients with anomic aphasia are fluent and are able to comprehend and repeat, but have difficulty in naming. This is the most common but least specific type of aphasia. Patients with any aphasia type as it develops or recovers may pass through a stage in which anomia is the primary deficit. In addition, patients with other types of hemispheric dysfunction may have anomia as an isolated deficit, so-called nonaphasic misnaming.

Other Aphasias

Other notable aphasia types include conduction, isolation of the speech area, transcortical, and subcortical aphasia (Enrichment Box 6–1).

OTHER HIGHER CORTICAL FUNCTION DEFECTS

Despite relatively normal speech and the absence of confusion or cognitive impairment, some patients have unusual behaviors related to focal pathology involving specific brain regions. These other abnormalities of higher cortical function include the apraxias, agnosias, and related exotic syndromes (Enrichment Box 6–2). It is important to recognize these abnormalities to avoid mistakenly concluding that the patient is demented or has a comprehension defect.

Abnormalities of Cranial Nerve Function

In the course of examining the cranial nerves, any number of findings may emerge. Space does not permit a description of much more than the most common abnormalities. Findings related to vision and oculo-

---

ENRICHMENT BOX 6–1

Lesions of the arcuate fasciculus, which joins the Wernicke area to the Broca area, produce conduction aphasia, an inability to repeat that is out of proportion to other language deficits. Conduction aphasia is one of the most commonly encountered types of disconnection syndrome.

Testing for repetition ability efficiently screens for aphasic disorders, since it is compromised in Broca aphasia (because of inability to utter words), Wernicke aphasia (because of inability to understand the command), and conduction aphasia (because of inability to link the two functions). Aphasias that spare repetition (e.g., transcortical motor, transcortical sensory, and isolation of the speech area, or transcortical mixed) occur infrequently.

Subcortical aphasia is due to a lesion involving the striatum or thalamus, and is often of a mixed type or is difficult to classify.

Apraxia refers to the inability to perform a motor activity in the presence of intact motor and sensory systems, comprehension, attention, and cooperation. Ideomotor apraxia refers to the inability to execute, on command, an act done with ease spontaneously, and may involve either midline movements (e.g., tongue protrusion) or limb movements (e.g., making a fist). Ideational apraxia is much less common than ideomotor apraxia and is variously defined as (1) the inability to use actual objects, or (2) the inability to carry out multistep activities even though the individual component execution is intact (e.g., lighting a pipe from the raw materials). Constructional apraxia describes an inability to appreciate relationships between form and space. Patients can draw straight lines but cannot synthesize them into a three-dimensional cube. Patients with dressing apraxia cannot don clothing properly.

Gerstmann syndrome, seen in lesions of the angular gyrus in the dominant parietal lobe, has four components: finger agnosia (inability to name, identify, or localize fingers), right–left disorientation, acalculia (possibly because of paraphasic substitution of numbers), and agraphia. Most patients have constructional apraxia as well. A single component of the syndrome does not reliably indicate parietal dysfunction, but if all four components occur, dominant parietal lobe abnormality is almost invariably present.

motor functions are discussed in Chapter 7. This section briefly discusses abnormalities of other cranial nerves that are seen regularly.

FACIAL WEAKNESS

Facial weakness is a relatively common clinical finding that can take several patterns (Table 6–2). Keep in mind the essential fact that the lower face is innervated only by the contralateral cerebral hemisphere, while the upper face receives innervation from both hemispheres. Therefore, a unilateral hemispheric lesion causes weakness primarily of the contralateral lower face with relative sparing of the upper face. This weakness is referred to as a central facial palsy. In contrast, a lower motor neuron, or peripheral, facial palsy paralyzes both the upper and lower face ipsilateral to the lesion. This abnormality occurs because each facial nerve carries all of the lower motor neuron fibers, which represent the final common pathway, to its half of the face, both upper and lower.

In addition, the facial musculature may be weakened by other processes. Patients with generalized peripheral neuropathies, particularly Guillain-Barré syndrome, may develop facial nerve involvement. It is usually bilateral and produces facial diplegia, which is paralysis of both sides

TABLE 6–2. REVIEW OF THE DIFFERENT PATTERNS OF FACIAL WEAKNESS AND POTENTIAL EXPLANATIONS

Weakness Pattern	Possible Responsible Conditions
Unilateral lower	Contralateral cerebral hemispheric lesion
Unilateral upper and lower	Ipsilateral facial nerve lesion (e.g., Bell palsy, cerebellopontine angle lesion, pontine stroke)
Bilateral upper and lower	Bilateral facial nerve lesions (e.g., Guillain-Barré syndrome, sarcoidosis)
	Myopathy (e.g., facioscapulohumeral or myotonic muscular dystrophy)
	Neuromuscular junction disorder (e.g., myasthenia gravis)*
	Large pontine lesion (e.g., locked-in syndrome)

*The weakness produced by neuromuscular junction disorders is often limited to eye closure, and this function must be specifically tested.

of the face, both upper and lower. Other disease processes can produce facial diplegia as well, especially sarcoidosis. Other conditions that may cause facial weakness include myasthenia gravis and certain myopathies.

DEAFNESS

Most hearing loss takes the form of bilateral, sensorineural deafness related to acoustic trauma or presbyacusis. When the hearing loss is very asymmetric, the physician should be concerned about a lesion of the acoustic nerve, such as a schwannoma. When hearing loss is associated with a history of tinnitus or vertigo, consider Ménière disease.

ABNORMALITIES OF THE LOWER CRANIAL NERVES

The key abnormalities most commonly encountered in examination of cranial nerves IX and X are suppression of the gag reflex and palatal deviation. A decreased gag reflex is a nonspecific and usually nonlocalizing finding, which is more likely to occur as a result of obtundation and depression of the level of consciousness than from a focal CNS lesion. The palate is innervated by both cerebral hemispheres; therefore, a unilateral supratentorial lesion does not produce unilateral palatal weakness. When palatal weakness is present, it is always the result of a lower motor neuron lesion. The lesion might involve the nucleus ambiguus in the medulla or the ninth and tenth nerves anywhere along their extramedullary course.

Weakness of the eleventh cranial nerve does not occur, for all practical purposes, from a CNS lesion. The cause is always at or distal to the nerve's exit from the skull through the jugular foramen. The most common pathological process involving the eleventh cranial nerve is overactivity of the sternomastoid and trapezius muscles as a result of focal dystonia (cervical dystonia or spasmodic torticollis).

A pathological condition involving the twelfth cranial nerve is rare. The lesion may be anywhere from the hypoglossal nucleus in the medulla through the intra- and extramedullary course of the nerve or anywhere along its extracranial pathway. Minimal deviation of the tongue may occur because of a contralateral hemispheric lesion, but this is never dramatic. Bilateral weakness, wasting, and fasciculations of the tongue are a common manifestation of amyotrophic lateral sclerosis (ALS).

Weakness

Weakness is a common abnormality, and can take many forms. It may be focal or generalized. When focal, weakness may follow the distribution of a structure in the peripheral nervous system, such as a peripheral nerve or spinal root. It may affect one side of the body in a "hemi" distribution. A hemi distribution may affect the arm, leg, and face equally on one side of the body, or one or more areas may be more involved than others. Recall from Chapter 5 that the corticospinal tract preferentially innervates certain muscle groups, and that these groups are often selectively impaired. When weakness is nonfocal, it may be generalized, predominantly proximal, or predominantly distal. These various patterns have differential diagnostic and localizing significance.

Identification of the process causing weakness is further aided by accompanying signs, such as reflex alterations and sensory loss. Table 6–3 reviews the features of upper motor neuron versus lower motor neuron weakness. Table 6–4 summarizes common patterns of weakness and their localization.

GENERALIZED WEAKNESS

The term "generalized weakness" implies that the weakness involves both sides of body, more or less symmetrically. When a patient has truly generalized weakness, bulbar motor functions, such as facial movements, speech, chewing, and swallowing are involved as well. When the bulbar functions are intact and there is weakness of both arms and both legs, the patient is said to have quadriparesis; if only the legs are involved, the patient has paraparesis. When weakness affects all four extremities, the likely causes are spinal cord disease, peripheral neuropathy, neuromuscular junction disorder, or myopathy.

TABLE 6–3. FEATURES OF UPPER MOTOR NEURON VERSUS LOWER MOTOR NEURON WEAKNESS

Feature	Upper Motor Neuron	Lower Motor Neuron
Weakness distribution	Corticospinal distribution; hemiparesis, quadriparesis, paraparesis, monoparesis, faciobrachial	Generalized, predominately proximal, predominately distal, or focal. No preferential involvement of corticospinal innervated muscles
Sensory loss distribution	Central pattern	None, stocking glove, peripheral nerve, or root distribution
Deep tendon reflexes	Increased unless very acute	Normal or decreased
Superficial reflexes	Decreased	Normal
Pathological reflexes	Yes	No
Sphincter function	Sometimes impaired	Normal (except for cauda equina lesion)
Muscle tone	Increased	Normal or decreased
Pain	No	Sometimes
Other CNS signs	Possibly	No

CNS = central nervous system.

When spinal cord disease is the culprit and the deficit is incomplete, more severe involvement of the muscles that are preferentially innervated by the corticospinal tract can frequently be discerned. Reflexes are usually increased (though in the acute stages they may be decreased or absent), sensation is usually altered (sometimes at a discrete spinal level), superficial reflexes disappear, and there may be bowel and bladder dysfunction. Generalized peripheral nerve disease tends to predominantly involve distal muscles, though there are exceptions. There is no preferential involvement of corticospinal innervated muscles, reflexes are usually decreased, sensory loss is frequently present, and bowel and bladder functions are not disturbed. When a neuromuscular junction disorder is the culprit, the weakness is likely to be worse proximally, sensation is spared, reflexes are normal, and there is usually involvement of bulbar muscles, especially with ptosis and ophthalmoplegia. When the problem is a primary muscle disorder, weakness is usually more severe proximally, reflexes are normal, sensation

TABLE 6–4. PATTERNS OF WEAKNESS WITH LESIONS AT DIFFERENT LOCATIONS IN THE NEURAXIS

Location of Lesion	Distribution of Weakness	Sensory Loss	Deep Tendon Reflexes	Possible Accompanying Signs
Middle cerebral artery	Contralateral arm and face > leg*	Y	↑	Aphasia, apraxia, visual field deficit, gaze palsy
Anterior cerebral artery	Contralateral leg > arm and face*	Y	↑	Cortical sensory loss contralateral leg, frontal lobe signs, sometimes incontinence
Internal capsule	Contralateral face = arm = leg*	N	↑	None (pure motor stroke)
Brainstem	Ipsilateral cranial nerve and contra-lateral body*	Y	↑	Variable, depending on level
Cervical cord (transverse)	Both arms and both legs*	Y	↑†	Bowel, bladder, or sexual dysfunction common
Thoracic cord (transverse)	Both legs*	Y	↑†	Bowel, bladder, or sexual dysfunction common
Cauda equina	Both legs, asym-metric, multiple root pattern	Y	↓	Occasional bowel, bladder, or sexual dysfunction; sometimes pain
Anterior horn cell	Focal early, generalized late	N	↑	Atrophy, fasciculations, bulbar weakness
Single nerve root	Muscles of the affected myotome	Y	↓	Pain
Plexus	Plexus pattern, complete or partial	Usually	↓	Pain is common, especially with brachial plexitis
Mononeuropathy	Muscles of the affected nerve	Usually	↓	Variable atrophy, variable pain
Polyneuropathy	Distal > proximal	Usually	↓	Variable pain, atrophy late
Neuromuscular junction	Bulbar, proximal extremities	N	Normal	Ptosis, ophthalmoparesis, fatigable weakness, fluctuating weakness
Muscle	Proximal > distal	N	Normal	Pain uncommon, many potential patterns (e.g., limb girdle, facioscapulo-humeral), pseudohyper-trophy, myotonia

Y = yes; N = no; ↑ = increased; ↓ = decreased.
*Extremity weakness occurs in a corticospinal tract distribution.
†Reflexes may be decreased acutely (spinal shock).

is normal, and, with only a few exceptions, bulbar function is spared except for occasional dysphagia.

Anterior horn cell disease is a special case. The most common condition by far to affect anterior horn cells is ALS, which characteristically involves both the upper and lower motor neurons. It produces a clinical picture of weakness and wasting, which results from involvement of the lower motor neurons in the anterior horn of the spinal cord, combined with weakness and hyperreflexia caused by involvement of the upper motor neurons in the cerebral cortex that give rise to the corticospinal tract. There is upper motor neuron weakness (cerebral cortex pathology) superimposed on lower motor neuron weakness (spinal cord pathology). The weakness tends to be asymmetric and associated with hyperreflexia. Any time that an extremity is both atrophic and hyperreflexic, the cause is likely to be ALS.

FOCAL WEAKNESS

When the arm and leg on one side of the body are weak, the patient is said to have a hemiparesis. This condition may range in severity from mild (manifested only as pronator drift and impairment of fine motor control) to total paralysis. Monoparesis is weakness of only one extremity, such as the leg contralateral to an anterior cerebral stroke. Reflexes, which are typically increased unless the process is acute, and accompanying sensory loss help identify such focal weakness as being central in origin.

A focal neuropathy, such as a radial nerve palsy, or a spinal root lesion, such as from a herniated disc, cause weakness limited to the distribution of the involved nerve or root. A complete plexopathy, such as brachial plexitis, may cause weakness of the entire limb, or weakness only in the distribution of specific plexus components. With these lower motor neuron conditions, reflexes are typically decreased and there is often accompanying sensory loss. Localization of focal weakness due to root, plexus, and peripheral nerve abnormalities requires intimate familiarity with peripheral neuroanatomy.

Anterior horn cell disease usually begins with focal weakness, often involving one hand or one foot. A multinerve, multiroot distribution of weakness, normal or increased reflexes, and a lack of sensory loss are usually the earliest symptoms. As the condition progresses, as it invariably does, the clinical picture evolves into one of generalized weakness, as described earlier.

Except for extraocular muscle involvement in myasthenia gravis, it is rare for a myopathy or neuromuscular junction disorder to cause focal weakness.

Other Motor System Abnormalities

The motor examination is not limited to an assessment of strength. It also includes evaluation of muscle tone and bulk and a search for the presence of abnormal involuntary movements (AIMs).

Muscle tone may be increased (hypertonia), decreased (hypotonia), or abnormal (dystonia). Hypertonia comes in two common variants: rigidity and spasticity. When increased tone occurs to more or less the same degree throughout the range of passive motion and is independent of the speed of movement, it is referred to as rigidity. When hypertonia is most marked near the middle of the range of motion and is more apparent with fast passive movement than with slow passive movement (i.e., rate dependent), it is referred to as spasticity. Rigidity may be associated with smooth resistance throughout the range, so-called leadpipe rigidity or Gegenhalten, or with a ratchety, jerky, tremulous variation in the hypertonia, so-called cogwheel rigidity. Spastic hypertonia is typically associated with increased deep tendon reflexes (DTRs), loss of superficial reflexes, and Babinski signs. Cogwheel rigidity occurs in Parkinson disease and related conditions. Gegenhalten is usually associated with other abnormal neurologic signs, depending on the etiology.

The term "dystonia" refers to various movement disorders associated with transient or sustained hypertonic conditions that do not fit into the other categories. The dystonias are further discussed in the following section (see abnormal involuntary movements).

Hypotonia occurs in two primary settings in the adult: myopathies and cerebellar disease. An infant with hypotonia is referred to as a "floppy baby." The differential diagnosis of infantile hypotonia is extensive, and the workup of a floppy baby is a frequent exercise in pediatric neurology.

Muscle mass or volume may be decreased (atrophy) or increased (hypertrophy). Neurogenic atrophy results from a lesion involving the anterior horn cells, nerve root, or peripheral nerve innervating a muscle and may be severe. Muscle diseases usually cause only mild to moderate atrophy of the involved muscles. Disuse atrophy occurs after immobilization, such as when a limb is in a cast, and is usually mild to moderate in severity and recovers quickly with resumption of use.

True muscle hypertrophy results from an increase in the size or number of muscle fibers. It most often occurs as physiologic hypertrophy from heavy use but can also occur in certain neuromuscular disorders. Pseudohypertrophy refers to a situation in which a muscle appears to be enlarged, but in fact there has been replacement of diseased muscle by fat and fibrous tissue. Enlarged calf muscles in patients with Duchenne's muscular dystrophy are a classic example of muscle pseudohypertrophy.

ABNORMAL INVOLUNTARY MOVEMENTS

AIMs occur in a host of neurologic conditions. AIMs come in a range of forms: tremor, chorea, muscle fasciculations, or myoclonic jerks. The only common characteristic is that the movements are spontaneous and not under volitional control. AIMs may be rhythmic or random, fleeting or sustained, predictable or unpredictable. AIMs may occur in isolation or be accompanied by other neurologic signs. Table 6–5 summarizes the features of AIMs.

Tremors are the most common type of AIM and result from many different conditions. They can be broadly grouped into those that are most prominent when at rest, when arms and hands are outstretched in a sustained posture, or when making a movement [as in doing the finger-to-nose (FTN) or finger-nose-finger (FNF) test]. The first type is referred to as a rest tremor, the second as a postural tremor, and the last as an intention tremor. Table 6–6 summarizes common tremors.

The most common rest tremor by far is the pill-rolling tremor of parkinsonism, whether caused by idiopathic Parkinson disease or other basal ganglia disorders, or induced by drugs such as phenothiazine. The tremor is most prominent with the patient perfectly relaxed and the hand resting in the lap. The tremor, unless severe, dampens on intention.

Essential tremor is a common cause of high-frequency tremor (see Part III). It is most prominent with the body part held in a sustained posture (postural tremor), it changes variably on intention, and it always subsides at rest. This type of tremor is usually seen to best advantage with the arms, hands, and fingers outstretched and the patient attempting to maintain that position.

A tremor that is most dramatic when the patient attempts to make a precise movement, as in doing the FTN test, is typical of ataxia, either cerebellar or sensory.

Dystonia refers to slow, sustained, cramp-like spontaneous movements, either constant or intermittent, generalized or focal. Focal varieties include an array of occupational dystonias, such as writer's

---

TABLE 6–5. CLASSIFICATION OF ABNORMAL INVOLUNTARY MOVEMENTS AS A SPECTRUM OF MOVEMENTS

Regular/predictable	Intermediate	Fleeting/unpredictable
Tremor	Most dystonias	Fasciculations
Hemiballism	Myokymia	Myoclonus
	Athetosis	Chorea

TABLE 6–6. POTENTIAL COMMON ETIOLOGIES FOR DIFFERENT TYPES OF TREMOR

Rest Tremor	Postural Tremor	Intention Tremor
Parkinson disease	Essential tremor	Cerebellar ataxia
Parkinsonism	Thyrotoxicosis	Sensory ataxia
	Certain drugs	

cramp. A relatively common form of focal dystonia is cervical dystonia, or spasmodic torticollis. This form of focal dystonia affects the neck muscles and produces either a sustained or jerky turning of the head to one side, often with an element of head tilt. "Torti" implies a twisting or turning movement; less common variants of cervical dystonia include retrocollis (extension movement) and anterocollis (flexion movement). Notoriously refractory to medical therapy, cervical dystonia is now often treated by the injection of infinitesimally small amounts of botulinum toxin to weaken the abnormally contracting muscles.

Other important types of AIMs include chorea, athetosis, hemiballismus, generalized dystonia, tics, tardive dyskinesias, and Gilles de la Tourette syndrome (Enrichment Box 6–3).

Sensory Loss

Sensory function is divided clinically into primary modalities and secondary or cortical modalities. The primary modalities include light touch, pressure, pain, temperature, joint position, sense, and vibration. The cortical modalities are those that require synthesis and interpretation of primary modalities by the sensory association area in the parietal lobe. These include such things as two-point discrimination, stereognosis, graphesthesia, and tactile localization. When the primary modalities are normal in a particular body region, but the cortical modalities are impaired, a parietal lobe lesion may be responsible. Cortical impairments are rare, and much more often the clinician is faced with interpreting abnormalities of the primary modalities.

The primary modalities may be impaired because of disease involving peripheral nerve, spinal root, or sensory pathways within the CNS. When some primary modalities are involved more than others are, the sensory loss is said to be dissociated. Recall from neuroanatomy that

ENRICHMENT BOX 6-3

Chorea refers to abnormal involuntary movements (AIMs) that are highly erratic, fleeting, unpredictable, and generally of small amplitude. These movements may affect any body part but are usually most prominent in the hands. Most cases are due to Huntington disease. Athetosis is a slower, writhing movement that primarily involves proximal extremity muscles and occurs most often in patients with cerebral palsy. Hemiballism refers to a dramatic neurologic syndrome of wild, flinging, incessant movements that occur on one side of the body; it is usually due to infarction or hemorrhage in the region of the contralateral subthalamic nucleus. Hemiballismus is difficult to treat, incredibly disabling, and sometimes fatal because of exhaustion and inanition.

Dystonia musculorum deformans is a type of generalized dystonia that most often affects children and adolescents, is frequently familial, and produces striking twists and torsions of the body, turning the unfortunate affected individual into a veritable human pretzel. Circus sideshows sometimes include dystonia musculorum deformans victims.

Tardive dyskinesias are AIMs that usually develop in patients who have received phenothiazine or related compounds, usually as treatment for major psychosis for prolonged periods. The movements primarily involve the mouth, tongue, and jaw with incessant chewing, smacking, licking, and tongue thrusting that is difficult to eradicate. Some patients are unaware they have these movements. Long-term dopamine receptor blockade likely leads to denervation hypersensitivity of the receptor. The movements frequently first appear when the dose of dopamine-blocking agent is reduced, and they can often be controlled, at least temporarily, by reinstituting or increasing the dose of the drug. Tardive dyskinesias are more prone to develop in older patients, especially women.

Tics are quick, irregular, repetitive movements. They are common and usually benign. Examples of simple motor tics include repetitive blinking, facial contortions, or shoulder shrugging. More complicated tics can occur, and tics can also involve the voice, producing bizarre vocalizations, such as barking and grunting. Patients affected with Gilles de la Tourette syndrome have multifocal tics and compulsive behavior, and they may utter profanity and obscenities over which they have no control, a feature referred to as coprolalia. The disease is hereditary, probably autosomal dominant with variable expressivity, and apparently causes dysfunction of dopamine receptors. The exaggerated, complex tics, together with the other features of the disease, can be disabling. It is likely that the noted English literary figure, Dr. Samuel Johnson, famously eccentric, suffered from Tourette syndrome.

the pathways conveying pain and temperature (the spinothalamic tracts or the anterolateral system) run in a different location than the pathways conveying touch, pressure, position, and vibration (the posterior columns and medial lemniscus). After running divergently through much of their central course, the sensory pathways converge again as they approach the thalamus and remain together in the thalamocortical projections. When the pathways are close together, such as in the peripheral nerve, spinal root, or thalamus, disease processes tend to affect all primary modalities to an approximately equal degree. When the pathways are remote from each other, such as in the spinal cord and brainstem, the disease process may affect one type of sensation and not another, producing dissociated sensory loss.

A common example of dissociated sensory loss is lateral medullary stroke, or Wallenberg syndrome. In this condition, infarction involves the lateral medulla, where the lateral spinothalamic tract ascends and where the spinal tract of the trigeminal nerve descends. Both the lateral spinothalamic tract and the descending spinal tract of the trigeminal subserve pain and temperature. In a Wallenberg stroke, a characteristic pattern of sensory loss occurs, which only involves pain and temperature and completely spares light touch. The pain and temperature loss affects the ipsilateral face because of involvement of the spinal tract of V and affects the contralateral body because of damage to the lateral spinothalamic tract.

A classic but uncommon cause of dissociated sensory loss is syringomyelia. A syrinx involves the central canal of the spinal cord, causing it to expand. The first structures to be involved are sensory fibers crossing in the anterior commissure, just anterior to the central canal. These pain and temperature sensory fibers synapse in the posterior horn on one side of the spinal cord and decussate to the other side of the spinal cord before ascending in the spinothalamic tract. Sensory fibers subserving light touch and pressure run in the posterior columns, well removed from the site of the syrinx. As a result, syringomyelia characteristically causes sensory loss to pain and temperature, with preservation of light touch.

Anterior spinal artery stroke, another cause of dissociated sensory loss, results in infarction of the anterior two-thirds of the cord. The posterior columns, perfused by the posterior spinal arteries, are spared. Patients have dense motor deficits and dense sensory loss to pain and temperature, but normal touch, pressure, position, and vibration sensations. Patients with Brown-Sequard syndrome have the most extreme dissociation of modalities, with sensory loss to pain and temperature on one side of the body below the lesion and loss to touch, pressure, position, and vibration on the other side of the body.

In contrast, disease processes affecting a peripheral nerve trunk or a spinal root tend to involve all of the sensory fibers traveling in that nerve or root. The sensory loss involves all modalities. Occasionally, generalized polyneuropathies may have a predilection for large or small fibers and can cause differential involvement of pain and temperature sensation as opposed to touch and pressure sensation. These neuropathies are uncommon and tend to be generalized. When there is marked sensory dissociation affecting one body region, the pathological condition is virtually always going to be in the CNS, specifically in those regions where the different sensory pathways run in widely divergent locations.

Joint position sense is tested by moving one of the patient's digits up and down and asking the patient to identify the direction of movement. Position sense is conveyed along large myelinated fibers in the peripheral nerve and posterior root. These fibers turn upward without synapsing in the spinal cord and pass upward in the posterior columns to finally synapse in the nucleus gracilis and nucleus cuneatus at the level of the lower medulla. The ability to perceive the vibration of a tuning fork is generally considered to follow essentially the same pathway.

Vibration is a sensitive modality because the nervous system must accurately perceive, transmit, and interpret a rapidly changing stimulus. One of the first functions impaired when there is demyelination in the nervous system, either peripheral or central, is the ability to follow a train of stimuli. Testing vibratory sensibility measures this functional ability, and loss of vibratory sensation is often a sensitive early indicator of dysfunction of the peripheral nervous system or the posterior columns, especially when there is any degree of demyelination.

The other consideration in elucidating the cause of sensory loss, in addition to the modalities involved, is the distribution of the abnormality. Deficits in a hemi distribution suggest CNS disease, likely either involving the cortex or the thalamus. Crossed deficits, affecting the face on one side and the body on the opposite side, suggest brainstem disease. Deficits involving both sides of the body below a certain level, for example, T5, suggest spinal cord disease. A spinal cord level with sacral sparing suggests intraparenchymal spinal cord pathological conditions rather than a myelopathy due to external pressure. Deficits caused by peripheral nerve disease typically involve the most distal body regions in a so-called stocking-glove distribution. Sensory loss because of dysfunction of a peripheral nerve, nerve root, or nerve plexus follows the innervation pattern of that particular structure. Figure 6–1 depicts commonly seen types of sensory loss.

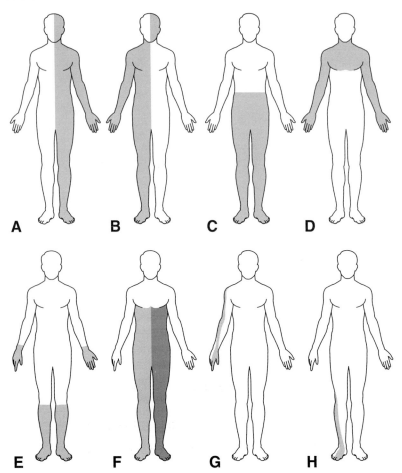

FIGURE 6–1 ■ Common patterns of sensory loss. (*A*) Hemisensory loss due to a hemispheric lesion. (*B*) Crossed sensory loss to pain and temperature due to a lateral medullary lesion. (*C*) Midthoracic spinal cord level. (*D*) Suspended, dissociated sensory loss to pain and temperature due to syringomyelia. (*E*) Distal, symmetric sensory loss due to peripheral neuropathy. (*F*) Crossed spinothalamic loss on one side with posterior column loss on the opposite side due to Brown-Sequard syndrome. (*G*) Dermatomal sensory loss due to cervical radiculopathy. (*H*) Dermatomal sensory loss due to lumbosacral radiculopathy.

Abnormal Reflexes

Reflexes may be abnormal because they are increased (hyperreflexia) or decreased (hyporeflexia). Hyperactive DTRs are a sign of CNS disease, specifically corticospinal tract dysfunction. Patients who have true pathologic hyperreflexia invariably have other accompanying signs of corticospinal tract dysfunction, such as increased tone or pathologic reflexes (e.g., Babinski sign). With pathologic hyperreflexia there is concomitant abolition or diminishment of the superficial reflexes (abdominals and cremasterics). Hyporeflexic (not hyporeflex*ive*) patients usually have peripheral neuropathy. Myopathies and neuromuscular junction disorders do not appreciably diminish the DTRs unless the weakness is extremely severe. These abnormal reflex patterns are summarized in Table 6–7.

The most important pathologic reflex is the extensor plantar response, or Babinski sign. There are other pathologic reflexes, but their significance is minor compared with the extensor plantar response. Other pathologic reflexes, such as the palmomental and Hoffman reflexes, are often seen in normal individuals. Reflexes such as the snout and grasp are more for clinical entertainment value than they are of any real utility. Only a pronounced asymmetry of a reflex such as the Hoffman or palmomental has any real significance, and this asymme-

TABLE 6–7. PATTERNS OF ABNORMAL REFLEXES IN DISEASE PROCESSES AFFECTING DIFFERENT PARTS OF THE NEURAXIS

Disease Location	Deep Tendon Reflexes	Superfical Reflexes	Pathological Reflexes
Central nervous system	Increased*	Decreased or absent	Yes
Nerve root	Focally decreased	Normal	No
Plexus	Focally decreased	Normal	No
Mononeuropathy	Focally decreased	Normal	No
Demyelinating polyneuropathy	Globally decreased	Normal	No
Axonal polyneuropathy	Distally decreased (length-dependent pattern)	Normal	No
Neuromuscular junction disorder	Normal†	Normal	No
Myopathy	Normal (unless weakness is very severe)	Normal	No

*Reflexes are increased unless the disease process is very acute, as in spinal shock, when the deep tendon reflexes may be suppressed.
†Reflexes are normal except in Lambert Eaton syndrome, when lower extremity deep tendon reflexes are usually decreased.

try generally does not occur without other, probably more impressive and significant, clinical signs.

Deficits of Cerebellar Function and Coordination

A lack of coordination is usually detected on the FTN or FNF, heel-to-shin, or rapid alternating movement (RAM) part of the examination. There are many potential causes. First, weakness and spasticity can cause incoordination and clumsiness. These deficits should not be mistaken for evidence of pathological findings elsewhere in the nervous system, especially the cerebellum. A good general rule is that the examiner should avoid drawing conclusions about the meaning of intention tremor and incoordination in a patient with any significant degree of weakness or spasticity. Assuming then that the examination shows no weakness and that the DTRs are normal or decreased, incoordination and awkwardness in such circumstances is usually due to cerebellar disease. The inability to make RAMs because of cerebellar disease is referred to as dysdiadochokinesia, but "impaired RAMs" or similar language is often favored by those reluctant to attempt to spell the technical term. (The ability to spell dysdiadochokinesia and tic douloureux is not strictly necessary for a career as a neurologist!)

The patient with impaired RAMs has difficulty with such standard tests as patting the palm of one hand alternately with the palm and dorsum of the other hand, or tapping out a complex rhythm, or tapping the foot in steady beat. Incoordination and decreased RAMs are usually accompanied by intention tremor (see ABNORMAL INVOLUNTARY MOVEMENTS). Error in judging distance when making a movement is dysmetria. The combination of incoordination, awkwardness, and errors in the speed, range, and force of movement, along with dysdiadochokinesia and intention tremor, is referred to as cerebellar ataxia.

Cerebellar disease may affect all or only a specific part of the cerebellum. The primary clinical manifestation of dysfunction of the flocculonodular lobe (archicerebellum, man the fish; see Chapter 3) is nystagmus and other abnormalities of extraocular movement. Dysfunction of the vermis (paleocerebellum, man the snake; see Chapter 3) produces gait and balance abnormalities ranging from slight widening of the base on walking in mild disease to total inability to sit or walk in severe disease. Disease of the cerebellar hemispheres (neocerebellum, man the monkey; see Chapter 3) produces appendicular ataxia. Cerebellar hemispheric deficits occur ipsilateral to the lesion because the pathways are uncrossed (or, more correctly, double crossed; see Chapter 2 for a discussion of the decussation of the superior cerebellar peduncle). The occurrence of cerebellar ataxia in a hemi distribution usually signals a unilateral, ipsilateral lesion of the cerebellum or cerebellar connections (e.g., cerebellar astrocytoma, multiple sclerosis, or lateral medullary stroke). Table 6–8 summarizes the clinical manifestations of disease of these parts of the cerebellum.

In summary, a patient with unilateral disease of a cerebellar hemisphere or its connections manifests intention tremor on FTN and heel-to-shin testing, clumsiness, and impaired ability to perform RAMs or tap a rhythm with hand or foot, all ipsilaterally. A patient with vermian disease (e.g., hereditary cerebellar degeneration, paraneoplastic processes, or alcoholic degeneration) has gait ataxia; when severe, standing and sitting balance are affected, leading to constant to-and-fro swaying referred to as titubation. A patient with disease of the flocculonodular lobe or its connections has nystagmus. Pancerebellar ataxia refers to the condition in which all of the preceding abnormalities occur together.

Incoordination may also result from a lack of proprioceptive input from the limbs, referred to as sensory ataxia. This type of ataxia can occur because of peripheral nerve disease that primarily affects sensory fibers or because of pathological conditions involving the dorsal root ganglia, the dorsal roots, or the posterior columns of the spinal cord. Incoordination due to sensory ataxia can closely mimic that of cerebellar ataxia (Table 6–9). The distinction between the two is made primarily by the associated findings (including an absence of findings that suggest the alternative possibility).

TABLE 6–8. CLINICAL MANIFESTATIONS OF DISORDERS OF THE CEREBELLUM RELATED TO THE DIFFERENT ZONES OF THE CEREBELLUM

Zone of Cerebellum	Clinical Manifestation	Possible Disorder
Flocculonodular lobe (archicerebellum)	Nystagmus; extraocular movement abnormalities	Drug intoxication
Vermis	Gait ataxia	Alcoholic degeneration
Hemisphere (neocerebellum)	Appendicular ataxia	Tumor, stroke
Pancerebellar	All of the above	Paraneoplastic

TABLE 6–9. ASSOCIATED FINDINGS HELPFUL IN DISTINGUISHING SENSORY ATAXIA FROM CEREBELLAR ATAXIA

Sensory Ataxia	Cerebellar Ataxia
Sensory loss, especially for joint position and vibration	Nystagmus, ocular dysmetria, and other eye movement abnormalities
Steppage gait	Reeling, ataxic gait
Decreased reflexes	Other signs of cerebellar disease (hypotonia, rebound, impaired check response)
Lack of evidence of CNS disease	Other evidence of CNS disease (spasticity, extensor plantar responses)

CNS = central nervous system.

TABLE 6–10. COMMON ORGANIC NEUROLOGIC ABNORMALITIES OF GAIT

Gait Disorder	Gait Characteristics	Usual Associated Findings
Spastic	Stiff legged, scissoring (wooden soldier)	Hyperreflexia, extensor plantar responses
Cerebellar ataxia	Wide based, reeling, careening (drunken sailor)	Heel-to-shin ataxia, other cerebellar signs
Sensory ataxia	Wide based, steppage	Positive Romberg, impaired joint position sense
Hemiparetic	Involved leg spastic, circumduction often with foot drop	Weakness, hyperreflexia, extensor plantar response
Parkinsonian	Small steps, flexed posture, shuffling, festination	Tremor, rigidity, bradykinesia
Marche a petit pas	Small steps, slow shuffling	Dementia, frontal lobe signs
Foot drop (unilateral or bilateral)	High-steppage pattern to clear the toes from the floor, double tap with toe strike before heel strike	Foot dorsiflexion weakness
Myopathic	Exaggerated "sexy" hip motion, waddling, lumbar hyperlordosis	Hip girdle weakness

Gait Abnormalities

Abnormalities of gait are a common clinical problem with numerous causes, both neurologic and nonneurologic. A careful general evaluation is always necessary to exclude a nonneurologic cause. The particular possibility of orthopedic or musculoskeletal disease must always be borne in mind when a patient has difficulty walking. More than one neurologic consultation has been requested in a patient who was unable to walk because of acute podagra. Hip fractures are common and easily missed.

Neurologic causes of an abnormal gait are also numerous, including disparate conditions as varied as foot drop caused by peroneal nerve palsy, myopathy, hydrocephalus, and cerebellar degeneration. The various gait abnormalities produce different findings of the gait itself on physical examination, such as a steppage pattern as opposed to a pelvic waddle. The differential diagnosis of the gait abnormality is also dependent on the history and the other clinical signs present. Some of the more common abnormal gait patterns are summarized in Table 6–10.

A problem arises with the use of the term "steppage," which in essence means that the patient is lifting one or both legs high during their respective stride phases. Patients with foot drop may do this to help the foot clear the floor and avoid tripping. Patients with sensory ataxia, classically tabes dorsalis, may also lift the feet up high and then slap them down smartly to improve proprioceptive feedback. Since both of these gaits are high stepping, they have been referred to as steppage gaits, but the causes and mechanisms are different. For a striking illustration of a tabetic gait in sequential photographs by Eadweard Muybridge in 1887, the best demonstration outside of flesh or film, see Lanska DJ, Goetz CG: Romberg's sign: Development, adoption, and adaptation in the 19th century. *Neurology* 55:1201–1206, 2000.

7

Neuro-ophthalmology

The brain devotes an enormous amount of its capacity to visual functions, and disorders of the afferent and efferent facets of vision comprise a vast and vital aspect of neurology. The following material provides an overview of this important area. The anatomy of the visual system is complex but important; the seemingly arcane details are clinically relevant.

Disorders of The Optic Disc

The myelinated axons forming the optic disc give the normal disc a yellowish white color. It is paler temporally where the papillomacular bundle, which carries 90% of retinal axons, enters (Figure 7–1). The normal disc is well demarcated against the surrounding retina, with arteries and veins crossing the margins and capillaries staining the surface a faint pink. The physiologic cup is an area in the center of the disc that is less pinkish than the disc periphery and shows a faint latticework due to the underlying lamina cribrosa.

The appearance of the disc may change with the circumstances. The disc may change color to abnormally pale in optic atrophy or to abnormally red with disc edema. The margins may become obscured because of disc edema or the presence of anomalies. Edema of the disc is nonspecific. It may reflect increased intracranial pressure, or it may occur because of optic nerve inflammation, ischemia, or other local processes. By convention, disc swelling due to increased intracranial pressure is referred to as papilledema; under all other circumstances the noncommittal terms "disc edema" or "disc swelling" are preferred.

Visual function provides a critical clue about the nature of disc abnormalities. Patients with acute papilledema and those with disc anomalies have normal visual acuity, visual fields, and color perception; impairment of these functions is the rule for patients with optic neuropathies

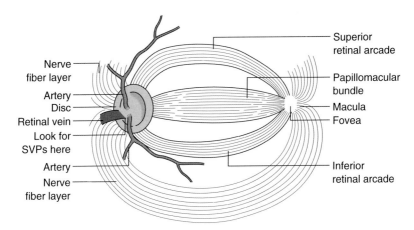

FIGURE 7–1. ■ The optic disc and associated structures. Axons destined to form the bulk of the fibers in the optic nerve arise from the macula, those from the nasal side form the papillomacular bundle, and those from other areas enter the disc as superior and inferior arcades. Spontaneous venous pulsations (*SVPs*) are best seen by looking at the tip of the column of one of the large veins on the disc surface.

of any cause. An important first step in evaluating a questionably abnormal disc is therefore a careful assessment of vision (see Chapter 5).

PAPILLEDEMA

Increased intracranial pressure exerts pressure on the intracranial portions of the optic nerves, impairing axoplasmic flow and producing axonal edema. The swollen axons impair venous return from the retina, engorging first the capillaries on the disc surface and then the retinal veins, ultimately causing splinter- and flame-shaped hemorrhages as well as cotton wool exudates in the retinal nerve fiber layer. The axonal swelling eventually leads to discernable elevation of the disc above the retinal surface.

There are four stages of papilledema: early, fully developed, chronic, and atrophic. Fully developed papilledema is easy to recognize, with elevation of the disc surface, humping of vessels crossing the disc margin, obliteration of disc margins, peripapillary hemorrhages, cotton wool exudates, engorged and tortuous retinal veins, and marked disc hyperemia.

The recognition of early papilledema is much more problematic, especially in patients with headache, altered mental status, or other neurologic symptomatology: a frequent clinical scenario (Enrichment Box 7–1). In chronic papilledema, hemorrhages and exudates resolve, leaving a markedly swollen "champagne cork" disc bulging up from the

ENRICHMENT BOX 7-1

Papilledema

Occasionally, the only way to resolve the question of early papilledema is by serial observation. The earliest change is loss of previously observed spontaneous venous pulsations (SVPs). Venous pulsations are best seen where the large veins dive into the disc centrally. The movement is a back and forth rhythmic oscillation of the tip or edge of the blood column, resembling a slowly darting snake's tongue, more than a side to side expansion of the vein. The presence of SVPs indicates an intracranial pressure less than approximately 200 mm H_2O, but since they are absent in 10%-20% of normal patients, only the disappearance of previously observed SVPs is clearly pathological. With developing papilledema, increased venous back pressure dilates the capillaries on the disc surface, transforming its normal yellowish pink to fiery red. Blurring of the superior and inferior margins evolves soon after. However, since these margins are normally the least distinct areas of the disc, blurry margins alone are not enough to diagnose papilledema. There is no alteration of the physiologic cup with early papilledema. With further evolution, splinter- or flame-shaped peripapillary hemorrhages and cotton wool exudates develop, along with engorgement and tortuosity of the retinal veins. Frank disc elevation then ensues as the fundus ripens into fully developed papilledema.

Papilledema ordinarily develops over days to weeks. With acutely increased intracranial pressure due to subarachnoid or intracranial hemorrhage, it may develop within hours. Measuring diopters of disc elevation ophthalmoscopically has little utility. Transient visual obscurations (momentary graying out or blacking out of vision) are a classic symptom of papilledema, especially in pseudotumor cerebri.

An old saw describes these conditions aptly. When the patient sees (has normal vision) and the doctor sees (observes disc abnormalities), it is papilledema. When the patient does not see (has impaired vision) and the doctor sees (observes disc abnormalities), it is papillitis. When the patient does not see (has impaired vision) and the doctor does not see (observes no disc abnormality), it is retrobulbar neuritis.

Pseudopapilledema

Drusen, or hyaloid bodies, of the optic nerve may elevate and distort the disc. On the disc surface, drusen have a highly refractile, "rock candy" appearance, but when "buried" beneath the surface may produce only disc elevation and blurred margins, causing confusion with papilledema. Myelinated nerve fibers occasionally extend beyond the disc margin into the retina, causing a striking disc picture but signifying nothing. Other causes of pseudopapilledema include remnants of the

(Continued)

primitive hyaloid artery (Bergmeister papilla), tilted discs, and extreme hyperopia.

Foster Kennedy syndrome

Disc edema in one eye and optic atrophy in the other eye can occur because an atrophic nerve head cannot develop papilledema in response to increased intracranial pressure. Foster Kennedy syndrome, a neurologic classic that is now a rarity, develops when an olfactory-groove or sphenoid-wing meningioma produces a chronic, compressive optic neuropathy on one side that results in optic atrophy. When the tumor reaches sufficient size, increased intracranial pressure develops, producing papilledema in the opposite eye but not in the atrophic eye. Optic atrophy in one eye with disc edema in the other eye is now much more commonly seen with anterior ischemic optic neuropathy (AION; pseudo-Foster Kennedy syndrome), which may affect the opposite eye weeks to months after an initial episode renders the originally affected disc atrophic.

plane of the retina. If unrelieved, impaired axoplasmic flow eventually leads to death of axons and visual impairment, and evolves into the stage of atrophic papilledema or secondary optic atrophy (see OPTIC ATROPHY). The visual fields undergo concentric constriction.

Changes ophthalmoscopically indistinguishable from papilledema occur when conditions primarily affecting the optic nerve cause disc edema. These optic neuropathies generally cause marked visual impairment, including loss of acuity, central or cecocentral scotoma, altered color perception, and an afferent pupillary defect (APD, or Marcus Gunn pupil). Optic neuritis and anterior ischemic optic neuropathy (AION) both cause impaired vision and disc edema. Optic neuritis with disc edema is sometimes called "papillitis." When optic neuritis strikes the retrobulbar portion of the nerve, marked visual impairment occurs but the disc appearance remains normal, since the pathology is posterior to the papilla (see Enrichment Box 7-1). Optic neuritis (papillitis or retrobulbar neuritis) may occur as an isolated abnormality, as a manifestation of multiple sclerosis (MS), or as a complication of a systemic illness. AION, essentially an infarction of the optic disc, generally occurs in older patients with small vessel disease; it is a feared complication of giant cell (temporal) arteritis.

PSEUDOPAPILLEDEMA

Some conditions affecting the nerve head cause striking disc changes of little or no clinical import. Routine ophthalmoscopy may unexpectedly reveal an abnormal-appearing disc in a patient with migraine or a seemingly benign neurologic complaint. Such patients generally have normal vision and no visual complaints. Common causes of pseudopapilledema include optic nerve drusen and myelinated nerve fibers (see Enrichment Box 7–1).

OPTIC ATROPHY

In optic atrophy, the disc is paler than normal and more sharply demarcated from the surrounding retina, sometimes having a "punched-out" appearance. Loss of axons and their supporting capillaries with replacement by gliotic scar produce the lack of color, which may vary from a dirty gray to stark white. Optic atrophy may follow another condition (optic neuritis, AION, or papilledema), in which case it is referred to as secondary or "consecutive" optic atrophy. Primary optic atrophy, appearing de novo, occurs as a heredofamilial condition (e.g., Leber's optic atrophy) or after toxic, metabolic, nutritional, compressive, or glaucomatous insult to the nerve.

Sometimes a patient may have disc edema in one eye and optic atrophy in the other eye, the Foster Kennedy syndrome (see Enrichment Box 7–1).

Pupils

NORMAL PUPILS

Pupillary size depends primarily on the balance between sympathetic and parasympathetic innervation and the level of ambient illumination. Anisocoria means that the two pupils are not of the same size (*an* = not, *iso* = the same, *cor* = pupil). Mild degrees of inequality, less than 1 mm of difference between the two sides, occur in 15%–20% of the population. With such physiologic anisocoria, the degree of inequality remains the same in light and dark.

The pupillary light reaction is mediated by the macula, optic nerve, chiasm, and optic tract. Just before reaching the lateral geniculate body, pupil afferents veer away from the optic tract to synapse in the pretectum. Extensive crossing occurs through the posterior commissure, explaining the bilaterality of the light reaction. Fibers project from the pretectum to the Edinger-Westphal subnucleus of the oculomotor nuclear complex in the midbrain. Parasympathetic pupillary efferents from the Edinger-Westphal subnucleus enter the third cranial nerve and travel through the cavernous sinus and along the inferior branch of cranial nerve III in the orbit to innervate the pupilloconstrictor muscle of the iris. Balancing parasympathetic tone from the Edinger-Westphal subnucleus are sympathetic fibers ascending from the superior cervical ganglion in the pericarotid sympathetic plexus surrounding the internal carotid artery.

Pupillary constriction also occurs as part of the near response, along with convergence and rounding up of the lens. Fibers mediating the near response are generally less vulnerable to most pathological processes, so that pupillary "light–near dissociation" (a better reaction to near than to light) occurs in a variety of conditions.

Pupils are normally larger in younger patients than in older patients and larger in patients with myopia than in patients with hyperopia. Normal pupils may display constant, small amplitude fluctuations in size, termed "hippus." Many systemically acting and locally acting drugs influence pupil size and reactivity.

A pupil may be abnormal because it is too large or too small or because it displays altered reactivity.

LARGE PUPILS

The two conditions that most commonly cause a large pupil are third cranial nerve palsy and Adie tonic pupil. In third cranial nerve palsy, the large pupil has impaired reactions to light and to near; abnormalities of extraocular movement and eyelid position generally betray the origin of the abnormal pupil. With total third cranial nerve palsy there is complete ptosis; lifting the eyelid reveals the eye resting in a down and out position (Enrichment Box 7–2). To see a simulation of a complete third cranial nerve palsy, visit the Web site *cim.ucdavis.edu/eyes*.

SMALL PUPILS

The pupils in the elderly are normally smaller than are those in younger patients. Many older patients use pilocarpine eye drops to manage chronic open-angle glaucoma. Many systemic drugs with anticholinergic effects, such as opiates, may symmetrically shrink the pupils. Important neurologic conditions causing an abnormally small pupil include Horner syndrome and neurosyphilis. The Argyll-Robertson (AR) pupil, a classic finding in tertiary neurosyphilis, is small (1–2 mm) and irregular in outline, and it displays light–near dissociation (i.e., it accommodates but does not react). AR pupils are generally bilateral but asymmetric. Lyme disease may produce AR-like pupils.

In full-blown Horner syndrome, sympathetic dysfunction produces ptosis, miosis, and anhidrosis. The ptosis is much milder than with third cranial nerve palsy and easily missed. The small pupil dilates poorly in the dark, so that pupillary asymmetry that is greater in the dark than in the light generally means Horner syndrome. Recall that physiologic anisocoria produces about the same degree of pupillary

Although third cranial nerve palsies often affect the pupil more than they affect other functions, ptosis and ophthalmoparesis is usually present. Since the pupillary parasympathetics occupy a position on the periphery of the third cranial nerve as it exits the brainstem, compressive lesions such as aneurysms generally affect the pupil prominently. Ischemic lesions tend to affect the interior of the nerve and spare the pupil, as in diabetic third cranial nerve palsies. This rule is not absolute: pupil-sparing third cranial nerve palsies have been reported with aneurysms (in up to 1% of cases), as have diabetic palsies involving the pupil. Lesions in the cavernous sinus may involve both the third cranial nerve and the sympathetics, leaving the pupil midsize and unreactive (Figure 7–2).

The patient who presents with a tonic pupil is typically a young woman who suddenly notes a unilaterally enlarged pupil, with no other symptoms. The pupillary reaction to light may appear to be absent, whereas the reaction to near, although slow, is better preserved. Once constricted, the tonic pupil re-dilates very slowly when the patient looks back at distance, perhaps causing a transient reversal of the anisocoria. The pupilloconstrictor eventually develops denervation supersensitivity; the pupil may then constrict to solutions of pilocarpine that are too dilute to affect a normal eye.

The term "tectal pupils" refers to the large pupils with light–near dissociation that are sometimes seen when lesions affect the pretectum or upper midbrain. Such pupils may accompany the impaired upgaze and convergence–retraction nystagmus of Parinaud syndrome. Only severe, bilateral lesions of the retina or anterior visual pathways, enough to cause near blindness, affect the resting pupil size. Deliberately or accidentally instilled mydriatics produce a dilated, fixed pupil. Such pharmacological blockade can be distinguished by the failure to respond to full-strength pilocarpine, which promptly constricts a large pupil of any other cause. The variably dilated, fixed pupils that reflect midbrain dysfunction in a comatose patient carry a bleak prognosis. Glutethimide intoxication, infamous for causing fixed pupils in drug-induced coma, has fortunately become rare.

asymmetry in the light and dark. In contrast, third cranial nerve palsy and Adie pupil cause greater asymmetry in the light because of the involved pupil's inability to constrict. Examining the eyes under light and dark conditions can help greatly in sorting out asymmetric pupils (Table 7–1). The causes of Horner syndrome are legion: brainstem lesions (especially of the lateral medulla), cluster headache, internal carotid artery thrombosis or dissection, cavernous sinus disease, apical

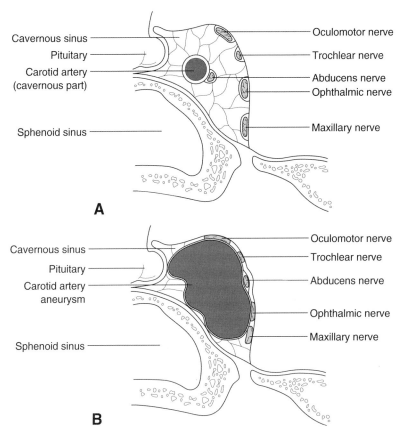

FIGURE 7–2. ■ (*A*) The cavernous sinus lies just lateral to the sella turcica. Within it lie the carotid artery and cranial nerves III, IV, and VI and branches of V. (*B*) Pathological findings involving the cavernous sinus are not rare and can usually be recognized by the pattern of cranial nerve involvement.

lung tumors, and other conditions. The tiny and minimally reactive pupils seen commonly in pontine hemorrhage may represent acute, severe, bilateral oculosympathetic paresis.

In Horner syndrome the lower lid is frequently elevated because of denervation of the muscles holding the lid down. Lower-lid elevation plus mild ptosis produces "apparent enophthalmos." Since the fibers mediating facial sweating travel up the external carotid, lesions distal to the carotid bifurcation produce no anhidrosis except for perhaps a small area of medial forehead. Pharmacological testing of the pupil is an important adjunct in the evaluation of Horner syndrome.

TABLE 7–1. BEHAVIOR OF UNEQUAL PUPILS IN LIGHT AND DARK CONDITIONS

Etiologic Factor	Ambient Light	Strong Light	Dark	Conclusion
Physiologic anisocoria	• ●	• •	● ●	Same relative asymmetry under all conditions
Right Horner syndrome	• ●	• •	• ●	More asymmetry in the dark; abnormal pupil can not dilate
Left third cranial nerve palsy	● •	● •	● ●	More asymmetry in the light; abnormal pupil cannot constrict

ABNORMALLY REACTIVE PUPILS

Disruption of the afferent or efferent limbs of the pupillary reflex arcs or disease of the brainstem pupil-control centers may alter pupil reactivity to light or near, as may local disease of the iris sphincter (e.g., old trauma). Disease of the retina does not affect pupil reactivity unless there is involvement severe enough to cause near blindness. Cataracts and other diseases of the anterior segment rarely impair light transmission enough to influence the pupil.

Because of the extensive side-to-side crossing of pupillary control axons through the posterior commissure, light constricts not only the stimulated pupil (the direct response) but also the pupil of the other eye (the consensual response). The eye with a severed optic nerve shows no direct response, but has a normal consensual response and constriction to attempted convergence; there is no anisocoria. The pupil frozen because of third cranial nerve palsy has no near response and no direct or consensual light response, but the other eye exhibits an intact consensual response on stimulation of the abnormal side.

Mild optic nerve dysfunction can often be detected with the swinging flashlight test. There is usually no detectable alteration in pupil reactivity to direct light stimulation, but alternately stimulating the two pupils by swinging a light back and forth between them can often detect a side-to-side difference. With stimulation of the good eye, both pupils constrict smartly; when the light is swung to the involved eye the brain detects a relative diminution in light intensity and dilates a bit in response. This paradoxical dilation of a light-stimulated pupil is an APD. It is an extremely useful and important neurologic sign.

The Eyelids

The normal upper eyelid in primary position crosses the iris between the limbus (junction of the cornea and sclera) and the pupil. With ptosis, the lid droops down and may cross at the upper margin of the pupil, or cover the pupil partially or totally. With complete ptosis, the eyelid is down and the eye appears closed. Patients with ptosis often display telltale wrinkling of the ipsilateral forehead as they attempt to hold the eye open by using the frontalis muscle. Ptosis may be unilateral or bilateral, partial or complete, and occurs in many neurologic conditions (Figure 7–3).

With eyelid retraction, the upper lid pulls back and frequently exposes a thin crescent of sclera between the upper limbus and the lid

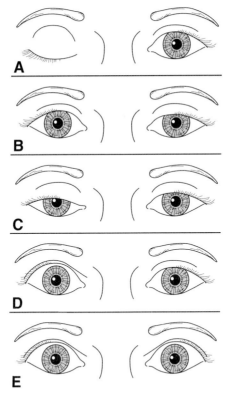

FIGURE 7–3. ■ Characteristics of different causes of abnormal lid position. (*A*) Right third cranial nerve palsy with complete ptosis. (*B*) Left Horner syndrome with drooping of upper lid and slight elevation of lower lid. (*C*) Bilateral, asymmetric ptosis in myasthenia gravis. (*D*) Right lid retraction in thyroid eye disease. (*E*) Bilateral lid retraction with a lesion in the region of the posterior commissure.

margin. Lid retraction is a classic sign of thyroid disease, but occurs in neurologic disorders as well.

The width of the palpebral fissures is normally equal on the two sides. Sometimes inequality results from subtle lid retraction on one side, not to be confused with ptosis on the other side. When in doubt, measure the width of the palpebral fissures with a ruler, in both primary position and in upgaze. In addition to observing the lid position at rest, notice the relationships of the lid to the globe during eye movement. The seventh cranial nerve, via contraction of the orbicularis oculi, closes the eye. Facial weakness never causes ptosis; in fact, the palpebral fissure on the weak side is often wider than normal, and unilateral widening of one palpebral fissure may be an early sign of facial palsy.

Mild to moderate unilateral ptosis occurs as part of Horner syndrome (see SMALL PUPILS), or with partial third cranial nerve palsy. In Horner syndrome, slight elevation of the lower lid may occur as well. Mild to moderate bilateral ptosis suggests a neuromuscular disorder, such as myasthenia gravis (MG), muscular dystrophy, or another myopathy. The ptosis in neuromuscular disease is frequently asymmetric and may be unilateral, although it tends to shift from side to side. The ptosis of MG characteristically fluctuates from moment to moment and is worsened by prolonged upgaze (fatigable ptosis). Cogan lidtwitch sign, characteristic of MG, consists of a brief overshoot twitch of lid retraction following sudden return of the eyes to primary position after a period of downgaze.

Ocular Motility

ORBITAL ANATOMY

The orbits lie in the skull divergently, making the anatomic axes of the eyes diverge slightly from the visual axes, which lie straight ahead for distance vision and convergently for near vision. In sleep and coma, the eyes rest in the divergent position of anatomic neutrality. In wakefulness, cerebral cortical activity that influences the extraocular muscles lines the eyes up for efficient vision. Phorias and tropias are manifestations of the latent or manifest tendency, respectively, of the eyes to drift away from the visual axis. For example, exotropia is an obvious outward ocular deviation (wall-eye); exophoria must be brought out by testing.

The medial and lateral recti adduct and abduct the eye. The medial rectus of one eye is "yoked" to the lateral rectus of the opposite eye to achieve conjugate lateral gaze. Yoked muscles are connected neurologically: they function as a team. The nervous system attempts to maintain visual fusion of images by controlling precisely the movements of the two eyes. Hering law, or the law of equal innervation, states that the same amount of innervation goes to an extraocular muscle and to its yoked partner.

The superior and inferior recti lie in the orbit and insert into the globe along the anatomic axis, exerting their maximally efficient pull when the eye is slightly abducted. The superior and inferior obliques insert into the globe at an angle of about 30° from medial to lateral; they exert maximal pull with the eye slightly adducted. The obliques insert posteriorly into the globe: the superior oblique pulls the back of the eye up, producing downgaze; the inferior oblique pulls the back of the eye down, producing upgaze. The superior oblique therefore works as a depressor of the adducted eye, and the inferior oblique works as an elevator. To achieve conjugate downgaze to one side, the superior oblique of the adducting eye is yoked to the inferior rectus of the abducting eye.

Because of the anatomic arrangement of the obliques and vertically acting recti, examination of extraocular movement should include gaze to the right and left, plus upgaze and downgaze in eccentric position to both sides: the six cardinal directions of gaze (Figure 7–4).

Chapter 2 discusses the anatomy of the visual system. See Enrichment Box 7–3 for further review of the anatomic details.

DISORDERED OCULAR MOTILITY

Patients may develop disordered ocular motility for a number of reasons. Acquired disorders typically produce diplopia. Causes are protean and include local disease in the orbit (e.g., blowout fracture), ocular myopathies [e.g., thyroid eye disease (TED)], impaired neuromuscular transmission (e.g., MG), palsies of individual cranial nerves alone or in combination (e.g., diabetic third cranial nerve palsy), and disease of the central oculomotor control pathways [e.g., internuclear ophthalmoplegia (INO) in MS]. Barely controlled phorias may decompensate and "break down," causing diplopia under conditions of fatigue, stress, or intoxication. A commonly heard but inaccurate clinical dictum is that monocular diplopia can only result from hysteria. Numerous organic lesions may produce monocular diplopia, including disease of the cornea, lens, media, macula, and central pathways.

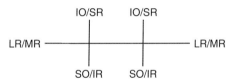

FIGURE 7–4. ■ The yoke muscles control extraocular movement in the six cardinal directions of gaze. *LR* = lateral rectus; *MR* = medial rectus; *IO* = inferior oblique; *SR* = superior rectus; *SO* = superior oblique; *IR* = inferior rectus.

ENRICHMENT BOX 7-3

Central visuomotor pathways

The frontal eye fields lie in area 8 of the frontal lobe, anterior to the motor strip, and control horizontal conjugate gaze to the opposite side. Fibers descend and decussate en route to the pontine lateral gaze center in the pontine paramedian reticular formation (PPRF; Figure 7–5). On activation, the pontine gaze center sends impulses to the adjacent sixth cranial nerve nucleus. The sixth cranial nerve nucleus sends a signal to the ipsilateral lateral rectus and simultaneously to the contralateral medial rectus subnucleus in the midbrain via the medial longitudinal fasciculus (MLF). A left frontal eye field–initiated command to look right is thus transmitted down to the right pontine lateral gaze center, which simultaneously influences the right sixth cranial nerve to contract the lateral rectus and the left third cranial nerve to contract the yoked medial rectus.

The supranuclear pathways subserving vertical gaze descend in the region of the rostral midbrain and pretectum. Upgaze and downgaze pathways occupy different positions, and abnormalities may affect one without the other.

There are four main eye movement control systems: saccadic, smooth pursuit, vergence, and vestibulo-ocular reflex. The frontal eye field to contralateral PPRF system controls saccadic eye movements, rapid small movements used to acquire a target. The smooth-pursuit system controls slower eye movements used to track a target once it is acquired. The vergence system controls the degree of convergence or divergence of the eyes, maintaining macular fixation no matter the distance to the target. The vestibular system has a large input into the oculomotor system to maintain proper eye orientation in relation to head and body position, thus maintaining the object of interest on the fovea despite head movements.

Diplopia is sometimes analyzed by using a red lens over one eye, by convention the right eye. "Labeling" the image from one eye with the red lens can help identify the faulty muscle. Good in theory, red lens testing is frequently less than satisfying in practice.

Peripheral Disorders Of Ocular Motility

Disturbances of ocular motility may result from processes involving the orbit that cause mechanical limitation of eye movement, or from ocular myopathies, neuromuscular transmission disorders, or a "palsy" of

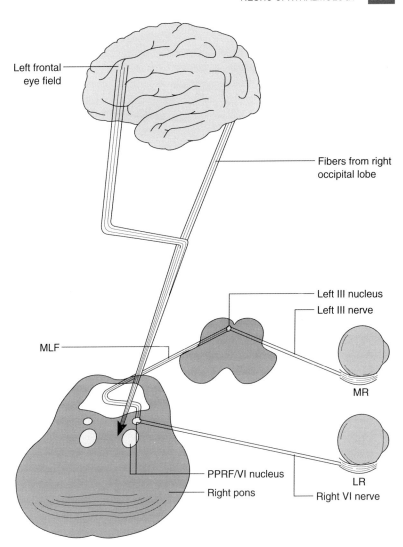

FIGURE 7–5. ■ The major suprasegmental oculomotor control pathways. The right pontine paramedian reticular formation (*PPRF*) receives input from the left frontal eye fields for saccadic movements and from the right occipital lobe for pursuit movements. The PPRF projects to the sixth cranial nerve (*VI*) nucleus, from which the sixth cranial nerve arises to control the right lateral rectus (*LR*). The sixth cranial nerve nucleus also gives rise to the medial longitudinal fasciculus (*MLF*), which decussates and ascends to the medial rectus subnucleus of the left third cranial nerve (*III*) nucleus, from which the third cranial nerve arises to control the left medial rectus (*MR*).

an individual nerve controlling extraocular movements. Forced ductions are used to detect mechanical limitations of eye movement (Enrichment Box 7–4).

Orbital disease Masses within the orbit may restrict normal movement of the globe, often causing telltale proptosis as well. Following trauma to the orbit, individual extraocular muscles may become entrapped by fracture fragments—the most classic example is entrapment of the inferior rectus by an orbital blowout fracture, producing a mechanical limitation of upgaze and vertical diplopia. Other examples of orbital disease include orbital pseudotumor, lymphoma, and rhabdomyosarcoma.

Muscle disease. Primary ocular muscle disease may cause impaired motility because of weakness or because of restriction of movement. Several myopathies and muscular dystrophies may affect eye muscles; chronic progressive external ophthalmoplegia associated with ragged red fibers on muscle biopsy is a typical example. TED is a common cause of ocular muscle dysfunction (see Enrichment Box 7–4).

Neuromuscular transmission disorders. MG, the most common neuromuscular transmission disorder, frequently involves the extraocular muscles, affecting any muscle or combination of muscles. Myasthenia causes fatigable weakness, which may develop with sustained eccentric gaze even when not present initially. Fluctuating ptosis and diplopia, and worsening symptoms toward the end of the day, are characteristic.

Individual nerve palsies. The same basic processes cause third, fourth, and sixth cranial nerve palsies, but with different frequencies. As many as 25% of cases are idiopathic, and of these 50% recover spontaneously. See Enrichment Box 7–4 for further details.

Oculomotor nerve palsy produces varying degrees and combinations of extraocular muscle weakness, ptosis, and pupil involvement. Third cranial nerve palsy is frequently an ominous sign, especially in the setting of alteration of consciousness. Uncal herniation from mass effect of any sort may result in compression as the temporal tip crowds through the tentorial hiatus and traps the third cranial nerve against the sharp edge of the tentorium. Posterior communicating or distal internal carotid aneurysms commonly cause third cranial nerve palsy (Figure 7–6).

Sixth cranial nerve palsies are common, and many resolve with no explanation. Elevated intracranial pressure often produces sixth cranial nerve palsies because of stretch of the nerve over the petrous ridge as

Forced ductions

Mechanically limited eye excursions exist for passive as well as active movements. Forced ductions involve pushing or pulling on the anesthetized globe to passively move it through the impaired range. An eye affected by ocular muscle weakness, myasthenia gravis (MG) or a sixth cranial nerve palsy, moves freely and easily throughout a full range. An eye affected by restrictive myopathy or an entrapped muscle cannot be moved passively any better than it can be moved actively.

Thyroid eye disease (TED)

TED commonly causes deposition of mucopolysaccharide in eye muscles, making them stiff and unable to relax during contraction of the antagonist. This sort of restrictive myopathy is easily confused with weakness of the antagonist (e.g., restrictive myopathy of the medial rectus simulating weakness of the lateral rectus). Forced ductions may rapidly clarify matters. The inferior rectus is frequently involved with TED, producing impaired upgaze on the affected side. TED bears no consistent relationship to thyroid gland activity, and may exist without the obvious accompaniments of proptosis, lid retraction, and chemosis, making the diagnosis difficult. The possibility of TED must be constantly borne in mind when dealing with ocular motility disturbances.

Individual nerve palsies

With third cranial nerve palsy, processes affecting the nucleus or fascicles within the brainstem generally produce accompanying neighborhood signs permitting localization (e.g., Weber or Benedikt syndrome). In its long course along the base of the brain, cranial nerve III may be affected in isolation. In the cavernous sinus or orbit, accompanying deficits that are related to involvement of other structures usually permit localization.

Patients with fourth cranial nerve palsies may not complain of diplopia, but rather of blurry vision or a vague problem when looking down, as when reading a book or descending stairs. They may tilt the head to the opposite side to eliminate diplopia, tucking the chin so the affected eye may ride up and into extorsion, out of the field of action of the weak superior oblique. Some fourth cranial nerve palsies, particularly in children, present with head tilt rather than diplopia. The Bielschowsky maneuver consists of tilting the head to each side, localizing the fourth cranial nerve palsy by the changes in diplopia that result. If diplopia improves with head tilt to the left and worsens with tilt to the right, the patient has a right fourth cranial nerve palsy.

Trauma is the most common cause of fourth cranial nerve palsies and the second most common cause of third cranial nerve palsies and sixth

(Continued)

cranial nerve palsies. Microangiopathic vascular disease due to diabetes or hypertension is the most common cause of third cranial nerve and sixth cranial nerve palsies. Aneurysms are an important cause of third cranial nerve palsies. Increased intracranial pressure may cause third cranial nerve palsies because of uncal herniation and sixth cranial nerve palsies as a nonspecific and nonlocalizing effect. Neoplasms may affect any of these nerves. A third cranial nerve palsy developing after trivial head trauma suggests the possibility of subclinical stretch due to an underlying mass. Basilar meningitis, migraine, viral infection, immunizations, cavernous sinus disease, sarcoid, vasculitis, and Guillain-Barré syndrome are rare causes.

the increased pressure forces the brainstem attachments inferiorly, a classic false localizing sign. Neighborhood signs (clinical findings indicative of dysfunction of nearby structures) usually permit localization when the nerve is involved in the brainstem, cavernous sinus, or orbit.

Since cranial nerve IV exits dorsally and arches around the edge of the tentorium before running forward, it has the longest course of any cranial nerve. It is also the most slender. These two factors likely explain its vulnerability to injury. The most common cause of fourth cranial nerve palsies is head trauma. Nontraumatic cases are usually idiopathic or congenital.

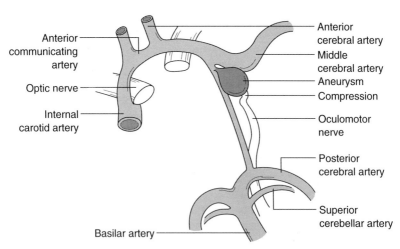

FIGURE 7–6. ■ Anatomy of the oculomotor nerve in relation to the major arteries at the base of the brain. An aneurysm arising from the posterior communicating artery is compressing and distorting the nerve.

Central Disorders Of Ocular Motility

Gaze palsies and gaze deviations. The frontal eye fields move the eyes into contralateral conjugate horizontal gaze. The eyes normally remain straight ahead because of a balance of input from the frontal eye fields in each hemisphere. Seizure activity in one frontal lobe drives the eyes contralaterally. In an adversive seizure, the eyes, and then the head, deviate to one side, after which the seizure may generalize. Sustained eye deviation can be a manifestation— rarely the only manifestation—of status epilepticus.

With destructive frontal lobe lesions, most often caused by stroke, the patient is unable to move the eyes contralaterally, termed "gaze palsy," or, if less severe, "gaze paresis." The intact, normal hemisphere maintains its tonic input, and the imbalance causes the eyes to move contralaterally toward the diseased side, termed "gaze deviation." Patients may have gaze palsy without gaze deviation. The presence of gaze deviation usually means gaze palsy to the opposite side, but may occasionally signal seizure activity (see preceding paragraph).

Similar considerations apply to disease of the pons. The pontine paramedian reticular formation (PPRF) governs ipsilateral, conjugate horizontal gaze. The PPRF "pulls" the eyes ipsilaterally, in contrast to the frontal eye fields, which "push" the eyes contralaterally. Destructive lesions of the PPRF impair the ability to gaze ipsilaterally, resulting in a gaze deviation toward the intact side as the normal PPRF pulls the eyes over. Fortunately, seizures do not affect the PPRF.

When faced with a patient whose eyes rest eccentrically to one side, the diagnostic possibilities are (1) frontal lobe seizure activity, (2) frontal lobe destructive lesion, and (3) pontine destructive lesion.

Patients with destructive frontal lesions gaze away from the side of the hemiparesis (e.g., right-hemisphere stroke causes left hemiparesis with left-gaze palsy and a compensatory right-gaze deviation away from the hemiparetic side). Patients with pontine strokes gaze toward the hemiparesis (e.g., right-pontine stroke causes left hemiparesis and right-gaze palsy and a compensatory left-gaze deviation toward the hemiparetic side).

Frontal-lobe gaze deviations are generally large amplitude, pronounced, and clinically obvious, whereas pontine gaze deviations tend to be subtle and easily missed. Frontal gaze deviations tend to resolve in a few days, but pontine deviations persist much longer, sometimes permanently. Epileptogenic gaze deviations are usually betrayed by a component of jerky eye movement and subtle twitches elsewhere, and are definitively demonstrated by electroencephalography.

Internuclear ophthalmoplegia. The medial longitudinal fasciculus (MLF) is an extensive and prominent brainstem pathway. One of its primary functions is to connect the sixth cranial nerve nucleus on one side with the third cranial nerve nucleus on the opposite side to maintain conjugacy of horizontal gaze. Signals from the sixth cranial nerve nucleus travel via the MLF, which crosses soon after beginning its ascent to the contralateral third cranial nerve complex. Lesions of the MLF disrupt communication between the two nuclei: hence the appellation INO.

Lesions of the MLF deprive the contralateral medial rectus of the command to contract when the PPRF and sixth cranial nerve nucleus act to gaze laterally. As a result, gaze to one side results in abduction of the ipsilateral eye, but no adduction of the contralateral eye. Typically, the abducting eye has nystagmus as well. Failure of the medial rectus to adduct is an isolated abnormality in the affected eye; normality of the lid, pupil, and vertical eye movements distinguish an INO from a third cranial nerve palsy. The earliest detectable sign of an INO may be slowness of adducting saccades compared with abducting saccades, as demonstrated by rapid refixation or an optokinetic nystagmus (OKN) tape. By convention, the INO is labeled by the side of the adduction failure; a right INO produces adduction failure of the right eye.

Many brainstem lesions can cause an INO, but the common conditions are MS and brainstem stroke. INOs due to MS are usually bilateral and seen in young patients, whereas those due to brainstem vascular disease are more often unilateral and seen in older patients. Beware of "pseudoINOs," caused by MG, Wernicke encephalopathy, TED, or partial third cranial nerve palsy.

Vertical Gaze Abnormalities

The pathways controlling up and down gaze course in the region of the rostral midbrain, pretectum, and posterior commissure. The rostral interstitial nucleus of the MLF acts more or less as the vertical gaze analogue of the PPRF. Two common disorders affecting vertical gaze are Parinaud syndrome and progressive supranuclear palsy (Enrichment Box 7–5).

Nystagmus and Other Ocular Oscillations

Nystagmus refers to rhythmic ocular oscillations. It is a complex topic. A whole host of conditions can cause nystagmus: ocular disease, drug effects, peripheral vestibular disease, and central nervous system (CNS) disease. Nystagmus may also be congenital. A few beats of nystagmus at the extremes of lateral gaze occur commonly in normal individuals and have no pathological significance.

The core feature of Parinaud syndrome is impaired upgaze. When patients attempt to look up, the eyes may spasmodically converge and retract backward into the orbits (convergence-retraction nystagmus). The convergence-retraction movements often readily appear during forced upward saccades in response to a down-moving optokinetic nystagmus (OKN) tape. Parinaud syndrome usually results from a mass lesion involving the region of the posterior third ventricle, such as a pinealoma. Sometimes, upgaze paresis is severe enough that the eyes are forced into sustained downgaze—a "setting sun sign"—seen in children with obstructive hydrocephalus ballooning of the posterior third ventricle and rostral aqueduct and in adults with thalamic hemorrhage.

In progressive supranuclear palsy, degenerative changes in the rostral brainstem and thalamus result in impairment first of downgaze, then of upgaze, and eventually in global gaze paresis. The gaze abnormalities are accompanied by Parkinsonian signs and a pronounced tendency to extensor axial rigidity.

When faced with a patient with nystagmus or similar movements, the usual clinical exercises are twofold: deciding if the nystagmus indicates neurologic pathology, and, if so, whether the pathology is central or peripheral. This discussion focuses on the types of nystagmus commonly encountered in neurologic practice and on the differentiation between nystagmus that likely signifies neurologic disease (neuropathological) and that which does not (nonneuropathological). Nystagmus is classified in multiple ways: pendular (both phases of equal amplitude and velocity) versus jerk (a fast phase and a slow phase); central versus peripheral; induced versus spontaneous; physiologic versus pathological; and localizing versus nonlocalizing. Further characterizations include rapid–slow, coarse–fine, manifest–latent, sensory–motor, and horizontal–vertical. By definition, nystagmus direction is the direction of the fast phase. Nystagmus severity may be divided into first, second, and third degree (Enrichment Box 7–6). Since pendular nystagmus rarely signifies neurologic disease, the following discussion is limited to jerk nystagmus. Table 7–2 summarizes important but infrequently encountered types of nystagmus and related movements.

NYSTAGMUS
End-Point Nystagmus
Many patients have fine, variably sustained nystagmus at the extremes of lateral gaze, especially with gaze eccentric enough to eliminate fixation by the adducting eye. In some normal patients, this physiologic

---

First-degree nystagmus is present only with eccentric gaze, (e.g., right-beating nystagmus on right gaze). Second-degree nystagmus is present in primary gaze and increases in intensity with gaze in the direction of the fast component (e.g., right-beating nystagmus in primary gaze increasing with gaze to the right). With third-degree nystagmus, the fast component continues to beat even with gaze in the direction of the slow component (e.g., right-beating nystagmus persisting even with gaze to the left).

---

end-point nystagmus appears with as little as 30° of deviation from primary position, often with greater amplitude in the abducting eye. Symmetry on right and left gaze, abolition by moving the eyes a few degrees toward primary position, and the absence of other neurologic abnormalities generally serve to distinguish end-point from pathological nystagmus. End-point nystagmus is the most common form seen in routine clinical practice.

Drug-Induced Nystagmus

Alcohol, sedative hypnotics, anticonvulsants, and other drugs commonly produce nystagmus. Such drug-induced nystagmus is typically symmetric and gaze evoked horizontally and vertically, especially in upgaze. Nystagmus that is more prominent than the few unsustained end-point jerks that are commonly seen usually proves to be a drug effect.

Optokinetic Nystagmus

OKN is a normal phenomenon sometimes affected by disease. OKN occurs whenever the eyes must follow a series of rapidly passing objects, such as telephone poles zipping by a car or train window. Clinical testing usually entails moving a striped tape in front of the patient and requesting him to "count" the stripes. In normal, alert individuals, an OKN tape induces brisk nystagmus with the fast phase in the direction opposite tape movement. The OKN tape can be a handy and useful bedside tool (Enrichment Box 7–7). It may localize hemianopias. It may crudely check visual acuity because the response is difficult to voluntarily suppress. It may provide a clue to the presence of psychogenic visual loss. The slowed adducting saccades of a subtle INO may be best appreciated by OKN testing. OKN forced upward sac-

TABLE 7–2. NYSTAGMUS AND SIMILAR MOVEMENTS

Nystagmus Type	Characteristics	Location of Pathological Condition	Possible Disease or Condition
Upbeat	Upbeating nystagmus in primary gaze	Cerebellar vermis (if nystagmus increases), or medulla (if it decreases) in upgaze	Cerebellar or medullary lesion, meningitis, Wernicke encephalopathy, rarely drug intoxication
Downbeat	Downbeating nystagmus in primary gaze, maximum in eccentric downgaze (downbeat in the corners)	Cervico-medullary junction	Arnold-Chiari malformation, basilar invagination, MS, foramen magnum tumor, spinocerebellar degeneration, rarely drug intoxication, Wernicke encephalopathy, vascular disease
Convergence–retraction	Convergence motions and simultaneous retraction of globes back into the orbits	Rostral midbrain, pretectum, posterior commissure, posterior third ventricle	Mass lesions, especially pinealoma; vascular disease; up herniation
Rebound	Horizontal nystagmus that briefly beats in opposite direction on return to primary position	Cerebellum or cerebellar connections	MS, chronic cerebellar disease
Ocular bobbing	Downward jerk with slow drift back to primary position	Pons (lesion usually massive and patient comatose)	Pontine hemorrhage or infarction
Ocular flutter	Rapid back-to-back saccades causing a quivering or shimmering movement	Cerebellum or brainstem cerebellar pathways, ? dentate nucleus	Same as for opsoclonus; flutter and opsoclonus are a continuum
Opsoclonus	Continuous, involuntary, random, chaotic saccades (dancing eyes, lightning eye movements)	Cerebellum or brainstem cerebellar pathways, ? dentate nucleus	In children, occult neuroblastoma (dancing eyes–dancing feet/opsoclonus–myoclonus); in adults, occult lung

(continued)

TABLE 7–2. NYSTAGMUS AND SIMILAR MOVEMENTS (CONTINUED)			
Nystagmus Type	Characteristics	Location of Pathological Condition	Possible Disease or Condition
			or breast carcinoma; encephalitis
Ocular dysmetria	Overshoot or undershoot on rapid refixation, requiring corrective saccades	Cerebellum or brainstem cerebellar pathways, ? dentate nucleus	MS

MS = multiple sclerosis.

cades may induce convergence retraction nystagmus in patients with Parinaud syndrome.

Congenital Nystagmus

A patient with a clear history of nystagmus present since infancy presents no neurologic diagnostic problem. However, occasionally patients with congenital nystagmus are unaware of its presence; when they appear later in life with neurologic complaints, sorting out the significance of the nystagmus may prove difficult (see Enrichment Box 7–7).

Neuropathological Nystagmus

Vestibular nystagmus. The vestibular system connects to the PPRF and the sixth cranial nerve nucleus in such a way that vestibular stimulation pushes the eyes conjugately contralaterally. Symmetric, equal activity of the vestibular systems on each side normally maintains the eyes in a straight-ahead, primary position. Vestibular imbalance causes the eyes to deviate toward the less active side as the "push" from the normal side overcomes the weakened "push" from the abnormal side. In an alert patient, the frontal eye fields saccade the eyes back toward primary position, creating the fast phase of vestibular nystagmus.

Ice-water irrigation of one ear inhibits vestibular function, and the normal unopposed vestibule then pushes the eyes toward the irrigated side. The cortical correcting saccade jerks in the opposite direction, yielding the well-known mnemonic "COWS" (cold opposite–warm same) to describe the fast phase of vestibular nystagmus. When the cor-

ENRICHMENT BOX 7–7

Optokinetic nystagmus (OKN)

The smooth-pursuit eye-movement system originates in the ipsilateral occipital lobe, projects corticocortical fibers to the ipsilateral frontal lobe, and descends in the internal sagittal stratum adjacent to the atrium of the lateral ventricle down to the ipsilateral pontine paramedian reticular formation (PPRF). Smooth pursuit to the right is controlled by the right occipital lobe in concert with the right PPRF. Quick refixation saccades back to the left are mediated by the right frontal eye fields, so the process of following a series of moving objects (as in OKN, or railroad nystagmus) is all accomplished in the same cerebral hemisphere. When testing for OKNs, the ipsilateral occipital lobe mediates pursuit of the acquired stripe. When ready to break off, the occipital visuomotor centers communicate with the ipsilateral frontal lobe, which then generates a saccadic movement in the opposite direction to acquire the next target.

Patients with hemianopsias due to occipital lobe disease have a normal OKN response, despite their inability to see into the hemifield from which the tape originates. Because of interruption of the OKN pathways in the internal sagittal stratum, patients with hemianopsias due to disease of the optic radiations in the parietal lobe have abnormally blunted or absent OKN responses. The pursuit function may work, but the frontal lobe never receives the message to generate a saccade into the blind hemifield. The OKN tape may draw the eyes over into full lateral gaze toward the side of the lesion with no contra-motion saccades.

The significance of OKN asymmetry lies in the vascular anatomy and the differing pathological conditions that affect the parietal and occipital lobes. Tumors are rare in the occipital lobe; they are much more common in the parietal lobe. Furthermore, the OKN pathways in the deep parietal lobe are outside the distribution of the posterior cerebral artery. Therefore, a patient with a hemianopsia and normal OKN responses is more likely to have an occipital lesion, and more likely to have had a stroke. With asymmetric OKNs, the lesion is more likely to reside in the parietal lobe, and more likely to be nonvascular, that is, a tumor (Cogan rule).

Congenital nystagmus

In distinguishing congenital from other types of nystagmus, the following features are helpful. Congenital nystagmus is most often horizontal jerk, and remains horizontal even in upgaze and downgaze; that is, it is not gaze evoked. This pattern is unusual in other forms of nystagmus. Patients often have a null point of least nystagmus intensity and best vision in slightly eccentric gaze. They may adopt a head turn or tilt to maintain gaze in this null zone. The nystagmus typically damps tex does not generate a correcting saccade, as in coma, only the tonic deviation develops; the eyes deviate toward the ice-water-irrigated ear.

Because of the influence of the three different semicircular canals, vestibular nystagmus may beat in more than one direction, the summation of which creates an admixed rotatory component rarely seen with other conditions. Vestibular nystagmus typically is fine, often present but easily overlooked in primary position. Third-degree nystagmus (fast component opposite to the direction of gaze; see Enrichment Box 7–6) rarely occurs with any other nystagmus type. Deafness and tinnitus also help mark nystagmus as peripheral.

Positional nystagmus. Degenerative changes in the otoliths frequently produce the syndrome of positional vertigo and nystagmus (see Chapter 12). In benign positional vertigo, nystagmus occurs after a latency of up to 30 seconds, beats with the fast phase toward the down ear, quickly fatigues despite holding the position, and adapts with repeated attempts to elicit it. Positional vertigo is a common condition. Although generally peripheral, it may occur with central disease (tumor, stroke, MS, degenerative disease) [see CENTRAL VERSUS PERIPHERAL NYSTAGMUS].

Gaze-evoked nystagmus. Any nystagmus not present in primary gaze but appearing with gaze in any direction with the fast phase in the direction of gaze is referred to as gaze-evoked nystagmus. Normal physiologic endpoint nystagmus is gaze evoked, but only present horizontally. Drug-induced nystagmus is gaze evoked, usually horizontally and in upgaze. Nystagmus with the same appearance in the absence of drug effects is nonspecific but usually indicates disease of the cerebellum or cerebellar connections.

Gaze-paretic nystagmus. Patients with incomplete gaze palsies or recovering complete palsies may, rather than having an absolute inability to gaze in a particular direction, achieve full lateral gaze transiently but not be able to maintain it. The eyes drift back toward neutral, then spasmodically jerk back in the desired gaze direction, producing gaze-paretic nystagmus.

CENTRAL VERSUS PERIPHERAL NYSTAGMUS

Distinguishing central nystagmus, due to CNS disease, from peripheral nystagmus, due to peripheral vestibular disease, is a common clinical problem. The most helpful features are the presence of aural symptoms and signs in peripheral nystagmus and the presence of CNS symptoms and signs in central nystagmus (Enrichment Box 7–8).

The Afferent Visual System

ANATOMY

The anatomy of the afferent visual system is summarized in Chapter 2. Enrichment Box 7–9 contains further details of clinical utility.

EVALUATION OF VISION

Clinically important parameters of visual function include acuity, color perception, subjective assessment of the brightness of an examining light, and pupillary reactivity. For neurologic purposes, only the pa-

---

ENRICHMENT BOX 7–8

Disease of the peripheral vestibular apparatus, or eighth cranial nerve, produces peripheral nystagmus. Disease of the central vestibular connections produces central nystagmus. The vestibular nuclei lie within the central nervous system (CNS) in the dorsolateral medulla; disease there may appear like either peripheral or central forms of nystagmus.

The vestibular apparatus pushes not only the eyes, but also the limbs and the body to the opposite side. Patients with peripheral nystagmus therefore display past pointing, deviation on walking with eyes closed, or falling, all in the direction of the slow phase. Failure to follow these rules, for example, past pointing in the direction of the fast phase, suggests a central lesion. Peripheral nystagmus is often positional. When it is, vertigo and vegetative symptoms in proportion to the nystagmus, latency to onset, fatigability, and adaptability all support a peripheral process (see positional nystagmus). Minimal vertigo with prominent nystagmus, or lack of latency, fatigability, and adaptability suggest a central process.

Peripheral nystagmus often has a rotary component, and the horizontal nystagmus beats in the same direction in all fields of gaze (it may even be third degree). Central nystagmus may change directions. Visual fixation inhibits peripheral nystagmus, but has no effect on central nystagmus.

The optic nerves are formed by the axons of retinal ganglion cells, which constitute the retinal nerve fiber layer as they stream toward the disc to exit through the lamina cribrosa. The macula lutea, the area of central fixation and most acute vision, consists entirely of cones. Axons from the macula form the dense papillomacular bundle, and enter the temporal aspect of the disc. Fibers from the temporal hemiretina arch around the macula and enter the disc as the superior and inferior retinal arcades (see Figure 7–1). The papillomacular bundle forms the bulk of the axons in the optic nerve, and runs as a compact bundle in the center of the optic nerve. The macula, not the disc, forms the center of the retina, and the macular fixation point, the fovea, is the center of the clinical visual field. Myelin in the optic nerve is central nervous system (CNS) myelin, formed by oligodendroglia.

After traversing the orbit and optic canal, the optic nerves join to form the chiasm. Fibers from the temporal retina continue directly back to enter the ipsilateral optic tract. Fibers from the nasal retina decussate to enter the opposite optic tract (Figure 7–7). In the process of decussating, fibers from the inferior nasal quadrant actually loop forward into the opposite optic nerve, forming von Willebrand knee, an important anatomic detail that helps the physician to understand the formation of a "junctional scotoma" (Figure 7–8).

The optic tracts extend from the chiasm to the lateral geniculate body. Pupillary afferents leave the tract just anterior to the geniculate to enter the pretectum (see pupils). The visual afferents synapse in the geniculate on second-order neurons that give rise to the geniculocalcarine pathway (optic radiations) [see Figure 7–7].

Leaving the lateral geniculate, the optic radiations pass through the retrolenticular portion of the internal capsule, then fan out. Inferior retinal fibers run forward in the temporal lobe to within 5–7 cm of the temporal tip, and then curve back, forming Meyer loop. Fibers from the superior retina run directly back in the deep parietal lobe in the external sagittal stratum. Approaching the occipital lobe, fibers from the upper and lower retina again converge. This divergence and convergence of fibers influences the congruity of visual field defects, which has localizing value.

The primary visual cortex, or calcarine area, lies in Brodmann area 17. The immediately adjacent areas 18 and 19 are visual association cortex and also the locus of the smooth-pursuit eye-movement centers.

The cavernous sinuses and carotid siphons lie just lateral to the chiasm on either side (see Figure 7–2). The circle of Willis lies above, sending numerous small perforators to supply the chiasm. The ophthalmic artery, the carotid's first intracranial branch, runs alongside

(Continued)

the optic nerve through the canal and orbit, and then gives off the central retinal artery, which pierces the nerve and runs forward onto the disc. The central retinal artery divides at the disc head into superior and inferior branches that supply the retina. Terminal branches of the ophthalmic artery, the posterior ciliary arteries, supply the disc with the central retinal artery, making only a minimal contribution.

The anterior choroidal artery off the terminal internal carotid and thalamoperforators off the posterior cerebral supply the optic tract. The geniculate is perfused by the anterior choroidal and thalamogeniculate branches from the posterior cerebral. Perhaps because of this redundant blood supply, vascular disease only rarely affects the optic tract or lateral geniculate. Meyer loop receives blood supply primarily from the inferior division of the middle cerebral artery, whereas the optic radiations in the parietal lobe are perfused via the superior division. The occipital lobe is supplied primarily by the posterior cerebral artery. Collaterals from the anterior and middle cerebral arteries may provide additional perfusion to the macular areas at the occipital tip. The parietal smooth-pursuit optomotor center and its projections are supplied by the middle cerebral artery.

Retinotopic anatomy

The organization of the visual afferent system is anything but random. Tight retinotopic correlation prevails throughout the system; each point on the retina has a specific representation in the optic nerve, the chiasm, the tract, the radiations, and the cortex. Upper retinal fibers remain upper in the optic nerve and chiasm. The decussations of upper and lower nasal fibers differ slightly, as detailed earlier. In the optic tract, the upper retinal fibers rotate to a medial position and the lower retinal fibers rotate to a lateral position. In the six-layered lateral geniculate, fibers from the ipsilateral temporal retina synapse in layers 2, 3, and 5, while fibers from the contralateral nasal retina synapse in layers 1, 4, and 6; upper retinal fibers remain medial and lower fibers remain lateral.

Leaving the geniculate, inferior retinal fibers arch anteriorly into the temporal lobe while superior fibers run in the deep parietal lobe. Thus, upper (retina) is upper and lower (retina) is lower in the radiations. In the calcarine cortex, upper retinal fibers end on the superior bank and lower fibers end on the inferior bank. The most peripheral parts of the retina are represented most anteriorly in the calcarine cortex; the closer a retinal point lies to the macula, the more posterior is its calcarine representation, culminating in the representation of the macula at the most posterior portion of the occipital pole. The nasal hemiretina extends farther forward than does the temporal (the temporal visual

(Continued)

field is more extensive than the nasal), creating a portion of retina for which no homology exits in the opposite eye. This unpaired nasal retina is represented in the most anterior portion of the calcarine cortex, near the area of the tentorium, creating an "isolated temporal crescent" in each visual field. Sparing or selective involvement of this isolated temporal crescent has localizing value.

tient's best, corrected visual acuity is pertinent. Refractive errors, media opacities, and similar optometric problems are irrelevant, and acuity is always measured by using the patient's accustomed correction. In the absence of correction, improvement of vision by looking through a pinhole (a small hole in an index card suffices) suggests impairment related to a refractive error. Neurologists generally assess vision with a "near" card. Though examination of distance vision is preferable, the requisite devices are generally not at hand. Vision worse than the measurable 20/800 is described as "counts fingers," "hand motion," "light perception only," or "no light perception."

Color plates formally and quantitatively assess color vision. Having the patient identify the colors in a fabric, such as a tie or dress, can provide a crude estimate. Color desaturation, or "red washout," describes a graying down or loss of intensity of red. The bright red cap on a bottle of mydriatic drops is a common test object. The patient compares

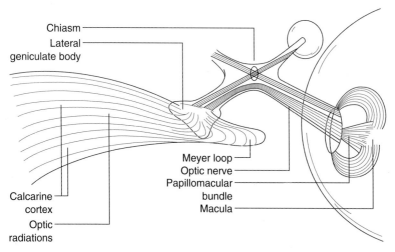

FIGURE 7-7. ■ Anatomy of the afferent visual system.

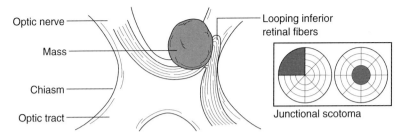

Optic nerve

Mass

Chiasm

Optic tract

Looping inferior retinal fibers

Junctional scotoma

FIGURE 7–8. ■ A mass impinges on the optic nerve at its junction with the chiasm, producing a junctional scotoma.

the brightness or redness in right versus left hemifields, temporal versus nasal hemifields, or central versus peripheral fields. No right–left or temporal–nasal desaturation to red occurs normally. Red does normally look brighter in the center of the visual field than it does off center; reversal of this pattern suggests impairment of central vision.

Patients may compare the brightness or intensity of an examining light in one eye versus the other. A diminution of brightness on one side suggests optic nerve dysfunction, and is sometimes referred to as a "subjective" Marcus-Gunn pupil or APD.

Clinicians use many different methods for visual field evaluation, depending on the circumstances. The time and energy expended on bedside, confrontation testing depends on the history and on the facilities available for formal field testing with tangent screen (central 30°) or perimetry (entire field). Even sophisticated confrontation testing cannot approach the accuracy of formal fields. For the patient with nothing in the history to suggest a visual system problem, or the possibility of a problem, a screening examination usually suffices. A screening visual field examination method is described in Chapter 5. This technique of small finger movements in the far periphery in both upper and lower quadrants is an excellent screen; when properly done, even binocularly, this method misses few hemianopias.

If there is any hint of abnormality, or if the patient has or could be expected to have a visual system problem, higher-level testing is in order. When examining the patient monocularly, techniques include having her assess the brightness and clarity of the examiner's hands as they are held in the right and left hemifields, in both upper and lower quadrants, or having her count fingers that are fleetingly presented in various parts of the field.

More exacting techniques compare the patient's field dimensions with those of the examiner by using various targets: fingers, the head of a cotton swab, pinheads, or similar objects. If the patient and examiner position themselves at the same eye level and gaze eyeball to eyeball over an 18- to 24-inch span, targets introduced midway between them should appear to both simultaneously in all parts of the field except temporally, where the examiner must simply develop a feel for the extent of a normal field.

For obtunded or uncooperative patients, paper money (the larger the denomination the better) makes a compelling target. Even if you have only a $1 bill, suggest to the patient that it might be $100-those who can will glance to see. Checking for a blink response to a threatening visual stimulus (e.g., an oncoming finger) provides a crude, last-resort method; movements should be slow and deliberate to avoid stimulating the cornea with an induced air current. Testing central fields can include having the patient gaze at the examiner's face and report any defects in visual perception, such as a missing or blurred nose. Having the patient survey a grid (Amsler grid, graph paper, or a quickly sketched home-made version) while fixing on a central point is a sensitive method to detect scotomas. Probing the central field with a small white or red object may detect moderate or large scotomas. With a cooperative patient, the physician can estimate the size of the blind spot.

By convention, visual fields are depicted as seen by the patient, that is, right eye drawn on the right. Violations of this rule occur sufficiently often that labeling notations are prudent.

ABNORMALITIES OF VISUAL FUNCTION
Visual Field Abnormalities

For neurologic purposes, visual field abnormalities can be divided into scotomas, hemianopias, altitudinal defects, and concentric constriction of the fields. Figure 7–9 depicts examples of different types of field defects.

A scotoma is an area of impaired vision in the field, with normal surrounding vision. With an absolute scotoma, there is no visual function within the scotoma to testing with all sizes and colors of objects. With a relative scotoma, visual function is depressed but not absent; smaller objects and colored objects are more likely to detect the abnormality. A central scotoma involves the fixation point and is seen in macular or optic nerve disease (it is typical for optic neuritis and can occur in vascular and compressive lesions). See Enrichment Box 7–10 for a discussion of other types of scotomas.

Hemianopia is impaired vision in half the visual field of each eye; hemianopic defects do not cross the vertical meridian. Hemianopias may be homonymous or heteronymous. A homonymous hemianopia causes impaired vision in corresponding halves of each eye; for example, a right homonymous hemianopia is a defect in the right half of

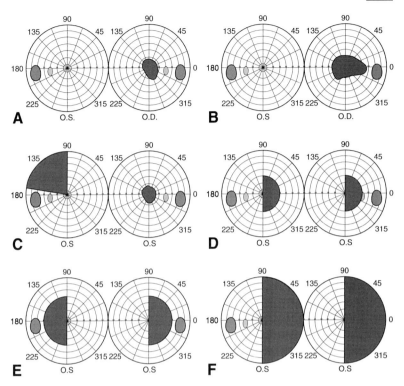

FIGURE 7–9. ■ Types of visual field defects. (*A*) Central scotoma. (*B*) Cecocentral scotoma. (*C*) Junctional scotoma. (*D*) Homonymous scotomas. (*E*) Heteronymous scotomas. (*F*) Right homonymous hemianopia. (*continued*)

each eye. A heteronymous hemianopia is impaired vision in opposite halves of each eye, the right half in one eye and the left half in the other.

A homonymous hemianopia may be complete or incomplete. If it is incomplete, it may be congruous or incongruous. With a complete hemianopia, congruity cannot be assessed; the only localization possible is to identify the lesion as contralateral and retrochiasmal. In congruous hemianopia, the patient has similarly shaped defects in each eye: the more congruous the field defect, the more posterior (closer to the occipital lobe) the lesion is likely to be. A patient with an incongruous hemianopia has differently shaped defects in the two eyes: the more incongruous the defect, the more anterior the lesion is. The most incongruous hemianopias occur with optic tract lesions. A superior quadrantopia implies a lesion in the temporal lobe that affects the Meyer loop (inferior retinal fibers); this type of lesion is termed "pie in the sky." An inferior quadrantopia implies a parietal

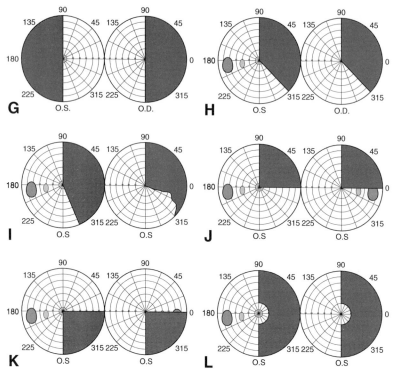

FIGURE 7–9. (Continued) ▪ (*G*) Bitemporal hemianopia. (*H*) Congruous right homonymous hemianopia. (*I*) Incongruous right homonymous hemianopia. (*J*) Right superior quadrantopia ("pie in the sky"). (*K*) Right inferior quadrantopia ("pie on the floor"). (*L*) Macular-sparing right homonymous hemianopia.

lobe lesion that affects superior retinal fibers; it is termed "pie on the floor." A macular-sparing hemianopia spares the area immediately around fixation; it implies an occipital lobe lesion (see Enrichment Box 7–10).

Heteronymous hemianopias are usually bitemporal; rarely are they binasal. A bitemporal hemianopia is usually due to chiasmatic disease, such as a pituitary tumor growing out of the sella turcica and pressing on the underside of the chiasm (Enrichment Box 7–10).

An altitudinal visual field defect involves the upper or lower half of vision, usually in one eye, and is usually due to retinal vascular disease (branch retinal artery occlusion or AION). Altitudinal defects do not cross the horizontal meridian.

Concentric constriction of the visual fields is a more or less sym-

Scotomas

A positive scotoma causes blackness or a sense of blockage of vision, as though an object were interposed; it suggests macular disease. A negative scotoma is an absence of vision, a "hole" or blank spot, as if part of the field had been erased; it suggests optic nerve disease. A paracentral scotoma involves the areas adjacent to the fixation point, and has the same implications as for a central scotoma. A cecocentral scotoma extends from the blind spot to fixation, and strongly suggests optic nerve disease. Any scotoma involving the blind spot implies optic neuropathy. An arcuate scotoma is a crescent defect arching out of the blind spot, usually due to optic neuropathy with the brunt of damage falling on the fibers forming the superior and inferior nerve fiber layer arcades. A junctional scotoma is an optic nerve defect in one eye (central, paracentral, or cecocentral scotoma) and a superior temporal defect in the opposite eye due to a lesion (usually a mass) involving one optic nerve near its junction with the chiasm. The lesion damages the inferior nasal fibers from the opposite eye (von Willebrand knee) as they loop forward into the proximal optic nerve on the side of the lesion (see Figure 7–8). Occipital pole lesions primarily affecting the macular area can produce contralateral homonymous hemianopic scotomas. Since the bulk of fibers in the chiasm come from the macula, early compression may preferentially affect central vision, producing bitemporal heteronymous scotomas; with progression of the lesion, a full-blown bitemporal hemianopia appears.

Macular sparing

The explanation for macular sparing is unknown. It may be due to dual representation of the macula in each occipital pole, to collateral blood supply from the anterior or middle cerebral artery, which protects the macular region from ischemia, or simply to the large extent of the cortical macular representation.

Bitemporal hemianopia

Bitemporal field defects can usually be detected earliest by demonstrating bitemporal desaturation to red. Because of the anterior inferior position of decussating inferior nasal fibers, lesions impinging from below produce upper temporal field defects that evolve into a bitemporal hemianopia. Lesions encroaching from above tend to cause inferior temporal defects initially. The defect is first and worst in the upper quadrants with infrachiasmatic masses (e.g., pituitary adenoma) and first and worst in the lower quadrants with suprachiasmatic masses (e.g., craniopharyngioma). Because of the large number of chiasmal fibers and their sensitivity to pressure, early chiasmal mass effect may produce bitemporal heteronymous paracentral scotomas. Patients with postfixed chiasms and pituitary tumors may present with optic nerve defects, and those with prefixed chiasms may present with optic-tract defects.

metric, progressive reduction in field diameter. It may occur with optic atrophy, especially when secondary to papilledema, late glaucoma, or retinal disease (retinitis pigmentosa). Concentric constriction of the fields is sometimes seen in hysteria. A suspicious finding is when the fields fail to enlarge as expected with testing at increasing distance ("tubular fields").

Examination of visual functions, including acuity, color vision, pupils, and visual fields usually suggests one of three possible lesion localizations: prechiasmal, chiasmal, or retrochiasmal. Prechiasmal lesions typically produce abnormalities in only one eye, with impaired acuity and pupillary abnormalities. Chiasmal lesions cause heteronymous hemianopias, most often bitemporal. Retrochiasmal lesions cause homonymous hemianopias, complete or incomplete; if the hemianopias are incomplete, they are either congruous or incongruous.

Prechiasmal Lesions

Most optic nerve dysfunction is due to demyelinating disease, inflammatory conditions, ischemia, or compression.

Optic neuritis. Inflammation or demyelination of the optic nerve can occur in a variety of conditions, including MS, postviral syndromes, sarcoidosis, collagen vascular disease, neurosyphilis, and others. Many cases are idiopathic. Optic neuritis occurs sometime during the course of MS in 70% of patients and is the presenting feature in 25% of them. Fifty percent to seventy percent of patients presenting with optic neuritis eventually develop other evidence of MS (Enrichment Box 7–11).

Anterior ischemic optic neuropathy. In AION, microangiopathy due to hypertension, diabetes, arteriosclerosis, atherosclerosis, or vasculitis (e.g., giant cell arteritis) produces occlusion of the short posterior ciliary arteries and infarction of all or part of the disc. Visual loss is sudden, painless, nonprogressive, and generally does not improve. Involvement of the opposite eye months to years later is common. Decreased acuity, impaired color perception, an inferior altitudinal field defect, and disc edema are the typical findings. Although there is no treatment that affects the outcome in the involved eye, recognition and management of underlying vasculitis may prevent a future attack in the other eye.

Compressive optic neuropathy. Compression, such as from an optic nerve meningioma, always figures prominently in the differential diagnosis of patients with optic neuropathy. Insidious visual loss producing decreased acuity; impaired color perception; and central, cecocentral, or arcuate scotoma is typical (see Enrichment Box 7–11).

Optic neuritis

Things that increase the likelihood of underlying multiple sclerosis (MS) in patients with optic neuritis include the presence of Uhthoff phenomenon, human leukocyte antigen-DR2 positivity, and a recurrent episode. Decreased acuity, impaired color perception, central or cecocentral scotoma, disc edema, and an APD are frequent findings. Visual loss in optic neuritis occurs suddenly and tends to progress over 1 or 2 weeks, with substantial recovery over 4–6 weeks. Severe visual loss acutely does not necessarily portend poor recovery.

Compressive optic neuropathy

With compressive optic neuropathy, lesions very near the chiasm may produce a junctional scotoma. Large, abnormal-appearing veins on the disc surface (opticociliary shunt vessels) provide a telltale clue to a compressive lesion. Common causes include optic nerve sheath meningiomas, pituitary tumors, and distal carotid aneurysms. Compressive neuropathies may evolve more acutely in patients with metastatic lesions, particularly lymphoma.

Other Optic Neuropathies

Numerous other conditions may affect the optic nerve, including glaucoma, Leber's and other hereditary optic atrophies, toxins and drugs, primary and metastatic tumors, malnutrition and deficiency states, neurodegenerative disorders, leukodystrophies, and congenital anomalies. Details are beyond the scope of this discussion.

Chiasmal lesions. Pituitary tumors, craniopharyngiomas, meningiomas, and carotid aneurysm are the lesions that commonly involve the chiasm. The chiasm lies about a centimeter above the diaphragma sella; therefore visual system involvement indicates suprasellar extension of a pituitary tumor, and is a late, not an early, manifestation of chiasmatic mass effect.

Retrochiasmal lesions. Optic tract and lateral geniculate lesions occur rarely, perhaps because of generous collateral blood supply, and are characterized by incongruous homonymous hemianopias.

In geniculocalcarine pathway lesions, temporal lobe pathological conditions typically produce contralateral superior quadrantopias and parietal lobe processes produce contralateral inferior quadrantopias. The more posterior the lesion, the greater the congruity of the field defect is. Parietal lesions are associated with asymmetric OKN responses. Occipital lesions tend to spare the macula and do not affect OKN responses. Bilateral occipital lesions may cause the syndrome of cortical blindness with denial of the deficit (Anton syndrome).

Most occipital lesions are vascular. Most temporal lobe lesions are neoplastic. Parietal lesions may be either. Trauma, vascular malformations, abscesses, demyelinating disease, and metastases can occur in any location.

8

Diagnostic Reasoning and Neurologic Differential Diagnosis

*"There are only two sorts of doctors: those who practise
with their brains and those who practise with their tongues."*
—*Sir William Osler*

Before discussing neurologic differential diagnosis, it may be useful to review general concepts of diagnostic reasoning. Establishing an accurate diagnosis is the cornerstone of effective clinical management, yet most physicians are left to stumble onto the principles of diagnostic reasoning on their own, because this important topic is seldom formally addressed in medical school.

There are usually two components to making a diagnosis: information gathering and hypothesis testing. Medical students learn to gather information ad nauseam—by doing a complete history and physical—but are often at a loss for what to do with it. The accomplished clinician uses a multifaceted diagnostic process: gathering information, or searching for clues; analyzing these clues for relevance, reliability, and significance; and using the clues to generate hypotheses that may explain the clinical facts. The clinician then tests the hypotheses to see which of them best matches clinical reality, rejecting those that do not until finally coming to closure by arriving at one best-fit hypothesis that becomes the diagnosis.

The generation and testing of hypotheses method requires experience and intimate familiarity with the subject. The inexperienced gravitate toward rote information gathering, in hopes the diagnosis will magically emerge. More experienced diagnosticians often eschew the gathering of information that does not aid in either generating or testing a hypothesis; less is more. Experts are also more flexible in modifying their initial diagnostic assumptions (Enrichment Box 8–1).

The list of hypotheses produced from information gathering is the

ENRICHMENT BOX 8-1

In a study of medical students confronted with contradictory evidence regarding an initial diagnostic assumption, the level of training influenced the response. Second-year students ignored the contradictory evidence or reinterpreted it to fit the original diagnostic hypothesis. Third-year students formed additional coexistent hypotheses to accommodate conflicting data. Fourth-year students generated several initial hypotheses and subsequently narrowed the possibilities by testing and rejecting rival hypotheses until arriving at a single coherent diagnostic explanation.

differential diagnosis. A test is then applied to disprove each hypothesis. The test might be a question posed to the patient, a search for a particular sign, or the request for a laboratory test or diagnostic procedure.

The average physician, when trying to make a diagnosis, keeps a mental list of differential diagnostic hypotheses. As each hypothesis is disproved, it is scratched from the list. Other possibilities are added as new information emerges. The list is dynamic, but the flux decreases as the physician approaches a conclusion. Many entities may cycle through the hypothesis list before coming to closure.

The hypotheses are commonly considered in order of probability. Sutton's law (attributed to Willie Sutton, an infamous bank robber) advises to "go for the money," that the most common diagnosis is most likely to be correct (Enrichment Box 8-2). Another important principle of diagnosis is Occam's razor, or the principle of parsimony, first articulated by William of Occam, which states that the most likely solution is the simplest. When applied to medical diagnoses, it means that the least complex diagnosis is most likely correct, or that the physician should never make two diagnoses when one will do (see Enrichment Box 8-2).

Another useful diagnostic aphorism is the so-called barking dog rule. This rule is derived from a Sherlock Holmes's story in which a dog did not bark when a horse was stolen in the night, implying that the thief was someone the dog knew well. As applied to differential diagnosis, the barking dog rule refers to something made most significant by its absence; for example, lack of fasciculations strongly challenges a diagnosis of amyotrophic lateral sclerosis (ALS).

Fisher's rules are clinical maxims collected from observations of C. Miller Fisher, a neurologist of legendary diagnostic acumen. Table 8-1 summarizes these and other maxims that are particularly helpful for developing clinical reasoning skills.

Errors in clinical diagnostic reasoning can lead to a variety of ad-

ENRICHMENT BOX 8-2

Sutton's law

When asked why he kept robbing banks despite being captured, Sutton reportedly replied, "because that's where the money is." Sutton's law has become a treasured diagnostic principle because odds favor a common disorder.

Occam's razor

Generally valid, Occam's razor must be tempered in older patients, who may well have more than one diagnosis. Sometimes Sutton's law and Occam's razor may lead a physician to think in opposite directions. Consider a case in which a young woman with headaches and white matter lesions was judged more likely to have two common but unrelated diagnoses [migraine and multiple sclerosis (MS)] rather than one rare but potentially unifying diagnosis (cerebral autosomal dominant arteriopathy with subcortical infarcts and leukoencephalopathy).

verse consequences. Common sources of error include the failure to recognize a possible diagnostic hypothesis and a faulty procedure for information gathering and processing. In a study of common errors in daily practice among neurology residents, the overall rate of diagnostic error and the frequency of diagnostic inaccuracy in various disease entities showed that the initial bedside diagnosis was correct for 67% of patients. The highest rates of inaccuracy were found in the diagnosis of subdural hematoma (SDH) [56%], myasthenia gravis (MG) [50%], subarachnoid hemorrhage (SAH) [42%], and Guillain-Barré syndrome (GBS) [40%] {Enrichment Box 8–3}. The causes of diagnostic inaccuracy were errors of reasoning (38%), an inadequate patient database (35%), and an inadequate fund of knowledge (27%).

We must accept the inevitability of diagnostic errors, while nonetheless trying to minimize them and to recognize, and admit, when an error has occurred. Methods to reduce diagnostic errors are discussed in Enrichment Box 8–4.

If the differential diagnosis is a list of hypotheses, where does the list come from? This varies with the level of experience of the physician and the complexity of the case. Diseases associated with a characteristic and unmistakable visual appearance may be recognized instantaneously ("augenblickdiagnose" is the German term for diagnosis in the blink of an eye). Pattern recognition suffices in straightforward cases, but the physician must be sensitive to significant deviations from the usual patterns that might signal an alternative diagnosis. In more complex cases, the tendency is to rely on a method of systematic analysis. This is frequently done in neurology.

TABLE 8–1. AXIOMS RELEVANT TO CLINICAL REASONING AND DIAGNOSTIC PRINCIPLES

Fisher's rules*

In arriving at a clinical diagnosis, think of the five most common findings (historical, physical findings, or laboratory) found in a given disorder. If at least three of these five are not present in a given patient, the diagnosis is likely to be wrong.

Resist the temptation to prematurely place a case or disorder into a diagnostic cubbyhole that fits poorly. Allowing it to remain unknown stimulates continuing activity and thought.

The details of a case are important; their analysis distinguishes the expert from the journeyman.

Pay particular attention to the specifics of the patient with a known diagnosis; it will be helpful later when similar phenomena occur in an unknown case.

Fully accept what you have heard or read only when you have verified it yourself.

Maintain a lively interest in patients as people.

Other axioms

When test results are equivocal, the best step is to repeat the testing later ("Susann's Law").[†]

When the diagnosis is in doubt, take another history.

Know the limits of the diagnostic tests; it is essential to know the likelihood of a false-negative test when interpreting the data.

If a diagnosis is not considered, it is not likely to be made: expand the differential diagnosis by systematic thinking or other methods.

Diagnosis by exclusion is treacherous if the differential diagnosis is incomplete.

Uncommon manifestations of common diseases are much more common than common manifestations of uncommon diseases.

*Caplan LR: Fisher's rules. *Arch Neurol* 39:389–390, 1982.
[†]Susann J: *Once Is Not Enough.* New York, William Morrow, 1973.

Neurologic Differential Diagnosis

Pathological processes behave in certain ways, depending on their location in the nervous system, and in certain other ways related to their inherent natures. Neurologists deal in two basic clinical exercises: differential diagnosis by location (where is the lesion in the nervous system?) and differential diagnosis by etiology (what is the lesion in the nervous system?). The anatomic diagnosis and the etiologic diagnosis aid and support each other. In general, the neurologic examination aids primarily in establishing the anatomic or localization diagnosis and the history aids in the etiologic diagnosis, but there is overlap.

ENRICHMENT BOX 8-3

Other conditions with a high rate of misdiagnosis included traumatic disorders (39%), herniation of intervertebral disc (33%), metabolic encephalopathy (30%), central nervous system (CNS) infection (30%), intracranial neoplasm (24%), drug overdose or intoxication (22%), and mixed neurologic and metabolic encephalopathy (21%).

In a prospective study of the accuracy of bedside diagnoses on a neurology service, patients were evaluated independently by a junior resident, a senior resident, and a staff neurologist. Each individual was required to make an anatomic and etiologic diagnosis based solely on the history and physical examination. In 40 patients with laboratory-confirmed final diagnoses, the clinical diagnoses of the junior residents, senior residents, and staff neurologists were correct for 65%, 75%, and 77% of them, respectively. The errors by the junior residents, <senior residents>, and (staff) were attributed to incomplete history and examination in 4 <1> (0), inadequate fund of knowledge in 4 <3> (3), and poor diagnostic reasoning in 6 <6> (6). Thus, experience beyond a certain level is not necessarily a cure for faulty reasoning.

Differential Diagnosis by Location

One way to organize anatomically is to start centrally or peripherally and to consider sequentially more peripheral or more central structures; for example, start by considering muscle disease, then neuromuscular junction (NMJ) disorders, then sequentially peripheral neuropathies, radiculopathies, myelopathies, and so forth up to the cerebral cortex. At each of these levels, disease processes tend to have

ENRICHMENT BOX 8-4

Suggestions to reduce diagnostic errors include the following. When the diagnosis is unclear, take another history (see Chapter 4, Re-taking the History). Do a careful complete physical examination; it often provides important clues to the correct diagnosis. Know the limits of the diagnostic tests, especially the likelihood of false negatives, but beware of overinterpretation and maintain skepticism. Avoid premature closure, accepting a diagnosis before it is fully verified. A knowledge of the natural history of the symptoms and the diagnoses under consideration can be a key diagnostic tool. If a diagnosis is not considered, it is not likely to be made; expand the differential diagnosis. Remember that psychosocial factors can generate or magnify symptoms. If the diagnosis remains in doubt, seek the advice of a colleague or a consultant.

characteristic clinical features, although with a degree of overlap. By trying to localize the disease process to one or two likely levels, such as muscle or NMJ, the physician can then think more systematically about the etiologic possibilities.

Sometimes manifestations of disease overlap in different locations, which can cause confusion. And some diseases simply do not follow the rules. A diabetic partial third cranial nerve palsy and extraocular muscle dysfunction caused by MG could be confused if the myasthenia caused weakness in a predominately third cranial nerve distribution, which it can do. Deafferentation due to peripheral nerve or posterior column disease can cause sensory ataxia that is difficult to distinguish from cerebellar disease. The differential between early GBS and early transverse myelopathy is notoriously difficult.

Assuming the process under consideration is indeed neurologic, the first major attempt at localization should be to decide whether the pathological process likely involves the peripheral nervous system (PNS) or the central nervous system (CNS). For purposes of this discussion, the PNS includes the NMJ and the muscle. If the evidence suggests the process probably involves the CNS, try to decide if it is likely above or below the foramen magnum. Clinical features that suggest these possibilities are summarized in Tables 8–2 and 8–3. For instance, other than for headache and thalamic pain syndromes, CNS disease is not often associated with pain. Likewise, muscle and NMJ diseases are usually painless, but processes that affect peripheral nerves and nerve roots are often painful. The presence of pain therefore makes a peripheral process more likely. Except for spinal shock or acute stroke, CNS disease usually produces increased reflexes, whereas the deep tendon reflexes in peripheral disease are usually normal or decreased. A Babinski sign is a strong indicator of CNS disease.

The findings in Tables 8–2 and 8–3 are not all absolute. For example, abnormal pupils usually indicate CNS disease, but some peripheral processes, for example, botulism, can affect the pupils. Other findings might have significance in proportion to degree. For example, chronic CNS disease that produces immobility might lead to disuse atrophy of muscles, but this is never more than mild. Severe atrophy is only seen in processes that involve the lower motor neuron, such as anterior horn cell disease, radiculopathy, plexopathy, or neuropathy.

The spinal cord and nerve roots are the boundary between the CNS and PNS, and recognition of pathological conditions involving these regions is one of the greatest challenges in clinical neurology. The nerve

TABLE 8–2. CLINICAL FEATURES THAT SUGGEST CENTRAL NERVOUS SYSTEM DISEASE VERSUS PERIPHERAL NERVOUS SYSTEM DISEASE

Central Nervous System Disease*	Peripheral Nervous System Disease†
Lack of pain	Pain
Hemi-distribution weakness	Symmetric, generalized weakness, very focal weakness (e.g., peripheral nerve distribution)
Hemi-distribution sensory loss	
Crossed or dissociated sensory loss (e.g., Brown-Séquard syndrome)	Stocking-glove sensory loss
Hyperreflexia or clonus	Dermatomal- or peripheral- nerve-distribution sensory loss
Muscle spasticity or hypertonia	Hyporeflexia
Babinski sign	Fluctuating weakness
Lhermitte sign	Myotonia
Abnormal involuntary movements (e.g., chorea)	Significant muscle atrophy
Seizures	Increased CK
Bowel, bladder, or sexual dysfunction	Abnormal EMG
Headache	
Meningeal signs	
Visual loss	
Abnormal pupils	
Crossed signs	
Cerebellar signs	
Presence of a bruit	
Altered mental status	
Dementia	
Focal cortical signs (aphasia, apraxia)	
Abnormal head or spine MRI	
Abnormal EEG	
Abnormal evoked potentials	

*The central nervous system includes the brain and spinal cord.
†The peripheral nervous system includes roots, plexus, peripheral nerves, neuromuscular junctions, and muscle.
CK = creatine kinase; EEG = electroencephalogram; EMG = electromyogram; MRI = magnetic resonance imaging.

TABLE 8–3. CHARACTERISTICS OF DISEASE ABOVE VERSUS BELOW THE FORAMEN MAGNUM

Above the Foramen Magnum	Below the Foramen Magnum
Hemi-distribution weakness or sensory loss	Bilateral weakness
	Bilateral sensory loss
Cranial nerve abnormalities	Prominent bowel, bladder, or sexual dysfunction
Altered mental status	
Dementia	Radicular pain
Focal cortical signs	Significant muscle atrophy
Seizures	Segmental hyporeflexia
Headache	Fasciculations
Vertigo	Typical spinal cord syndrome (transverse cord, central anterior cord, Brown-Séquard, conus medullaris, or cauda equina syndrome)
Cerebellar signs	
Nystagmus	
	Spinal sensory level
	Sacral sparing
	Lhermitte sign

roots, from a practical standpoint, are part of the PNS, although strictly speaking, peripheral myelin does not begin until the neural foramen. But the nerve roots run a variably long intradural course before exiting, and they lie in close proximity to the spinal cord during part of their course. Disease processes involving one or more roots and the adjacent spinal cord are not uncommon, for example, a radiculomyelopathy due to a large cervical disc herniation. Lesions of the cauda equina and conus medullaris may cause bowel, bladder, and sexual dysfunction. The rate of mislocalization (misjudgment in deciding on the location of disease) in spinal cord, cauda equina, conus medullaris, and nerve root syndromes is higher than for most other neurologic conditions.

The general rules in Tables 8–2 and 8–3 are useful and largely accurate. But knowledge of the exceptions to the rules distinguishes the novice from the expert. For example, mild to severe mental retardation can occur in association with some muscle diseases (neonatal myotonic, Duchenne, and Fukuyama congenital muscular dystrophy). Tremor can occur in some peripheral neuropathies. Bowel and bladder control difficulties are a common feature of amyloid neuropathy. A rare patient with a cerebral hemisphere lesion can present with wrist drop that mimics radial nerve palsy. It is a growing collection of experience with these exceptions that marks the seasoned practitioner. Nevertheless, the elements listed in Tables 8–2 and 8–3 are a good, general guide that will seldom lead the physician far astray. See Enrichment Box 8–5 for an example of the reasoning process.

Some neurologic signs and symptoms occur commonly in both CNS and PNS diseases, and arriving at the correct diagnosis sometimes depends much more on analyzing the associated findings than the presenting manifestation. Table 8–4 lists conditions that occur frequently in both central and peripheral disease.

The following sections discuss the typical clinical manifestations of disease at the various locations in the nervous and neuromuscular systems. Table 8–5 shows one scheme for locations where disease might occur in neurologic patients. Tables 8–6 through 8–20 summarize etiologic possibilities for disease at each of these locations.

CEREBRAL HEMISPHERE DISORDERS: CORTICAL VERSUS SUBCORTICAL

Characteristic of hemispheric pathology is a "hemi" deficit: hemisensory loss, hemiparesis, hemianopsia, or perhaps hemi seizures. Within this framework, disease affecting the cerebral cortex behaves differently from disease of subcortical structures, such as the basal ganglia, thalamus, deep white matter, and internal capsule. Since the cortex mediates higher cortical functions, patients with cortical involvement may have aphasia, apraxia, astereognosis, impaired two-point discrimination, memory loss, cognitive defects, focal seizures, or other abnor-

---

ENRICHMENT BOX 8–5

Consider dysphagia. It can occur in central diseases, such as brainstem stroke, brainstem tumor, amyotrophic lateral sclerosis (ALS), or pseudobulbar palsy. However, it is a common manifestation of certain peripheral processes, such as polymyositis, myasthenia gravis (MG), and some muscular dystrophies. If a patient with dysphagia has associated hemi-distribution sensory loss, an abnormally small pupil on one side (due to Horner syndrome), dissociated sensory loss involving pain and temperature but sparing touch, and incoordination on one side of the body, the most likely diagnosis is a brainstem stroke (Wallenberg syndrome). But if the patient has bilateral ptosis, normal pupils, diplopia, and symmetric proximal weakness, the most likely diagnosis is MG, a peripheral process.

> **TABLE 8–4. ABNORMALITIES THAT OCCUR COMMONLY IN BOTH PERIPHERAL AND CENTRAL NERVOUS SYSTEM DISEASE**
>
> Abnormal pupils
>
> Ptosis
>
> Diplopia
>
> Dysphagia
>
> Dysarthria
>
> Facial weakness
>
> Extremity weakness
>
> Sensory loss
>
> Difficulty walking

malities that reflect the essential integrative role of the cortex. If the process affects the dominant hemisphere, the patient may have considerable language dysfunction in the form of aphasia, alexia, or agraphia. With disease of the nondominant hemisphere, the patient may have disturbances of higher cortical function involving things other than language, such as apraxia.

If the disease affects subcortical structures, the clinical picture includes the hemi distribution of dysfunction but lacks those elements that are typically cortical: language disturbance, apraxia, and dementia. Lesions of the internal capsule produce hemiparesis without aphasia, apraxia, or visual field cut (e.g., "pure motor stroke"). Lesions of the thalamus cause isolated hemisensory loss.

Ancillary tests usually most helpful in the workup of suspected hemispheric disease include imaging studies, cerebrospinal fluid (CSF) analysis, electroencephalogram, and studies to rule out an embolic source.

BASAL GANGLIA DISORDERS

Except for acute hypertensive hemorrhage, the common diseases of the basal ganglia cause movement disorders such as Parkinson disease or Huntington chorea. Movement disorders may be hypokinetic or hyperkinetic, which indicate whether movement is in general decreased or increased. Parkinson disease causes akinesia, bradykinesia, and rigidity. Huntington disease, in contrast, causes increased movements that are involuntary and beyond the patient's control (chorea). Tremor is a frequent accompaniment of basal ganglia disease.

TABLE 8–5. CENTRAL AND PERIPHERAL LOCATIONS OF DISEASE IN NEUROLOGIC PATIENTS

Central nervous system
  Above the foramen magnum
    Supratentorial
      Cerebral hemisphere
      Basal ganglia
    Infratentorial
      Brainstem
      Cranial nerve
      Cerebellum
  Below the foramen magnum
    Spinal cord
Peripheral nervous system
    Nerve root
    Plexus
    Peripheral nerve
    Neuromuscular junction
    Muscle
Supporting elements
    Meninges and ventricular system
    Vascular system
    Skull and vertebral columns
Multifocal or diffuse

Ancillary tests usually most helpful in the workup of suspected basal ganglia disease include imaging, and occasionally copper studies (to exclude Wilson disease) or genetic analysis.

BRAINSTEM DISEASE

Brainstem disease processes tend to have a characteristic clinical signature. The classic distinguishing feature of brainstem pathology is that deficits are "crossed." The major long motor and sensory tracts decussate in the lower medulla, but the cranial nerve nuclei in the brainstem innervate structures ipsilateral to their location. For instance, in the right side of the pons lie the cranial nerve nuclei for VI

TABLE 8–6. ETIOLOGIC CATEGORIES FOR DISORDERS AFFECTING THE CEREBRAL HEMISPHERES

Etiologic Category	Condition
Tumor	Metastasis, glioma, meningioma, lymphoma, congenital tumors, limbic encephalitis as a remote effect, radionecrosis, radiation-induced neoplasms
Drugs or alcohol	ETOH dementia, Wernicke-Korsakoff disease; some of the many drugs that can cause encephalopathy include antiepileptic drugs, cimetidine, penicillin, lithium, metrizamide, methotrexate, and MAO inhibitors
Imbalance	Hypernatremia, hyponatremia, hypoglycemia, hyperglycemia (with or without ketosis), hypercalcemia, hypothyroidism, vitamin B_{12} deficiency
Mass lesion	Tumor, abscess, hematoma (intracerebral, epidural, subdural), gumma, toxoplasmosis, parasitic cyst
Seizure or sleep disorder	Many insults or lesions can cause seizures; narcolepsy or cataplexy; other sleep disorders can cause excessive sleepiness and other symptoms
Trauma	Closed head injury, hematoma, penetrating wounds, chronic traumatic encephalopathy, diffuse axonal injury, delayed cerebral edema, postconcussion syndrome
Degenerative	Alzheimer and other dementias, ALS, corticobasal degeneration, progressive supranuclear palsy, Lewy body disease
Migraine	Migraine with aura
Demyelinating disease	MS, ADEM, leukodystrophies
Congenital	Many; for example, encephalocele, porencephaly, agenesis of the corpus callosum, microcephaly, macrocephaly, hydrocephalus, Sturge-Weber, neural-tube-closure defects, Down syndrome dementia
Bleeding	Hypertensive hemorrhage, trauma, aneurysm, vascular malformation, amyloid angiopathy, bleeding dyscrasia
Stroke or TIA	Atherosclerosis, lacunar disease, embolism, vasculitis, arterial dissection, cryptogenic infarction
Hereditary	Sickle cell disease, other hemoglobinopathies, neurocutaneous syndromes, protein C or S deficiency, antithrombin III deficiency, MERRF, MELAS, lipidosis, porphyria
Psychiatric	Depressive pseudodementia, psychosis, neurosis, affective disorder, catatonia
Systemic	Many; especially heart disease (especially atrial fibrillation), hepatic encephalopathy

(continued)

TABLE 8–6. ETIOLOGIC CATEGORIES FOR DISORDERS AFFECTING THE CEREBRAL HEMISPHERES (*CONTINUED*)

Etiologic Category	Condition
Infectious	Abscess, toxoplasmosis, cysticercosis, echinococcosis, malaria, syphilis, viral encephalitis, HIV dementia, atypical mycobacteria, Rocky Mountain spotted fever, Creutzfeldt-Jakob disease, new-variant Creutzfeldt-Jakob disease (human "mad cow disease"), Gerstmann-Sträussler-Scheinker disease, subacute sclerosing panencephalitis, progressive multifocal leukoencephalopathy, Whipple disease
Toxin	Many; for example, lead encephalopathy, mercury (mad hatter syndrome), organic solvent encephalopathy
Inflammatory	Vasculitis, cerebritis (e.g., SLE), Behçet syndrome
Autoimmune	Lupus cerebritis
Other	Cerebral edema, hydrocephalus syndromes

ADEM = acute disseminated encephalomyelitis; ALS = amyotrophic lateral sclerosis; ETOH = ethyl alcohol; HIV = human immunodeficiency virus; MAO = monoamine oxidase; MELAS = mitochondrial encephalomyopathy, lactic acidosis, and stroke-like episodes; MERRF = myoclonic epilepsy with ragged red fibers; MS = multiple sclerosis; SLE = systemic lupus erythematosus; TIA = transient ischemic attack.

and VII, in proximity to the right corticospinal tract that is destined to decussate in the medulla to innervate the left side of the body. Thus, the patient harboring a lesion in the right pons will have cranial nerve findings on the right, such as sixth or seventh cranial nerve palsy, with a hemiparesis on the left.

This crossed deficit is often associated with symptoms reflecting dysfunction of other posterior fossa structures or their connections. These structures include the vestibular nuclei and cerebellum; patients with brainstem disease often have dizziness, unsteadiness, imbalance, incoordination, and difficulty walking. Vertigo, ataxia, nausea, and vomiting all suggest a posterior fossa localization. Pharyngeal muscles are innervated by neurons in the brainstem, and thus patients with posterior fossa disease sometimes have dysphagia. Disordered eye movements that reflect dysfunction of cranial nerves III, IV, and VI or their connections may produce a clinical complaint of diplopia or a limitation of extraocular movement on examination, or both. Unless the process has impaired the reticular activating system, these patients are

TABLE 8–7. ETIOLOGIC CATEGORIES FOR DISORDERS AFFECTING THE BASAL GANGLIA

Etiologic Category	Condition
Tumor	Glioma, paraneoplastic opsoclonus or myoclonus
Drugs or alcohol	Many; for example, phenothiazine-related agents, reserpine, tremorogenic agents (albuterol, lithium, terfenadine)
Imbalance	Kernicterus
Mass lesion	Tumor, hematoma, abscess
Seizure or sleep disorder	NA
Trauma	Head injury, pugilistic (chronic traumatic) encephalopathy ("punch drunk")
Degenerative	Parkinson disease and variants (striatonigral degeneration, Parkinson dementia complex of Guam, dentatorubropallidoluysian atrophy), corticobasal degeneration, senile chorea or tremor, progressive supranuclear palsy, Lewy body disease
Migraine	NA
Demyelinating disease	NA
Congenital	Status marmoratus, athetotic or dystonic cerebral palsy
Bleeding	Hypertensive hemorrhage, arteriovenous malformation, bleeding dyscrasia
Stroke or TIA	Lacunar infarction
Hereditary	Familial tremor, Huntington disease, Wilson disease, neuroacanthocytosis (may be familial or sporadic), Hallervorden-Spatz disease, Tourette syndrome
Psychiatric	Psychogenic movement disorders
Systemic	Acquired hepatocerebral degeneration, systemic lupus erythematosus (chorea)
Infectious	Sydenham chorea, CNS Whipple disease, Creutzfeldt-Jakob disease, toxoplasmosis, postencephalitic Parkinson disease
Toxin	MPTP, manganese
Inflammatory	Behçet syndrome
Autoimmune	Sydenham chorea
Other	Essential tremor, chorea gravidarum, hyperexplexia, essential myoclonus, paramyoclonus multiplex, postanoxic myoclonus, Meige syndrome, focal or occupational dystonias, torticollis syndromes, restless legs syndrome, paroxysmal choreoathetosis

CNS = central nervous system; MPTP = methylphenyltetrahydropyridine; NA = not applicable; TIA = transient ischemic attack.

TABLE 8–8. ETIOLOGIC CATEGORIES FOR DISORDERS AFFECTING THE BRAINSTEM

Etiologic Category	Condition
Tumor	Glioma, medulloblastoma, ependymoma, metastasis
Drugs or alcohol	Central pontine myelinolysis
Imbalance	Hyponatremia (central pontine myelinolysis), Wernicke syndrome
Mass lesion	Abscess, posterior fossa subdural hematoma, cerebellar hematoma
Seizure or sleep disorder	NA
Trauma	Rare
Degenerative	Olivopontocerebellar atrophy, multisystem atrophy, amyotrophic lateral sclerosis, progressive bulbar palsy, progressive supranuclear palsy
Migraine	Basilar artery migraine
Demyelinating disease	MS, acute demyelinating encephalomyelitis, central pontine myelinolysis
Congenital	Dandy-Walker syndrome, syringobulbia, Arnold-Chiari malformations
Bleeding	Hypertensive pontine hemorrhage, bleeding dyscrasia
Stroke or TIA	Brainstem infarct, basilar stenosis, top-of-basilar syndrome, embolism
Hereditary	Spinocerebellar atrophy syndromes, Kennedy disease
Psychiatric	NA
Systemic	Very few
Infectious	Tuberculoma, Gerstmann-Sträussler-Scheinker syndrome (mimics olivopontocerebellar atrophy)
Toxin	Trichloroethylene
Inflammatory	Brainstem encephalitis, vasculitis
Autoimmune	Postviral or postvaccinial demyelinating syndrome
Other	Herniation syndrome

MS = multiple sclerosis; NA = not applicable; TIA = transient ischemic attack.

TABLE 8–9. ETIOLOGIC CATEGORIES FOR DISORDERS AFFECTING CRANIAL NERVES

Etiologic Category	Condition
Tumor	Schwannoma, meningioma, neurofibroma, pituitary adenoma, optic nerve glioma, leukemic infiltrates, numb chin or numb cheek syndrome, meningeal carcinomatosis
Drugs or alcohol	Alcohol or tobacco amblyopia, methyl alcohol and other toxic optic neuropathies, ototoxic drugs
Imbalance	Vitamin deficiency optic neuropathy, Wernicke syndrome
Mass lesion	Tumors, aneurysms (vertebrobasilar system, especially top-of-basilar syndrome), cranial nerve palsy due to increased intracranial pressure
Seizure or sleep disorder	NA
Trauma	I, II, III, IV, VI, VII cranial neuropathies as a complication of head injury
Degenerative	Chronic progressive external ophthalmoplegia syndromes, Ménière disease
Migraine	Ophthalmoplegic migraine
Demyelinating disease	Multiple sclerosis, Devic disease
Congenital	Moebius syndrome, Duane syndrome, pseudopapilledema
Bleeding	Aneurysmal mass effects, pituitary apoplexy
Stroke or TIA	Diabetes mellitus, vasculitis, amaurosis fugax, anterior ischemic optic neuropathy, cavernous sinus thrombosis
Hereditary	Melkersson-Rosenthal syndrome, Leber optic atrophy
Psychiatric	NA
Systemic	Diabetes mellitus (diabetic cranial nerve palsies), sarcoid, connective tissue diseases, many others
Infectious	Meningitis, Lyme disease (Bannwarth syndrome: multiple cranial neuropathies due to Lyme disease), toxoplasmosis (optic nerve), botulism, herpes zoster (including postherpetic neuralgia), syphilis, malignant external otitis
Toxin	Ototoxic drugs, trichloroethylene
Inflammatory	Sarcoid, temporal arteritis, Miller-Fisher syndrome, Tolosa-Hunt syndrome, Raeder syndrome, Guillain-Barré syndrome
Autoimmune	Connective tissue diseases
Other	Bell palsy, Behçet syndrome, analgesia dolorosa, post lumbar puncture cranial nerve palsy, trigeminal neuralgia, glossopharyngeal neuralgia, herniation syndrome

NA = not applicable; TIA = transient ischemic attack.

TABLE 8–10. ETIOLOGIC CATEGORIES FOR DISORDERS AFFECTING THE CEREBELLUM

Etiologic Category	Condition
Tumor	Metastasis, glioma, ependymoma, medulloblastoma, ependymoma, paraneoplastic cerebellar degeneration
Drugs or alcohol	Alcoholic cerebellar degeneration, PCP abuse, organic solvent abuse, numerous medications (e.g., phenytoin, carbamazepine, lithium, benzodiazepines, antineoplastic agents, especially 5FU and cytosine arabinoside)
Imbalance	Hypothyroidism
Mass lesion	Tumor, abscess, hematoma
Seizure or sleep disorder	NA
Trauma	Posterior fossa subdural hematoma
Degenerative	Many; idiopathic spinocerebellar degenerations, multisystem atrophy, olivopontocerebellar atrophy
Migraine	Basilar artery migraine (Bickerstaff)
Demyelinating disease	MS, acute demyelinating encephalomyelitis (includes postinfectious and postvaccinial syndromes)
Congenital	Arnold-Chiari malformations, Dandy-Walker cyst, cerebral palsy
Bleeding	Cerebellar hemorrhage, bleeding dyscrasia
Stroke or TIA	PICA, AICA, or SCA ischemia
Hereditary	Inherited ataxias and spinocerebellar degeneration (several subtypes), ataxia telangiectasia, MERFF, Hartnup disease, lipidoses, Wilson disease, von Hippel-Lindau disease, Leigh syndrome
Psychiatric	NA
Systemic	Whipple disease, connective tissue disorders
Infectious	Abscess, progressive multifocal leukoencephalopathy, viral infection ("cerebellitis"), especially ECHO virus, Creutzfeldt-Jakob disease, Gerstmann-Sträussler-Scheinker syndrome, cysticercosis, echinococcus
Toxin	Many; for example, mercury, organic solvents, especially toluene
Inflammatory	Vasculitis, Behçet syndrome
Autoimmune	Paraneoplastic syndromes
Other	Late-onset sporadic cerebellar ataxia

AICA = anterior inferior cerebellar artery; 5FU = 5-fluorouracil; MERRF = myoclonic epilepsy with ragged red fibers; MS = multiple sclerosis; NA = not applicable; PICA = posterior inferior cerebellar artery; SCA = superior cerebellar artery; TIA = transient ischemic attack.

TABLE 8–11. ETIOLOGIC CATEGORIES FOR DISORDERS AFFECTING THE SPINAL CORD

Etiologic Category	Condition
Tumor	Metastases, glioma, meningioma, lymphoma, paraneoplastic myelopathy
Drugs or alcohol	Vaccination, nitrous oxide, heroin, alcohol
Imbalance	Vitamin B_{12} deficiency
Mass lesion	Spinal hematoma, abscess or tumor, intraspinal cyst, arachnoid cyst
Seizure or sleep disorder	NA
Trauma	Traumatic myelopathies, posttraumatic syringomyelia
Degenerative	Degenerative spine disease (cervical spondylosis) ALS, primary lateral sclerosis
Migraine	NA
Demyelinating disease	Multiple sclerosis, transverse myelitis, postvaccination myelitis, acute demyelinating encephalomyelitis, Devic disease
Congenital	Syringomyelia, myelomeningocele and other dysraphic states (occult spinal dysraphism), tethered cord, intraspinal cysts, diastematomyelia, developmental tumors (lipoma, teratoma)
Bleeding	Epidural or subdural hematoma, arteriovenous malformation, bleeding dyscrasia
Stroke or TIA	Anterior spinal artery occlusion; complications of aortic aneurysm surgery
Hereditary	Hereditary spastic paraplegia, hereditary motor sensory neuropathy types 2 and 5, achondroplasia, Friedreich ataxia, progressive spinal muscular atrophy syndromes, Kennedy disease, hexosaminidase A deficiency, mucopolysaccharidoses (especially Hurler syndrome)
Psychiatric	NA
Systemic	Connective tissue disease, cancer, AIDS, systemic vasculitis
Infectious	HTLV-I, herpes zoster, spinal epidural abscess, HIV-related chronic progressive myelopathy, tetanus, viral myelitis, mycobacteria, toxoplasmosis, Creutzfeldt-Jakob disease, parasites, neurosyphilis, polio (including postpolio syndrome)
Toxin	Lathyrism, N_2O abuse
Inflammatory	Idiopathic acute transverse myelitis, sarcoidosis, Behçet syndrome

(continued)

TABLE 8–11. ETIOLOGIC CATEGORIES FOR DISORDERS AFFECTING THE SPINAL CORD (*CONTINUED*)	
Etiologic Category	**Condition**
Autoimmune	Multiple sclerosis, stiff-man syndrome
Other	Radiation myelopathy, decompression sickness, intraspinal injections

AIDS = acquired immunodeficiency syndrome; ALS = amyotrophic lateral sclerosis; HIV = human immunodeficiency virus; HTLV-I = human T-cell lymphotrophic virus type I; NA = not applicable; N$_2$O = nitrous oxide; TIA = transient ischemic attack.

normal mentally, awake, alert, and able to converse (though perhaps dysarthric); they are not demented, confused, or aphasic.

Ancillary tests usually most helpful in the workup of suspected brainstem disease include imaging studies, evoked potentials, CSF analysis, and sometimes electromyography (EMG).

CRANIAL NERVE DISEASE

Sometimes a disease process selectively involves one, or occasionally more than one, cranial nerve. The long tract abnormalities, vertigo, ataxia, and similar symptoms and findings that are otherwise characteristic of intrinsic brainstem disease are lacking. Common cranial neuropathies include optic neuropathy due to multiple sclerosis (MS), third cranial nerve palsy as a result of aneurysm, and Bell palsy. Involvement of more than one nerve occurs in conditions such as Lyme disease, sarcoidosis, and lesions involving the cavernous sinus.

Ancillary tests usually most helpful in the workup of suspected cranial nerve disease include imaging studies, CSF analysis, evoked potentials, and EMG.

CEREBELLAR DISEASE

Patients with cerebellar dysfunction suffer from various combinations of tremor, incoordination, difficulty walking, dysarthria, and nystagmus, depending on the parts of the cerebellum involved. Disease involving the cerebellar connections in the brainstem causes abnormalities indistinguishable from disease of the cerebellum itself. The term ataxia essentially means incoordination, and can be caused by disease involving other parts of the nervous system, including the PNS, posterior columns of the spinal cord, and frontal lobe. Cerebellar ataxia is a specific type of ataxia seen with cerebellar disease; it has specific fea-

TABLE 8–12. ETIOLOGIC CATEGORIES FOR DISORDERS AFFECTING NERVE ROOTS

Etiologic Category	Condition
Tumor	Nerve sheath tumors, especially neurofibroma; cauda equina syndrome
Drugs or alcohol	NA
Imbalance	NA
Mass lesion	Tumor, herniated nucleus pulposus, osteophytic spur
Seizure or sleep disorder	NA
Trauma	Herniated nucleus pulposus, osteophytic spur, root avulsion
Degenerative	Degenerative disk disease and degenerative joint disease are contributory to most radiculopathies
Migraine	NA
Demyelinating disease	AIDP/CIDP
Congenital	Tethered cord
Bleeding	Hematoma (rare)
Stroke or TIA	NA
Hereditary	NA
Psychiatric	NA
Systemic	Diabetes (lumbosacral radiculoplexopathy)
Infectious	Lyme disease, Herpes zoster (including postherpetic neuralgia), CMV
Toxin	NA
Inflammatory	AIDP/CIDP, arachnoiditis
Autoimmune	AIDP/CIDP

AIDP/CIDP = acute/chronic inflammatory demyelinating polyradiculoneuropathy; CMV = cytomegalovirus; NA = not applicable; TIA = transient ischemic attack.

tures that usually allow the clinician to separate it from the other causes of ataxia. When cerebellar ataxia results from dysfunction of the cerebellar connections in the brainstem, there are usually other brainstem signs.

Ancillary tests usually most helpful in the workup of suspected cerebellar disease include imaging studies, CSF analysis, antineuronal antibodies, genetic studies, and sometimes evoked potentials.

TABLE 8–13. ETIOLOGIC CATEGORIES FOR DISORDERS AFFECTING THE BRACHIAL OR LUMBOSACRAL PLEXUS

Etiologic Category	Condition
Tumor	Nerve sheath tumors, Pancoast tumor, metastases (especially with breast, colon), lymphoma, radiotherapy
Drugs or alcohol	Immunizations, interleukin-2, interferon, heroin, botulinum toxin
Imbalance	NA
Mass lesion	Tumors
Seizure or sleep disorder	NA
Trauma	Traction injuries, especially motorcycle accidents, shoulder dislocation, external pressure (e.g., "Posey palsy"), penetrating wounds, cardiac surgery, internal jugular line placement, complication of first-rib resection for thoracic outlet syndrome, obstetrical or birth injury to child: brachial plexus (Erb palsy, Klumpke palsy), obstetrical or birth injury to mother: lumbar plexus
Degenerative	NA
Migraine	NA
Demyelinating disease	NA
Congenital	Erb palsy, Klumpke palsy (usually birth injuries)
Bleeding	Retroperitoneal hemorrhage, usually due to anticoagulants, can cause lumbosacral plexopathy
Stroke or TIA	NA
Hereditary	Hereditary neuralgic amyotrophy, hereditary neuropathy with liability to pressure palsy, Ehlers-Danlos syndrome
Psychiatric	NA
Systemic	Diabetes (lumbosacral radiculoplexopathy); collagen vascular disease, especially SLE, vasculitis; post liver transplant; aortic aneurysm (lumbar); sarcoid; amyloid
Infectious	Lyme disease, immunizations, viral infection, retroperitoneal abscess
Toxin	Some drugs (see DRUGS OR ALCOHOL)
Inflammatory	Neuralgic amyotrophy, (also known as brachial plexitis, Parsonage-Turner syndrome)
Autoimmune	Postinfectious or postvaccinial neuralgic amyotrophy, serum sickness
Other	Bradley syndrome (lumbar)

NA = not applicable; SLE = systemic lupus erythematosus; TIA = transient ischemic attack.

TABLE 8–14. ETIOLOGIC CATEGORIES FOR DISORDERS AFFECTING PERIPHERAL NERVES

Etiologic Category	Condition
Tumor	Nerve sheath tumors (schwannomas, neurofibromas, malignant nerve sheath tumors), paraneoplastic effects, neurolymphomatosis
Drugs or alcohol	Alcoholic neuropathy, chemotherapy, antiretroviral treatment, many others (see Toxin)
Imbalance	Hypothyroidism, low vitamin B_{12}, nutritional deficiency, deficiency of vitamins B_1 or E, excess or deficiency of vitamin B_6
Mass lesion	Nerve sheath tumors
Seizure or sleep disorder	NA
Trauma	Traumatic mononeuropathy; acute and chronic forms; injury by IM injections (injection palsy)
Degenerative	NA
Migraine	NA
Demyelinating disease	AIDP/CIDP and variants, osteosclerotic myeloma
Congenital	See Hereditary
Bleeding	Compression mononeuropathy due to hematoma
Stroke or TIA	Nerve infarction (e.g., vasculitis)
Hereditary	Charcot-Marie-Tooth disease, hereditary sensory neuropathy, a(alpha/beta)lipoproteinemia, Fabry disease, amyloidosis, Refsum disease, porphyria, mucopolysaccharidosis (carpal tunnel syndrome), others
Psychiatric	NA
Systemic	Paraneoplastic effects, connective tissue disease, sarcoid, diabetes mellitus, critical illness polyneuropathy, uremia, malnutrition, amyloid, paraproteinemias (MGUS, POEMS), acromegaly
Infectious	Leprosy, HIV, Lyme disease, diphtheria
Toxin	Heavy metals, many industrial and environmental poisons (lead, arsenic, methylbutylketone, n-hexane, and acrylamide), pharmaceutical agents (cancer chemotherapy, isoniazid, metronidazole, disulfiram, nitrofurantoin, pyridoxine, amiodarone, antiretroviral agents, nitrous oxide, and many others), ciguatera toxin, tetrodotoxin, saxitoxin
Inflammatory	AIDP/CIDP and variants, mononeuritis multiplex, vasculitic neuropathy, primary or secondary, sarcoidosis

(continued)

TABLE 8–14. ETIOLOGIC CATEGORIES FOR DISORDERS AFFECTING PERIPHERAL NERVES (*CONTINUED*)

Etiologic Category	Condition
Autoimmune	AIDP/CIDP and variants
Other	Causalgia/reflex sympathetic dystrophy/complex regional pain syndrome, neuromyotonia, painful legs and moving toes

AIDP/CIDP = acute/chronic inflammatory demyelinating polyradiculoneuropathy; HIV = human immunodeficiency virus; IM = intramuscularly; MGUS = monoclonal gammopathy of unknown significance; NA = not applicable; TIA = transient ischemic attack.

SPINAL CORD DISEASE

Instead of having decreased reflexes, as with peripheral neuropathy, patients with spinal cord disease tend to have increased reflexes because of loss of upper motor neuron modulation. Patients with acute myelopathies, such as spinal cord injury, often go through a period of spinal shock when reflexes are depressed. As the spinal shock phase resolves over several days to several weeks, or if the myelopathy evolves slowly such as with cord compression, the characteristic finding is hyperreflexia. With most myelopathies, there is symmetric involvement below a particular level. For example, with a problem at T8, the patient has symmetric weakness in both legs (paraparesis). A lesion at C3 causes symmetric weakness of all four extremities (quadriparesis). Patients with spinal cord disease also tend to develop sphincter dysfunction. Bladder dysfunction is often an early and prominent symptom; always ask about bladder problems when thinking about the possibility of a spinal cord process. Thus, the hallmarks of spinal cord disease are symmetry of the process below a certain level, increased reflexes together with the development of pathological reflexes such as the Babinski sign, and the involvement of bowel and bladder. Patients with peripheral nerve disease rarely have bowel and bladder problems. In addition to weakness below the level of the lesion, patients with spinal cord lesions may also have paresthesias, numbness, tingling, and sensory loss. A discrete sensory "level," usually on the trunk, is one of the most telltale signs of a transverse myelopathy (see Chapter 6, Figure 6–1C).

Ancillary tests usually most helpful in the workup of suspected spinal cord disease include imaging studies, CSF analysis, vitamin B level, and evoked potential studies.

TABLE 8–15. ETIOLOGIC CATEGORIES FOR DISORDERS AFFECTING THE NEUROMUSCULAR JUNCTION

Etiologic Category	Condition
Tumor	Thymoma (myasthenia gravis), carcinoma of the lung (Lambert-Eaton myasthenic syndrome)
Drugs or alcohol	Many drugs affect neuromuscular transmission, including antiarrhythmics, numerous antibiotics, morphine, paralytic agents (curare, vecuronium), barbiturates, and other tranquilizers
Imbalance	Hypermagnesemia
Mass lesion	NA
Seizure or sleep disorder	NA
Trauma	NA
Degenerative	NA
Migraine	NA
Demyelinating disease	NA
Congenital	Congenital myasthenic syndromes
Bleeding	NA
Stroke or TIA (ischemic event)	NA
Hereditary	See CONGENITAL
Psychiatric	"Neurasthenia" (may simulate)
Systemic	Thyroid disorders, connective tissue disease often associated
Infectious	Botulism
Toxin	Curare, botulism, tick paralysis, black-widow-spider bites, some snake bites
Inflammatory	NA
Autoimmune	Myasthenia gravis, Lambert-Eaton myasthenic syndrome, penicillamine, transient neonatal myasthenia gravis

NA = not applicable; TIA = transient ischemic attack.

TABLE 8–16. ETIOLOGIC CATEGORIES FOR MUSCLE DISEASE

Etiologic Category	Condition
Tumor	Rhabdomyosarcoma, paraneoplastic myopathy
Drugs or alcohol	Alcoholic myopathy, toxic myopathy, neuroleptic malignant syndrome, drug-induced malignant hyperthermia, steroid myopathy, critical illness myopathy, numerous other drug-induced myopathies (including chloroquine, AZT, statins, colchicine, eosinophilia myalgia syndrome, injection fibrosis), drug-induced rhabdomyolysis
Imbalance	Hypokalemia, hypo/hyperthyroidism, Cushing syndrome, metabolic myopathy, hyperparathyroidism
Mass lesion	NA
Seizure or sleep disorder	Postseizure rhabdomyolysis, chronic fatigue syndrome or fibromyalgia (often associated with sleep disturbance)
Trauma	Traumatic rhabdomyolysis, crush injuries, overexertion
Degenerative	Dystrophies; inclusion body myositis; proximal myotonic myopathy; chronic progressive external ophthalmoplegia syndromes
Migraine	NA
Demyelinating disease	NA
Congenital	Congenital myopathies (central core, myotubular)
Bleeding	Muscle hematoma
Stroke or TIA	Muscle infarction (diabetics most commonly)
Hereditary	Hereditary myopathies including muscular dystrophies (myotonic, Duchenne-Becker, FSH, limb girdle the most common), periodic paralysis syndromes, metabolic myopathies, mitochondrial myopathies, myotonia congenita, glycogen storage diseases, paramyotonia syndromes, distal myopathies
Psychiatric	Diffuse, chronic myalgias
Systemic	Sarcoid, connective tissue diseases, steroid therapy
Infectious	HIV-related myopathy, trichinosis, *Staphylococcus aureus,* mycobacteria, viral myositis
Toxin	Toxin-induced rhabdomyolysis (see DRUGS OR ALCOHOL)
Inflammatory	Polymyositis or dermatomyositis; inclusion body myositis, vasculitis
Autoimmune	Polymyositis or dermatomyositis, inclusion body myositis, vasculitis
Other	Fibromyalgia, chronic fatigue syndrome, continuous-muscle-fiber-activity syndromes, cramp disorders

AZT = zidovudine; FSH = follicle-stimulating hormone; HIV = human immunodeficiency virus; NA = not applicable; TIA = transient ischemic attack.

TABLE 8–17. ETIOLOGIC CATEGORIES FOR MULTIFOCAL OR DIFFUSE DISORDERS

Etiologic Category	Condition
Tumor	Gliomatosis or lymphomatosis cerebri, metastases
Drugs or alcohol	many; for example, alcohol, amiodarone, colchicine, chemotherapeutic agents
Imbalance	Most imbalances have multiple or diffuse effects
Mass lesion	Abscesses, metastases
Seizure or sleep disorder	some patients have multiple seizure types
Trauma	Multiple injuries, especially physical abuse, battering (child, spouse, or elder)
Degenerative	Amyotrophic lateral sclerosis, sporadic "spinocerebellar" degenerations, multisystem atrophy (striatonigral degeneration, olivopontocerebellar degeneration, Shy-Drager syndrome)
Migraine	NA
Demyelinating disease	Multiple sclerosis, acute disseminated encephalomyelitis, leukodystrophies, Devic disease, progressive multifocal leukoencephalopathy
Congenital	Many congenital syndromes involve multiple defects
Bleeding	Hemangioblastoma (von Hippel-Lindau disease), multiple aneurysms, bleeding dyscrasia
Stroke or TIA	Embolism, multi-infarct dementia
Hereditary	Many inborn metabolic errors and storage diseases (e.g., adrenoleukodystrophy, adrenomyeloneuropathy, MELAS, Machado-Joseph disease, lipidosis, leukodystrophy, hereditary ataxia syndromes, Lafora disease)
Psychiatric	Hysteria, malingering
Systemic	Heart disease, especially atrial fibrillation, subacute bacterial endocarditis, myxoma; connective tissue disease; anticardiolipin syndrome; thrombotic thrombocytopenic purpura
Infectious	Abscess, neurosyphilis, tuberculosis, some fungal infections, Creutzfeldt-Jakob disease, new-variant Creutzfeldt-Jakob disease (human "mad cow" disease), subacute sclerosing panencephalitis, Rocky Mountain spotted fever, Whipple disease
Toxin	Many toxins have multiple effects (e.g., lead and arsenic can both cause encephalopathy and neuropathy)
Inflammatory	Vasculitis
Autoimmune	Anticardiolipin syndrome
Other	Chronic fatigue syndrome

MELAS = mitochondrial encephalomyopathy; NA = not applicable; TIA = transient ischemic attack.

TABLE 8–18. ETIOLOGIC CATEGORIES FOR DISORDERS AFFECTING THE MENINGES OR VENTRICULAR SYSTEM OR FOR CAUSING ISOLATED ABNORMALITIES OF INTRACRANIAL PRESSURE

Etiologic Category	Condition
Tumor	Meningioma, carcinomatous or lymphomatous meningitis, choroid plexus papilloma, colloid cyst of the third ventricle, leptomeningeal gliomatosis
Drugs or alcohol	NSAIDs and other agents causing aseptic meningitis (Bactrim, IVIG, INH, Imuran, OKT-3, and others)
Imbalance	Hypothyroidism, hyperthyroidism, and diabetes may change CSF protein
Mass lesion	Gumma
Seizure or sleep disorder	Postictal pleocytosis
Trauma	CSF rhinorrhea or otorrhea, leptomeningeal cyst
Degenerative	NA
Migraine	Abnormal CSF may occur in complicated migraine
Demyelinating disease	NA
Congenital	Meningocele, arachnoid cyst, hydrocephalus
Bleeding	Subdural or epidural hematoma, dural arteriovenous malformation, bleeding dyscrasia
Stroke or TIA	NA
Hereditary	NA
Psychiatric	NA
Systemic	Meningitis in connective tissue disorders (e.g., systemic lupus erythematosus, vasculitis, sarcoid)
Infectious	Meningitis (bacterial; viral; mycobacterial; fungal, especially cryptococcus), syphilis, Lyme disease, rickettsia, parasites
Toxin	Drugs (see DRUGS OR ALCOHOL), chemical meningitis, lead intoxication (increased intracranial pressure, abnormal CSF)
Inflammatory	Recurrent meningitis (Mollaret and similar syndromes), arachnoiditis, Vogt-Koyanagi-Harada syndrome, Behçet syndrome, inflammatory pseudotumor cerebri
Autoimmune	Connective tissue disorders
Other	Epidural lipomatosis, normal pressure hydrocephalus or other common hydrocephalus syndromes, pseudotumor cerebri, eclampsia, postlumbar puncture headache

CSF = cerebrospinal fluid; INH = isoniazid; IVIG = intravenous immunoglobulin; NA = not applicable; NSAID = nonsteroidal antiinflammatory; OKT-3 = anti-CD3 monoclonal antibody; TIA = transient ischemic attack.

TABLE 8–19. ETIOLOGIC CATEGORIES FOR DISORDERS AFFECTING THE VASCULAR SYSTEM

Etiologic Category	Condition
Tumor	Malignant angioendotheliomatosis, lymphomatoid granulomatosis
Drugs or alcohol	Amphetamines, cocaine, oral contraceptives, heroin, LSD, IV drug abuse of any type
Imbalance	Dehydration (venous occlusion)
Mass lesion	NA
Seizure or sleep disorder	NA
Trauma	Arterial dissection due to head or neck injury
Degenerative	Atherosclerosis, amyloid angiopathy, giant aneurysm
Migraine	Hemiplegic migraine, basilar artery migraine, completed stroke
Demyelinating disease	NA
Congenital	Saccular aneurysm, arteriovenous malformation, Sturge-Weber syndrome, fibromuscular dysplasia
Bleeding	Bleeding dyscrasia, aneurysms, arteriovenous malformations, carotid cavernous fistula
Stroke or TIA	NA
Hereditary	Hemoglobinopathies, factor V Leiden deficiency protein C deficiency, protein S deficiency, antithrombin III deficiency, homocystinuria, neurofibromatosis, MELAS, Fabry disease, CADASIL
Psychiatric	NA
Systemic	Anticardiolipin syndrome, polycythemia, hyperviscosity syndromes, thrombocytosis, thrombotic thrombocytopenic purpura, cardiac embolic source (e.g., valvular disease, endocarditis, atrial myxoma, patent foramen ovale)
Infectious	Mycotic aneurysm, subacute bacterial endocarditis, syphilis, cerebral malaria, varicella zoster virus, aspergillosis
Toxin	NA
Inflammatory	Granulomatous angiitis of the nervous system, systemic vasculitis (temporal arteritis, polyarteritis nodosa, Wegener granulomatosis, Churg-Strauss vasculitis, Takayasu arteritis, Behçet syndrome, thrombotic thrombocytopenic purpura)
Autoimmune	Anticardiolipin syndrome and other connective tissue disorders

(continued)

TABLE 8–19. ETIOLOGIC CATEGORIES FOR DISORDERS AFFECTING THE VASCULAR SYSTEM (*CONTINUED*)

Etiologic Category	Condition
Other	Asymptomatic bruit, carotid sinus syncope, carotidynia, sinus thrombosis, venous and sinus occlusion, marasmus, pregnancy, hypertensive encephalopathy, fibromuscular dysplasia, moyamoya disease, radiation vasculopathy

CADASIL = cerebral autosomal dominant arteriopathy with subcortical infarcts and leukoencephalopathy; IV = intravenous; LSD = lysergic acid diethylamide; MELAS = mitochondrial encephalomyopathy, lactic acidosis, and stroke-like episodes; NA = not applicable; TIA = transient ischemic attack.

NERVE ROOT DISEASE

Most radiculopathies are due to disc herniations or spondylosis. Occasionally such disparate conditions as diabetes, viral infection (especially herpes zoster or cytomegalovirus), or Lyme disease can present as a radiculopathy or polyradiculopathy. The patient typically has a motor or sensory deficit, or both, and a depressed deep tendon reflex in the distribution of one or more roots. When caused by disc disease or spondylosis, there is usually pain and limitation of motion of either the neck or lower back along with signs of root irritability, such as a positive straight-leg-raising test.

Ancillary tests usually most helpful in the workup of suspected nerve root disease include EMG and imaging studies.

PLEXUS DISEASE

Diseases involving the brachial plexus are much more common than those involving the lumbosacral plexus. Patients with plexus disorders have a clinical deficit that mirrors the involved structures; the clinical complaints and deficits typically reflect involvement of more than one nerve in a single extremity. A knowledge of plexus anatomy is vital to deciphering the deficit. Most brachial plexopathies result from trauma, especially from motorcycle accidents. Inflammatory disorders of the brachial plexus (neuralgic amyotrophy, also called brachial plexitis or Parsonage-Turner syndrome) are notoriously painful. Plexus involvement may occur with tumors, especially Pancoast tumor, carcinoma of the breast, and tumors in the pelvis.

Ancillary tests usually most helpful in the workup of suspected plexopathy include EMG and imaging studies.

TABLE 8–20. ETIOLOGIC CATEGORIES FOR DISORDERS AFFECTING THE SKULL AND VERTEBRAL COLUMN

Etiologic Category	Condition
Tumor	Dermoid, epidermoid, chondroma, chondrosarcoma, clivus chordoma, metastasis
Drugs or alcohol	NA
Imbalance	Metabolic bone disease
Mass lesion	Intracranial extension of skull tumor (e.g., dermoid)
Seizure/sleep disorder	NA
Trauma	Fractures, dislocations
Degenerative	Basilar impression, platybasia
Migraine	NA
Demyelinating disease	NA
Congenital	Acrocephalosyndactyly, craniosynostosis, aneurysmal bone cyst, brachycephaly, microcephaly, anencephaly, various types of skull deformities, Arnold-Chiari malformations, Crouzon syndrome, Klippel-Feil syndrome, cervical block vertebrae, basilar impression, platybasia
Bleeding	NA
Stroke or TIA	NA
Hereditary	Achondroplasia, ankylosing spondylitis, osteopetrosis
Psychiatric	NA
Systemic	Subluxation of C1–2 is a common complication of rheumatoid arthritis and Down syndrome, Paget disease
Infectious	Osteomyelitis, Pott disease
Toxin	NA
Inflammatory	NA
Autoimmune	NA
Other	Fibrous dysplasia, musculoskeletal low back pain

NA = not applicable; TIA = transient ischemic attack.

PERIPHERAL NERVE DISEASE

Peripheral nerve diseases are divided into polyneuropathies (all the nerves are affected) and mononeuropathies. In multiple mononeuropathy (mononeuritis multiplex), more than one nerve is affected but not all (see Part III). With a mononeuropathy, symptoms and signs are specifically related to the affected nerve. Patients with a polyneuropathy often have symptoms of distal weakness: trouble turning keys in locks, trouble handling small objects, and weakness of the feet and ankles with a tendency to stub the toe because of foot drop or to sprain the ankle because of ankle instability. Patients commonly have paresthesias, numbness, and sometimes burning pain in the feet. Patients with myopathy or NMJ disorders have no sensory complaints or abnormalities; if a patient has sensory symptoms or findings, these localizations can be excluded. Examination of a patient with polyneuropathy usually discloses predominantly distal weakness, and sensory loss in a "stocking-glove distribution" (see Chapter 6, Figure 6–1E). This is referred to as a "dying-back" pattern, wherein the nerve dysfunction is roughly proportional to the axon length; the longest fibers in the body are most affected, producing a distal emphasis of signs and symptoms.

Another common manifestation of nerve disease is depression of reflexes. With an ordinary axonal polyneuropathy (a primary problem with the axon itself), the most distal reflexes disappear first, so patients tend to lose the ankle jerks. As the disease progresses, knee jerks and then upper extremity reflexes fade. Patients with demyelinating polyneuropathies, which typically affect all the nerves simultaneously, tend to lose all reflexes at once. GBS is a common example. The patient may have hyporeflexia or areflexia early on, even before noticeable weakness.

Ancillary tests usually most helpful in the workup of suspected peripheral neuropathy include clinical laboratory assessment (e.g., vitamin B_{12} level, thyroid function tests, antinuclear antibody, and others), nerve conduction studies, needle EMG, lumbar puncture, occasionally nerve biopsy, and genetic analysis.

NEUROMUSCULAR JUNCTION DISORDERS

NMJ diseases include MG, Lambert-Eaton syndrome, botulism, hypermagnesemia, and others. The most common condition by far is MG. Patients with NMJ disorders usually have proximal muscle weakness, which can simulate a myopathy, but in addition usually have bulbar involvement. Most commonly patients have weakness of eye movement that causes double vision, or ptosis of one or both eyelids. They may have trouble talking and swallowing, with a tendency to nasal regurgitation of fluids. Such symptoms and signs of bulbar weakness are one of the main differentiating features between an NMJ disease and a myopathy.

Ancillary tests usually most helpful in the workup of suspected NMJ disease include nerve conduction tests with repetitive stimulation, routine EMG, single-fiber EMG, and serologic testing for anti-acetylcholine receptor antibodies.

MUSCLE DISEASE

Muscle diseases include muscular dystrophies and inflammatory, metabolic, and congenital myopathies, to list a few. Patients with muscle disease usually have symmetric, proximal weakness. They have trouble getting up from a chair, difficulty getting out of a car, and difficulty raising their arms overhead. Patients often have difficulty with everyday grooming activities, such as shaving or handling hair and makeup. Early on, patients with muscle disease switch from tub baths to showers because they cannot get out of the tub. Patients may or may not have muscle pain, tenderness, or soreness; usually they do not. The examination typically reveals proximal weakness that reflects the clinical complaint. In contrast, peripheral nerve disease tends to produce distal weakness. While a good general rule is that muscle disease causes proximal weakness and generalized peripheral nerve disease causes distal weakness, there are exceptions. For instance, myotonic dystrophy is a common muscular dystrophy that produces distal weakness, and GBS is a common peripheral nerve disease that frequently produces proximal weakness.

Ancillary tests usually helpful in the workup of suspected muscle disease include serum creatine kinase, EMG, muscle biopsy, and genetic analysis.

DISORDERS OF THE MENINGES AND VENTRICULAR SYSTEM

Many conditions can affect the meninges, including infections, neoplasia, sarcoidosis, extracerebral fluid collections, and others. The most common disorders are infections and SDHs. Meningitis usually presents with evidence of infection and increased intracranial pressure, but some meningeal infections may be extremely indolent, lacking the classic signs associated with infection. Chronic meningitis can also present as dementia or altered mental status (AMS). Abnormalities of the ventricular system can occur with congenital anomalies, such as aqueductal stenosis, or with acquired conditions such as normal pressure hydrocephalus. Dilatation of the ventricular system may cause head enlargement in children. In adults such conditions usually present with evidence of increased intracranial pressure or with dementia, AMS, gait problems, or difficulty with bladder control.

The ancillary tests most helpful in the workup of a suspected meningeal process are imaging studies and CSF analysis.

DISORDERS OF THE VASCULAR SYSTEM

Diseases affecting the vascular system typically present as an ischemic or hemorrhagic event, either single or multiple. The usual clue to a vasculopathy is the occurrence of multiple events involving different parts of the nervous system. Other presentations, such as dementia, can occur as well. Obviously, atherosclerosis and hypertensive arteriosclerosis are the most common examples of disease processes primarily affecting the vascular system but there are others, such as vasculitis, amyloid angiopathy, moyamoya disease, Takayasu disease, and anticardiolipin syndrome.

Ancillary tests usually most helpful in the workup of suspected diffuse vascular disease are imaging studies (including angiography), sedimentation rate, blood work, and studies to rule out cardiac disease.

DISORDERS OF THE SKULL AND VERTEBRAL COLUMN

Disorders of the skull and vertebral column range from the mundane and minimally significant, such as spina bifida occulta, to the horrific, such as disfiguring craniosynostosis syndromes. The most common conditions are due to trauma, such as skull or spinal fractures. Occasionally patients with bony tumors may present with localized pain. Sometimes bony lesions are picked up as incidental findings on radiographic studies done for other reasons. Congenital and developmental skeletal disorders may be immediately obvious at birth, such as myelomeningocele, or present well into adulthood, such as occult spinal dysraphism.

Pathological findings of the skull and spine may be limited to a bony abnormality, such as a linear skull fracture or spondylolysis, or may also involve neural structures, such as a depressed skull fracture or diastematomyelia. In the absence of trauma, the challenge is to remember to consider the possibility of a congenital or developmental skull or spinal disorder, even in the adult patient.

The ancillary test usually most helpful in the workup of suspected bony disease is an imaging study.

MULTIFOCAL OR DIFFUSE DISORDERS

Some disease processes are diffuse or multifocal, producing dysfunction at more than one location, or involving a "system." For example, Devic disease, a form of MS, characteristically affects both the spinal cord and the optic nerves; that is, it is multifocal. ALS is a system disorder causing diffuse dysfunction of the entire motor system from the spinal cord to the cerebral cortex, sparing sensation and higher cortical function.

The full array of ancillary tests may be required in the workup of patients with a suspected multifocal or diffuse process.

Differential Diagnosis by Etiology

From a differential diagnostic standpoint, it is usually most helpful to think first about the "where," the localization of the disease process in the nervous system, and secondarily about the "what," the etiology. If the "where" exercise concludes that the patient has cerebral hemispheric disease, then muscular dystrophy, MG, and GBS will not rank high on the differential diagnostic list of etiologic possibilities; those processes do not cause dysfunction in that location. Knowing the likely location of the pathological process generally places the condition into a broad differential diagnostic category. Occasionally the "what" is obvious, such as stroke or CNS trauma, and the diagnostic exercise focuses mostly on the "where."

The best learning approach to the consideration of possible causes for a disease process in a particular location is to think first about broad categories of disease (such as neoplasia, degenerative disease, vascular disease, trauma, and so forth) and move into a specific etiologic diagnosis secondarily. It helps the novice to consciously think in such a systematic fashion. Experienced clinicians often use this sort of exercise when the diagnosis is not immediately obvious through "augenblickdiagnose," or pattern recognition, but the mental processing is so fast the operation may seem to be at an almost subconscious level. The more challenging the case, the greater the likelihood that the clinician will consciously resort to systematic analysis. Some cases defy even the systematic scrutiny of an astute and experienced clinician. One of the enduring attractions of neurology is the humility it engenders in its practitioners.

Many physicians use mnemonics or other systems to cue disease categories. There are numerous possible systems, the most effective being highly idiosyncratic. Creating an individualized mnemonic is by far the best way to sear these categories into memory. The truly effective mnemonics are ridiculous, obscene, set to music, or a combination of these features.

Most mnemonic systems that are used for general medicine do not incorporate some of the etiologic disease categories essential to neurology. These special neurologic disease categories include migraine, degenerative diseases, demyelinating diseases, mass lesions, and seizures and other paroxysmal disorders.

The following neurologic mnemonic is offered, which includes these uniquely neurologic disease categories. The format is that of a limerick. Each word in the limerick is designed to cue the disease category as a rhyme, sound alike, or other trigger. "Migraineuse" is French for "a woman who suffers from migraine." As a crude device, this limerick can be sung, more or less, to the tune of "The Mexican Hat Dance."

A neurologic disease category mnemonic

Two drunk imbalanced masseuses
Seized three degenerate migraineuses
Ms. Congeniality bled

Stroking her psyche said
I tolerate flaming abuses

Form a mental picture of two intoxicated, mentally imbalanced masseuses assaulting three morally degenerate ladies who have migraine. One is conked on the head and bleeds, then, stroking her psyche, says the final sentence. The disease categories these words are intended to cue are as follows. More detail is included in subsequent sections.

Two = tumor, neurologic syndromes related to neoplasms, both direct and indirect

Drunk = alcohol, drugs or other exogenous substances, including medications

Imbalanced = imbalances in body constituents (e.g. electrolytes, hormones, vitamins)

Masseueses = mass lesions

Seized = seizures, including all ictal and para-ictal phenomenon, as well as sleep disorders

Three = trauma

Degenerate = degenerative diseases

Migraineuses = migraine, including all variants and related syndromes

Ms. = multiple sclerosis and other demyelinating diseases

Congeniality = congenital disorders

Bled = hemorrhagic conditions

Stroking = ischemic cerebrovascular disease

Her = heredofamilial conditions

Psyche = psychiatric disease

Said = systemic diseases, neurologic complications of

I = infections and parainfectious syndromes

Tolerate = toxins

Flaming = inflammatory diseases, noninfection related

Abuses = antibody mediated and other autoimmune conditions

Tables 8–6 through 8–20 summarize possible etiologic categories for disease processes at various locations in the nervous system, beginning centrally with the cerebral hemispheres and moving progressively peripherally with muscle disorders. The order is arbitrary. The intent is to encourage systematic analysis and to provide a checklist, albeit incomplete, of disease processes likely to affect each part of the nervous system. Certain conditions overlap to a degree by logically fitting into more than one etiologic category. This is not a bad thing, and overlap and redundancy are favored when an option appears.

The following paragraphs summarize the typical clinical behavior of diseases in the etiologic categories used in the mnemonic. These disorders are covered in more detail in Part III. This section is intended to provide only a broad overview of the general clinical behavior of different types of diseases. Some entities mentioned in the tables are beyond the scope of this book and require a look at more detailed sources for further information.

TUMOR

Tumor should trigger a consideration of the direct effects of a neoplasm (e.g., a patient with a focal deficit due to a primary brain tumor) and the possibility of a remote effect of a systemic cancer (e.g., cerebellar degeneration due to carcinoma of the ovary). There is no essential difference between the clinical examinations of a patient with a left hemispheric syndrome due to glioblastoma multiforme and of a patient with the same syndrome due to middle cerebral artery stroke, but there is usually a difference in onset and progression. In contrast to the abrupt onset of vascular disease, tumors tend to have a gradual onset and a progressive course, usually over weeks to months. The history of progression is key. Metastatic brain tumors are much more common than primary lesions, and metastatic lesions are often multiple. Slow-growing tumors, such as meningiomas and low-grade gliomas, frequently present with seizures. More rapidly growing tumors, such as high-grade gliomas, are more likely to present with a progressive neurologic deficit. While most patients with a brain tumor have headache, it is not usually severe and only rarely does a patient with a tumor present because of headache.

In addition to metastatic deposits, systemic neoplasms can cause remote neurologic effects. The possibility of such a paraneoplastic syndrome often prompts a workup for an occult neoplasm in patients who primarily have neurologic complaints and findings.

ALCOHOL AND DRUGS

The term "drunk" is intended to trigger consideration of both the direct intoxicating effects of chemical substances and their complications. This includes substances of abuse and medicinal agents.

The direct intoxicating effects of alcohol are well known and obvious. In addition, chronic alcoholics are at risk of developing a host of neurologic complications, ranging from peripheral neuropathy to cerebellar degeneration. Not only alcoholics and young drug abusers taking "recreational" agents, but also older patients taking prescription and nonprescription medications may develop neurologic side effects and complications. Drugs and alcohol sometimes prove to be a factor in the most apparently unlikely circumstances.

IMBALANCES

Imbalance of body constituents, hyper- or hypo- natremia/calcemia/ glycemia/kalemia, as well as vitamin deficiency and overactivity or underactivity of various hormones, can lead to a number of neurologic syndromes. Metabolic disturbances tend to have fairly characteristic and typical clinical features, depending on the element (e.g., seizures with hyponatremia, muscle weakness with hypokalemia). Laboratory assessment is the key to diagnosis. The challenge lies in thinking to order the relevant laboratory test.

Patients with endocrine diseases often have neurologic complications. Hypothyroidism can present as progressive cerebellar ataxia, dementia, myopathy, or peripheral neuropathy. Hyperthyroidism can present as AMS, coma, or a syndrome resembling ALS. Hyperparathyroidism can cause a neuromuscular disease simulating myopathy. Hyperadrenalism and hypoadrenalism can both have prominent neurologic manifestations. There is seemingly no end to the neurologic complications of diabetes mellitus.

This element of the mnemonic overlaps with and serves as a crosscheck on "systemic diseases," since these neurologic syndromes are in essence neurologic complications of systemic disease. These conditions are relatively common.

MASS LESIONS

Mass lesions, or "space-occupying lesions" primarily cause focal deficits. The term "mass effect" refers to pressure exerted by a spaceoccupying lesion, such as a tumor, on other structures, causing intracranial tissue shifts, headache, papilledema, or other evidence of increased intracranial pressure. Mass effect is often due at least as much to the associated cerebral edema as to the lesion itself. Not all mass lesions cause mass effect. Indolent tumors that infiltrate but cause little edema are space occupying but produce little secondary mass effect. Patients with primary and metastatic tumors, abscesses, and other mass lesions are not uncommonly thought at first to have suffered a stroke.

SEIZURES AND SLEEP DISORDERS

Seizures are very common, and the topic can become complex. The most prevalent seizures in adults are generalized tonic clonic events. If witnessed, the diagnosis can usually be made by observer description. Such ictal events are unfortunately only the tip of the iceberg in terms of the potential neurologic manifestations of seizure disorders. Seizures may present in many other ways, such as with a postictal neurologic deficit

(Todd paralysis) or with a postictal stupor, in which the preceding seizure was not apparent. Rare patients in apparent coma suffer from subclinical status epilepticus. Seizure disorder is a routine consideration in the differential diagnosis of unexplained loss of consciousness. Atypical ictal events and postictal syndromes should be considered in patients with difficult-to-explain neurologic syndromes.

Sleep disorders may also present in many ways rather than with a complaint related to sleep, and the possibility of a sleep disorder is sometimes not at all apparent initially.

TRAUMA

Trauma is obvious most of the time, but relatively minor trauma may sometimes have neurologic sequelae. For example, older patients may develop a chronic SDH as a result of trivial and often unrecalled trauma, such as a bump on the head of which they have no recollection. The "trauma" may sometimes be a sneeze or an awkward movement, for example, in radiculopathy patients. Chronic low-grade repetitive trauma, as in repetitive motion injuries may be implicated in many entrapment neuropathies. So a traumatic cause is not necessarily excluded by the absence of an obvious history of trauma or external wounds.

DEGENERATIVE DISEASE

The term "degenerative disease" is applied to conditions for which we presently have an inadequate etiologic understanding, such as Alzheimer disease, ALS, or Parkinson disease. Although slower, the time course of degenerative disease resembles that of tumor in its inexorable progression. The tumor patient usually progresses over weeks to months, whereas the patient with a degenerative disease progresses over months to years. The diagnosis in degenerative disease usually lies in steady clinical progression, a recognizable clinical syndrome, and the exclusion of all else.

MIGRAINE

As with seizure disorders, the headache in migraine is only part of the disorder. Migraine may do many other things, and the diagnosis may be difficult, especially when the headache is only a minor component of the disorder. Migraine may mimic transient ischemic attack (retinal, hemispheric, or vertebrobasilar), cause stupor and alteration of consciousness, cause completed stroke, or present with ophthalmoplegia. Recognizing migraine as the underlying etiologic factor in such circumstances is often challenging.

MULTIPLE SCLEROSIS AND OTHER DEMYELINATING DISEASES

MS is the only common demyelinating disease, and the term "demyelinating disease" is essentially a euphemism for MS. Most MS patients have episodic disease with exacerbations and remissions over time, producing a fluctuating clinical coarse. Another demyelinating disease seen occasionally is acute disseminated encephalomyelitis. Although demyelinating peripheral neuropathies, such as GBS, are common, the term "demyelinating disease" as commonly used is restricted to CNS processes.

CONGENITAL DISORDERS

Pediatricians tend to see most congenital disorders, but adult patients sometimes present with congenital malformations. For instance, the Arnold-Chiari malformation consists of a hindbrain malformation with the cerebellar tonsils herniated into the foramen magnum. Although most patients present as newborns with associated myelomeningocele, occasional patients without associated myelomeningocele present as adults. The possibility of a congenital or developmental disorder must often be entertained even in adult patients.

HEMORRHAGIC CONDITIONS

Posttraumatic hemorrhage is common, and the trauma is usually obvious. Spontaneous hemorrhage may cause either a neurologic deficit, or pain, or both. Intracranial bleeding causes headache; intraspinal bleeding, which is much less common, causes backache. The deficit depends on where the hemorrhage occurs. Major intracranial hemorrhage is often associated with alteration of consciousness. With intracranial bleeding, the diagnosis is usually obvious on initial imaging studies, although computed tomography may miss cases of SAH and subacute SDH.

STROKE (ISCHEMIC EVENT, COMPLETED STROKE, OR TIA)

Ischemic vascular disease is primarily characterized by its tempo. The patient, although feeling otherwise well, experiences the sudden onset of a neurologic deficit, or discovers a deficit on awakening. The patient then usually stabilizes and often gets better, sometimes back to normal or nearly so. With TIAs, the deficit may resolve rapidly, over minutes to hours. Uncomplicated hemispheric ischemic lesions do not cause alteration of consciousness. Patients with very large hemispheric infarctions may develop obtundation and coma as cerebral edema evolves after the first 1–2 days, but not acutely. Loss of consciousness is not a typical feature of TIA, and prominent alteration of consciousness early in the course of a focal deficit makes a simple ischemic lesion much less likely.

HEREDOFAMILIAL DISORDERS

Inherited disease is most often seen in pediatric neurologic practice, but occasionally adult patients present with a genetic disorder (e.g., Huntington chorea). The diagnosis usually rests on the family history and clinical suspicion, though increasingly sophisticated genetic testing is becoming available.

PSYCHIATRIC DISEASE

Psychiatric disease as an etiologic category requires a caveat. Physicians, particularly when young and inexperienced, and particularly when confronted with an enigmatic patient, sometimes conclude that the problem must lie in the emotions of the patient rather than in an ailment or malady. The problem, in fact, may lie in the attitude of the physician rather than in the emotions of the patient. Many diseases, particularly neurologic diseases, may present with puzzling manifestations, which seem all the more so if the physician has not encountered the entity before. This tendency to assume puzzling symptoms have an emotional basis is particularly prominent when dealing with young female patients, and seems to affect female physicians no less noticeably than male physicians. Concluding the patient is hysterical can have dire consequences. Neurologic illnesses often initially diagnosed as hysteria, malingering, depression, anxiety, or another "functional" disorder include MG, MS, porphyria, GBS, and botulism (Enrichment Box 8–6). Failure of the doctor to fathom the patient's complaint does not mean the patient is crazy. When tempted to resort to such a conclusion, especially in the emergency room, relegate it to the bottom of your list of hypotheses until and unless evidence to the contrary becomes overwhelming, and a psychiatrist concurs that the patient has psychopathology sufficient to explain the clinical presentation. Adopt the axiom, "there are no hysterics in the emergency room." Emotional disease does occur and can be associated with neurologic complaints, but it should be a diagnosis of last resort, particularly for trainees.

SYSTEMIC DISORDERS

A great many systemic illnesses have neurologic complications, and on occasion a patient with systemic illness presents with the neurologic manifestations of the disease. Examples of neurologic complications of systemic illness include the peripheral neuropathy of systemic lupus erythematosus, the myopathy of scleroderma, the NMJ disturbance associated with carcinoma of the lung, hepatic encephalopathy, the facial nerve palsy of sarcoidosis, the focal seizures of nonketotic hyperosmolar hyperglycemia, and the myelopathy of pernicious anemia. Always bear in mind the possibility that the patient may not have a primary neu-

It has been estimated that the average patient with myasthenia gravis (MG) sees five to seven physicians before the correct diagnosis is made. Similar difficulties with diagnosis occur with multiple sclerosis (MS). It is axiomatic that the porphyric patient sees, in sequence, the surgeon, the psychiatrist, and then the neurologist. In one cooperative study on plasmapheresis in Guillain-Barré syndrome (GBS), young women with the illness were diagnosed as hysterical four times more frequently than men or older women; the average patient with GBS is sent home from the emergency room several times before the correct diagnosis is made. Patients with GBS have died while the physicians caring for them continued to presume the shortness of breath and paresthesias represented hyperventilation. According to the Centers for Disease Control and Prevention, the leading misdiagnoses in botulism are acute abdomen, pharyngitis, brainstem stroke, and hysteria. Malpractice litigation, sometimes with psychiatrists as codefendants, has involved patients who were diagnosed as hysterical or "functional" and who proved to have such things as cervical spine injury, hematomyelia, vertebral artery dissection with brainstem stroke, brainstem encephalitis, toxoplasmosis, Lyme disease, subarachnoid hemorrhage (SAH), transverse myelitis, vasculitis, and tuberous sclerosis. Patients have died while carrying an erroneous diagnosis of hysteria.

rologic disease, but rather, a neurologic complication of a systemic process. The systemic disease may not be at all obvious initially, hence the importance of the neurologist being a passable general internist.

INFECTIONS AND PARAINFECTIOUS SYNDROMES

Patients with an infectious process in the nervous system tend to have the same signs as patients with infection elsewhere: fever, increased white blood cell count, and so forth. Special features must be borne in mind. Only about half of the patients with a bacterial brain abscess have fever or an elevated white blood cell count. Patients with tuberculous or fungal meningitis may also have little evidence of systemic infection. Prion and chronic viral infections behave atypically, often simulating degenerative disease.

TOXIN EXPOSURE

Although drugs and medications can be considered toxins on occasion, the term is generally applied to agents with which a patient might have been poisoned, deliberately or accidentally. Particular syndromes, such as a peripheral neuropathy, raise the possibility of toxin exposure most often. Potential toxins include lead, arsenic, n-hexane (in patients who spray glue or model airplane paint into a paper sack and sniff it, so-called huffer's neuropathy), methylbutyl ketone (used in plastic manufacturing), toluene (also from huffing spray paint), carbon monoxide, organophosphate pesticides, and numerous others. The clue is generally a history of potential exposure in the workplace or a clinical syndrome known to be toxin induced. The key to the diagnosis is suspecting the possibility and doing the medical detective work to uncover the exposure.

INFLAMMATORY DISEASE

Noninfectious inflammatory diseases that may involve the nervous system include such things as sarcoidosis, vasculitis, and connective tissue disorders. There may or may not be evidence of a systemic disease process. Vasculitis can on occasion be limited to the CNS or to the PNS. Some patients with sarcoidosis present with a neurologic syndrome with scant evidence of systemic disease. Behçet disease is essentially a chronic vasculitis that may have prominent neurologic features.

AUTOIMMUNE DISORDERS

Many neurologic patients have an autoimmune disease, either as a primary neurologic process or as a complication of a systemic disease. MG, inflammatory myopathies, inflammatory neuropathies, and MS are all conditions of known or probable autoimmune origin. The key to recognition lies in recognizing a pathoanatomic location of disease known to be susceptible to autoimmune processes, such as the NMJ, and ordering the appropriate laboratory tests. The diagnosis may at times be very difficult.

9

Neurodiagnostic Testing

After completion of the history, the general physical and neurologic examinations, the formulation of a working differential diagnosis, and the performance of routine laboratory work, the next step in the workup of a neurologic patient is often to obtain specialized tests. These specialized tests include neuroimaging studies, electrophysiologic studies, examination of the cerebrospinal fluid (CSF), and certain blood tests. The anatomic localization derived from the history and neurologic examination determines which area(s) to image. Imaging the head is ineffective if the problem lies in the spinal cord.

Neuroimaging Studies

Radiographic imaging studies are mainstays of neurologic diagnosis in diseases involving the central nervous system (CNS), including the spinal cord and spinal roots. A significant number of patients with head injuries have an associated cervical spine injury. Plain films of the cervical spine, therefore, are a necessary part of the acute management of head and neck injuries. Except in cases of acute trauma, plain film studies have been largely supplanted by the more advanced techniques of computed tomography (CT) and magnetic resonance imaging (MRI).

COMPUTED TOMOGRAPHY

In a CT scan (Figure 9–1), an x-ray beam is transmitted from an x-ray delivery source to a detection source that lies 180° away on the opposite side of the patient. The beam source then rotates in a circle around the patient, transmitting beams from slightly different angles in succession to the detector. This process is repeated until the beam has been transmitted in increments throughout a 360° arc.

A computer then uses this information to calculate the density of a small portion of the imaged substance at each point where the beams

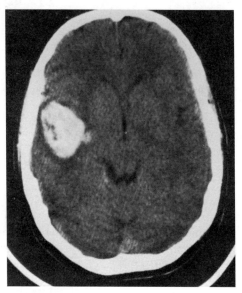

FIGURE 9–1. ■ Unenhanced computed tomography (CT) scan of the brain demonstrating a large intracerebral hemorrhage in the right Sylvian region. The bright appearance is typical of acute bleeding on CT scan. Compare this with the bright appearance of abnormal myelin on magnetic resonance imaging (MRI) in Figure 9–3. The appearance is similar but the pathophysiology is completely different. (Reprinted with permission from Wagle WA: Neuroradiology. In *Clinical Neurology*, Edited by Joynt RJ. Philadelphia, Lippincott Williams & Wilkins, 1992, p 101.)

intersect. This small piece of imaged substance is referred to as a pixel. The smaller the pixel, the more refined the final image. The size of the pixel is determined by several factors, including the sophistication of the system and the number of beams transmitted to obtain the image.

The current generation of CT scanners has two outstanding characteristics: small pixel size and fast scan time. The resolution allows the appreciation of fine detail. The rapid scan time makes CT ideal for dealing with acutely ill, injured, or uncooperative patients.

Additional information can often be obtained by repeating the CT scan after administration of intravenous radiographic contrast material. A small but finite incidence of complications is related to contrast administration, including allergic reactions, renal failure, and most commonly, nausea and vomiting. Contrast-enhanced CT is done much less often since MRI became available.

Once the computerized information is stored, CT images can be reconstructed in several ways. Sagittal and coronal images may be produced even though the scan is done axially. The computer settings may be manipulated to allow detection of tissues of various densities; these are referred to as window settings. With certain window settings, all of the brain tissue becomes a vague, monotonous mélange, while bony detail becomes very discrete. This is visualization by using bone windows, and is often used in a search for skull fractures, metastatic lesions, and other osseous abnormalities. By using tissue windows, the bony detail is less apparent and the CNS structures are better visualized.

The CT absorption coefficients of various tissues form a gray scale in which the appearance varies from black to white with many shades in between. The range of absorption coefficients is summarized in Table 9–1.

CT is frequently used to detect acute intracerebral hemorrhage in patients who have stroke syndromes before they are treated with tissue plasminogen activator and similar agents. Table 9–2 summarizes clinical situations in which CT may be preferable to MRI.

MAGNETIC RESONANCE IMAGING

MRI has largely supplanted CT scanning as the neuroimaging procedure of choice in most circumstances. MRI is possible because of the interrelatedness of electricity and magnetism. Flowing electrical current creates a magnetic field, and a moving magnet creates electrical current. Water protons are highly polar and behave like tiny magnets. The spinning motion of these tiny magnets creates electrical signals, which can be detected by the imaging equipment.

Under normal circumstances, the water protons in tissue have a random orientation. When placed in a strong magnetic field, these polar

---

TABLE 9–1 CT ABSORPTION COEFFICIENT RANGE FOR VARIOUS TISSUES

Darkest
- Air
- Fat
- Cerebrospinal fluid
- Brain
- Extravasated blood
- Contrast medium
- Bone

Lightest

CT = computed tomography.

TABLE 9–2 CIRCUMSTANCES IN WHICH COMPUTED TOMOGRAPHY (CT) OR MAGNETIC RESONANCE IMAGING (MRI) MAY BE MORE USEFUL

CT Preferable	MRI Preferable
Acute trauma	Contrast allergy
Ventilated patient	Renal insufficiency
Uncooperative patient	Evaluation of most parenchymal processes
Agitated patient	Evaluation of the meninges
Claustrophobic patient	Evaluation of the spinal cord
Suspicion of subarachnoid hemorrhage	
Suspicion of intracerebral hemorrhage	
Patient with pacemaker or other implanted device	
Patient with ferromagnetic aneurysm clip	
Evaluation of middle ear and paranasal sinuses	
Evaluation of skull base	
Evaluation of bony detail	

water protons line up in the same plane. During an MRI scan, the patient is placed in a strong magnet that creates the main magnetic field. Another magnet, referred to as the resonance frequency (RF) magnet, or the coil, is then used to produce a brief pulse of magnetic activity, the RF pulse, which causes the protons to tilt 90° from their original plane.

Different coils are used to image different tissues. There is a body coil, a head coil, and so forth. After the coil delivers the RF pulse, images are taken at varying time intervals. The RF pulse is repeated at intervals; the interval between repetitions is called the repetition time (TR). At a point after each repetition of the RF pulse, an imaging sample is taken; this is referred to as the echo time (TE). Two imaging protocols are commonly used, T1 and T2. A short TR and a short TE produce a T1-weighted image (Figure 9–2), whereas a long TR and a long TE produce a T2-weighted image (Figure 9–3). T1- and T2-weighted images are distinct in appearance. With CT and MRI, the density of various tissues lies on a gray scale. However, with MRI the scale for T1 images is different from the scale for T2 images. Table 9–3 summarizes the appearance of common components on T1 versus T2.

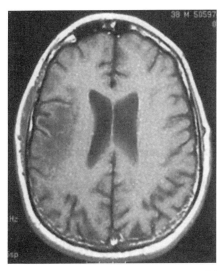

FIGURE 9–2. ■ T1-weighted magnetic resonance imaging (MRI) in a patient with progressive multifocal leukoencephalopathy, demonstrating a large area of signal abnormality in the subcortical white matter of the right hemisphere. The ventricles and sulci are dark as is the area of abnormal signal. (Reprinted with permission from Bradley WG, Brant-Zawadzki M, Cambray-Forker J: *MRI of the Brain I, The Lippincott Williams & Wilkins MRI Teaching File,* 2nd ed. Philadelphia, Lippincott Williams & Wilkins, 2001, p 6.)

The magnetic characteristics of a water proton depend on the environment in which it resides. The magnetic characteristics of the water protons in CSF differ from those of the water protons in white matter, gray matter, and other tissues. The water protons in the bed of a tumor or region of infarcted brain have magnetic characteristics that are distinct from the water protons in normal brain tissue. This disparity between the magnetic characteristics of water protons in various types of tissue allows for the differentiation of tissues by MRI.

The dissimilar appearances of a lesion on T1 versus T2 imaging permit speculation about the nature of the pathological process. This is one major advantage of MRI over CT. In CT, a lesion may be identified but not much information about its nature can be obtained. With MRI, not only can the lesion be identified, but also a reasonable guess can often be made about its nature. An abscess has different characteristics than a tumor or an infarct, for example.

A useful crude way to remember the T1 and T2 appearances of a pathological process is to focus on the CSF. On a T2-weighted image, the CSF is bright white. The ventricles, filled with bright CSF, are easy to locate for orientation, and they identify an image as being T2 weighted.

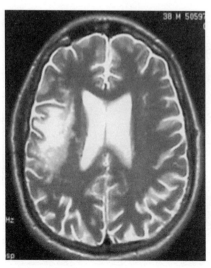

FIGURE 9–3. ■ T2-weighted magnetic resonance imaging (MRI) through the same level as in Figure 9–2. The cerebrospinal fluid-containing spaces are bright, as is the area of signal abnormality. Areas of cerebral edema are usually apparent as increased signal on T2 images before they are obvious on T1 images. (Reprinted with permission from Bradley WG, Brant-Zawadzki M, Cambray-Forker J: *MRI of the Brain I, The Lippincott Williams & Wilkins MRI Teaching File,* 2nd ed. Philadelphia, Lippincott Williams & Wilkins, 2001, p 6.)

Most acute pathological processes in the brain produce a degree of edema, which is an increase in water content. Edema fluid resembles CSF in its water content, and is also bright on T2 images. Acute or subacute pathological processes can thus be identified by finding the T2-weighted images and looking for areas of increased T2 signal that produce bright areas in the brain parenchyma.

One of the newest MRI techniques is diffusion-weighted imaging (DWI). This technique analyzes the diffusion of water molecules through tissue. The images can be obtained rapidly. Areas where water diffusion is compromised, such as where there is low blood flow in an acute ischemic lesion, show up as intensely bright areas on DWI. This permits the detection of acute ischemic lesions, and differentiates between old strokes and fresh strokes. DWI has proved extremely useful in the management of patients with acute cerebrovascular disease.

Special methods for MRI can also be used to visualize blood vessels to perform magnetic resonance arteriography (MRA). These MRA techniques depict flowing blood as bright white against a dark back-

TABLE 9–3 RELATIVE BRIGHTNESS OR DARKNESS OF VARIOUS TISSUES ON T1- AND T2-WEIGHTED MRI

Tissue	T1	T2
Fat	White	Dark
Bone	Black	Black
White matter	Light	Dark
Gray matter	Intermediate	Intermediate
CSF	Dark	White
Gadolinium	Light	Light
Edema	Dark	Light
Tumor	Dark	Light
MS plaque	Dark	Light
Acute or subacute infarct	Dark	Light
Calcification	Dark	Dark
Acute hemorrhage	Dark	Black
Old hemorrhage	Light	Light

CSF = cerebrospinal fluid; MRI = magnetic resonance imaging; MS = multiple sclerosis.

ground. One of the primary uses of MRA is to noninvasively evaluate a suspected pathological condition at the carotid bifurcation. MRA of the circle of Willis can detect some aneurysms and evaluate the intracranial vasculature.

ANGIOGRAPHY

When MRA does not provide sufficient detail, angiography is used. This involves arterial puncture, usually of the femoral artery, and then insertion of a catheter and selective injection of contrast into various vessels of the neck or aortic arch. Angiography is less often necessary with the increasing sophistication of noninvasive techniques.

MYELOGRAPHY

Myelography involves spinal puncture, usually lumbar but occasionally cervical, and injection of contrast material to outline the spinal cord and nerve roots. It is often followed by CT scanning to produce a CT myelogram. For evaluating spinal disc disease, the detail provided by CT myelography is often better than that of MRI.

ULTRASONOGRAPHY

Ultrasonography is a noninvasive technique that uses sound waves to image tissues, primarily blood vessels in adult neurologic patients. The technique is similar to sonar. Echocardiography uses similar methods to evaluate the heart. Doppler ultrasonography evaluates the auditory characteristics of the flow in a blood vessel, and ultrasound imaging provides a visual representation of the vessel. Duplex ultrasonography combines both of these techniques. In the vernacular, the term "Doppler" usually means duplex ultrasonography.

The bony cranium does not transmit sound waves and ultrasound has only limited usefulness in imaging inside the calvarium in adults. With special transducers applied to the thinnest part of the temporal bone, transcranial Doppler can be used to evaluate the flow in the major arteries at the base of the brain. Transcranial Doppler is used most often to evaluate patients who have undergone a stroke and to detect vasospasm in patients with subarachnoid hemorrhage.

Electrophysiologic Studies

Electrophysiologic testing involves recording electrical potentials from brain, nerve, or muscle. The tests done most often are the electroencephalogram (EEG), evoked potentials, the electromyogram (EMG), and sleep studies. EEG is a completely noninvasive test that involves recording spontaneously occurring electrical potentials from the brain by using scalp recordings. Evoked potential studies involve delivering a stimulus—visual, auditory, somatosensory, or other—and recording the resulting potential from the CNS. EMG consists of two parts: nerve conduction studies and needle electromyography. Nerve conduction studies are performed by electrically stimulating a nerve and recording a nerve or muscle action potential induced by the stimulus. Needle electromyography involves insertion of a needle electrode into a muscle to record the resting electrical activity, the activity after manipulation of the needle, and the activity after voluntary contraction. Sleep studies involve recording electrophysiologic parameters, such as EEG and surface EMG, in combination with other physiologic measurements such as respiratory excursion and blood oxygenation.

ELECTROENCEPHALOGRAM

EEG records the electrical activity from the most superficial layers of the cerebral cortex—only the first few millimeters. The patterns seen on EEG are markedly dependent on the state of arousal of the subject. Four categories of EEG frequencies are seen in clinical recordings: beta, alpha, theta, and delta, from fastest to slowest.

In normal subjects during quiet wakefulness with the eyes closed, the dominant rhythm over the posterior head region is alpha. Faster frequencies are present more anteriorly. In sleep, the alpha rhythm disappears and the EEG is dominated by slower rhythms. During deep sleep, also known as slow-wave sleep, the dominant rhythms are in the delta range.

In normal individuals, the amplitudes and frequencies of the EEG waves are symmetric over the two hemispheres. Another characteristic of a normal EEG is that the electrical activity is variably synchronous or regular. The EEG is more or less rhythmic, meaning that definite patterns of activity can be discerned. The regularity may cause an EEG pattern approaching that of a sine wave. At other times, the EEG activity is extremely asynchronous. When an EEG loses its normal pattern of rhythms it is said to be dysrhythmic. The term dysrhythmia connotes a disturbance in the normal pattern of EEG rhythms; dysrhythmia may be classified as mild, moderate, or severe. When very mild, dysrhythmia may involve nothing more than loss of the normal level of integration and synchronization. A sharp wave may be looked on as a moderate level of dysrhythmia, and a spike as a severe level of dysrhythmia.

Types of Electroencephalogram Abnormality

There are two basic types of EEG abnormality: too fast and too slow. Waves that are too fast have a higher frequency in relation to amplitude than is normally encountered in the EEG. These are sharp waves or spikes, and often imply an underlying seizure tendency. The waves that are too slow have a frequency less than that expected for the patient's state of arousal. Frequencies that might be perfectly normal in a sleeping patient are abnormal in a patient who appears awake or confused.

In addition to the classification of wave forms that are too fast or too slow, EEG abnormalities may be viewed as diffuse, involving both hemispheres, or focal, involving either all or part of one hemisphere.

There are thus four basic types of EEG abnormality: focal too slow, diffuse too slow, focal too fast, and diffuse too fast. Each of these patterns has distinctly different diagnostic implications (Table 9–4). Figures 9–4 through 9–7 demonstrate examples of each of these types of EEG abnormality. Hyperventilation and photic stimulation are commonly used to bring out EEG abnormalities that might otherwise be missed.

EEG is vastly more complex than this simple explanation indicates. Some neurologists do as much as 1 year of additional training to achieve proficiency in EEG. This introduction to EEG should nonetheless help the reader to clarify some of the basic principles involved in interpreting EEG results.

TABLE 9–4 FOUR PATTERNS OF ELECTROENCEPHALOGRAM ABNORMALITY

Abnormality	Illustrative Clinical Condition
Diffuse too slow	Metabolic encephalopathy
Diffuse too fast	Active clinical seizure
Focal too slow	Structural lesion (e.g., tumor, infarct)
Focal too fast	Interictal spike or sharp wave

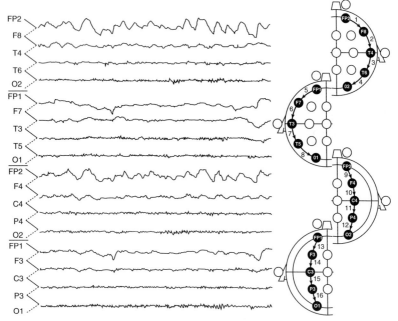

FIGURE 9–4. ▪Electroencephalogram (EEG) demonstrating a pattern of focal too slow. Tracings 1–4 and 9–12 are from the right side of the brain. Tracings 5–8 and 13–16 are from the left side. Lines 4, 8, 11, 12, 15, and 16 show fairly normal EEG activity. The activity coming from the right frontal region is high-voltage focal slow activity due to a tumor. Compare lines 1, 2, 9, and 10 (activity from the right frontal region) with lines 5, 6, 13 and 14 (activity from the left frontal region), which show only minor slowing related to eye movement. (Reprinted with permission from Fisch BJ: *Spehlmann's EEG Primer,* 2nd ed. New York, Elsevier, 1991, p 343.)

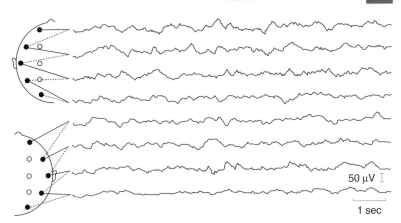

FIGURE 9–5. ■Electroencephalogram (EEG) demonstrating a pattern of diffuse too slow. All of the activity is high voltage and slow, with an absence of normal rhythms. (Reprinted with permission from Fisch BJ: *Spehlmann's EEG Primer,* 2nd ed. New York, Elsevier, 1991, p 363.)

Uses of Electroencephalogram

One of the most common uses of EEG is to evaluate a patient who has suffered one or more episodes of loss of consciousness. The finding on EEG of rhythms that are too fast increases the likelihood that the patient's episodes are seizure related.

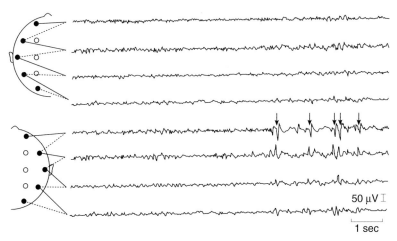

FIGURE 9–6. ■Electroencephalogram (EEG) demonstrating a pattern of focal too fast. The activity indicated by the arrows is interictal high-voltage spikes due to an underlying seizure focus in the right anterior temporal region. (Reprinted with permission from Fisch BJ: *Spehlmann's EEG Primer,* 2nd ed. New York, Elsevier, 1991, p 264.)

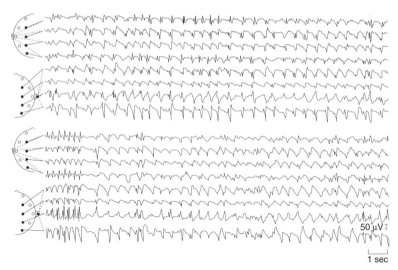

FIGURE 9–7. ■ Electroencephalogram (EEG) demonstrating a pattern of diffuse too fast. The EEG is filled with high-voltage spikes recorded during a generalized seizure. (Reprinted with permission from Fisch BJ: *Spehlmann's EEG Primer,* 2nd ed. New York, Elsevier, 1991, p 296.)

EEG is also used to look for evidence of focal structural abnormalities, although less so in the current era of sophisticated neuroimaging than in the past. Focal structural pathological conditions generally produce EEG abnormalities that are too slow and that are limited to a focal region of the brain (i.e., the focal slow pattern). EEG is also used to evaluate patients who have altered mental status (AMS) or confusional states. When AMS is due to a metabolic derangement, such as hepatic encephalopathy, uremia, or drug intoxication, the EEG is typically diffusely too slow. Rarely, a patient with AMS may have subclinical seizures, in which case the EEG demonstrates a diffuse, too fast pattern. When AMS is due to a structural brain lesion, the EEG may show focal slowing that usually corresponds well to the site of the underlying lesion. Patients with psychogenic unresponsiveness ("hysterical coma") appear to be in coma, but the EEG demonstrates normal waking rhythms.

The EEG is often used to evaluate patients with suspected brain death. Patients who are brain dead have no functioning cerebral cortex, and their EEG is totally devoid of recordable electrical activity (electrocerebral silence). The pattern of electrocerebral silence can also occur with hypothermia and drug intoxication; therefore, these possibilities must be eliminated before a diagnosis of brain death can be made. Very high gains and other methods to help detect minimal residual electrical activity are used for brain death recordings. As a result of these techniques, the recording of artifacts in the environment is a major problem, and they may be mistaken for cerebral electrical activity.

EVOKED POTENTIALS

The ongoing background activity of the EEG is quasi-random. A stimulus delivered to a sensory system—auditory, visual, or somatosensory—produces a response that changes the electrical activity of the cortex as the wave of depolarization is processed. This signal occurs in a fixed time relationship to the delivery of the stimulus. These are evoked potentials. Their amplitude is small, about the same level as the background EEG. Consequently, these potentials are easily lost in the background. A technique of computer averaging is used to detect evoked potentials. Numerous stimuli are delivered; in the case of the somatosensory evoked potentials (SEPs), the number of stimuli required to produce a discernible response may number in the thousands. Because the evoked potential occurs in a fixed time relationship to the delivery of the stimulus, as opposed to the quasi-random background activity that bears no fixed time relationship to the stimulus, the averaging technique allows the evoked response to emerge from the background. The background activity, being random, is canceled out over many sweeps, whereas the evoked response, being constant, is repetitive and reinforced. The evoked response is the signal, the background activity is the noise, and averaging extracts the signal from the noise. This basic technique is used for all evoked potentials.

The visual evoked potential (VEP) is produced by delivering a visual stimulus, a flash of light, or an alternating pattern checkerboard. The stimulus for an auditory evoked potential (AEP) is delivered as clicks or tones through headphones. The stimulus for an SEP is delivered as electrical shock to one or more peripheral nerves. These stimuli produce evoked potentials that are best seen over certain head regions: occipital lobe for VEP, parietal lobe for SEP, and brainstem for AEP.

Evoked potential studies are clinically useful because the latency of the response, measured from the time of delivery of the stimulus to the detection of response over the brain, is directly related to the speed of conduction through the relevant pathways. When disease is present involving the pathways, the speed of conduction slows, increasing the latency of the potential. Evoked potential studies are most often used in the workup of patients with suspected multiple sclerosis (MS). The demyelination caused by MS may markedly slow or block conduction in white matter pathways. Past episodes of demyelination may leave residual slowing, although clinical recovery appears complete. Since the diagnosis of MS is based in part on having lesions in multiple locations in the nervous system (the disease is called multiple sclerosis for a reason), evoked potential studies can sometimes detect a "clinically silent" lesion and help to establish the presence of disease in different locations. For instance, an abnormal VEP, even in the absence of clinical evidence of optic nerve disease, may be a useful marker of dissemination in the patient who has myelopathy.

ELECTROMYOGRAM

EMG consists of two different components: nerve conduction studies (electroneurography) and needle electromyography. The shorthand designation EMG is customarily used to denote both procedures. The information obtained from nerve conduction studies differs from, but complements, that of needle EMG.

EMG is used to evaluate patients with a variety of clinical problems, and the study can help to differentiate between diagnostic possibilities. A common use of EMG is to help distinguish pain caused by a musculoskeletal problem from pain caused by radiculopathy. Patterns of abnormality seen in common clinical situations are shown in Table 9–5.

Nerve Conduction Studies

In a nerve conduction study, an electrical stimulus is delivered percutaneously to a peripheral nerve and a response is then recorded from either the nerve itself in the case of sensory potentials, or from the muscle that the nerve innervates in the case of motor potentials. The sensory potentials are called sensory nerve action potentials or compound nerve action potentials, and the motor potentials are referred to as compound muscle action potentials (CMAPs). Three different types of measurements are made: latency, amplitude, and conduction velocity. The latency is the time from the delivery of the stimulus to the occurrence of the sensory or motor potential. The amplitude is the size of the potential. The conduction velocity is the time required for the stimulus to travel between two points. To obtain a conduction velocity, the physician determines the latency difference between two sites along the course of the nerve, for instance, the latency of the median nerve at the elbow minus the latency of the median nerve at the wrist. The distance between the wrist and elbow is then measured over the skin surface with a tape measure. A simple calculation of time and distance then produces a value for the nerve conduction velocity.

Nerve conduction studies are primarily used in the evaluation and management of patients with peripheral nerve disease, including those with mononeuropathies (e.g., carpal tunnel syndrome) and polyneuropathies (e.g., diabetic neuropathy). Peripheral nerve disease produces two basic patterns of abnormality in nerve conduction studies: demyelination and axon loss. Demyelination produces slow-

TABLE 9–5 PATTERNS OF ABNORMALITY ON ELECTROMYOGRAM IN VARIOUS CLINICAL CIRCUMSTANCES

Condition	Motor NCS	Sensory NCS	Repetitive Nerve Stimulation	Needle Examination Recruitment	Needle Examination Fibrillation Potentials
Myofascial or musculoskeletal pain	N	N	N	N	Absent
Radiculopathy with axon loss	N	N	N	N or neuropathic	Present
ALS	N or mildly slow	N	N	Neuropathic	Present
Demyelinating polyneuropathy	Very slow	Abnormal	N	Neuropathic	Equivocal
Axonal polyneuropathy	N or mildly slow	Abnormal	N	Neuropathic	Present
Neuromuscular junction disorder	N	N	Abnormal	N	Absent
Bland myopathy	N	N	N	Myopathic	Absent
Myonecrotic myopathy	N	N	N	Myopathic	Present

ALS = amyotrophic lateral sclerosis; N = normal; NCS = nerve conduction studies.

ing of nerve conduction velocities with relative preservation of amplitude. This is because the disease process affects the myelin sheath, but spares the axon. As a result, there is no loss of muscle or nerve fibers and motor and sensory amplitudes are preserved. Loss of myelin, however, produces dramatic interference with the conduction properties of the peripheral nerve, causing slowing of conduction velocity. In contrast, axon loss causes decreased motor and sensory amplitudes without dramatic change in conduction velocities. This is because some axons die, producing loss of muscle and nerve fibers and hence a decreased amplitude of the response. The surviving axons, however, conduct normally as long as they are able to conduct. This produces an all-or-nothing situation in which conduction in the surviving axons is normal, providing a normal conduction velocity, but amplitudes are decreased, reflecting the loss of nerve and muscle fibers. There are thus two patterns of abnormality: slow conduction velocity with normal amplitudes in demyelinating neuropathies, and normal or nearly normal conduction velocities with low amplitudes in axon-loss neuropathies.

The two basic types of nerve conduction abnormality can occur in one of three distributions: mononeuropathy, multiple mononeuropathy, and polyneuropathy. A mononeuropathy involves one nerve, such as in unilateral carpal tunnel syndrome. A multiple mononeuropathy involves more than one nerve but not all of the nerves, as might occur if the patient has radial nerve palsy on one side and peroneal nerve palsy on the opposite side. A polyneuropathy involves all of the nerves. Axonal polyneuropathies, however, continue to have a distal emphasis in many cases, so that involvement is not necessarily the same in all segments of all nerves. Table 9–6 demonstrates possible etiologic factors for these different conduction abnormality patterns.

A specialized type of nerve conduction study, repetitive stimulation, is used to evaluate patients with suspected neuromuscular transmission disorders, such as myasthenia gravis. Repetitive stimulation studies are done by delivering a train of stimuli to a nerve while recording from a muscle innervated by that nerve. The train of stimuli is delivered at various frequencies. The pattern of change in the CMAP is assessed as it occurs in response to each stimulus in the train. In a normal person at most frequencies, there is no change in the CMAP amplitude. Patients with neuromuscular transmission disorders may demonstrate an increase or a decrease in CMAP amplitude during the course of the train of stimuli. The pattern of increase or decrease in CMAP amplitude depends on the frequency of the train and the type of neuromuscular transmission disorder.

TABLE 9–6 PATTERNS OF NERVE CONDUCTION STUDY ABNORMALITIES AND DISTRIBUTIONS IN ILLUSTRATIVE CONDITIONS

Condition	Demyelinating Pattern	Axon Loss Pattern
Mononeuropathy	Carpal tunnel syndrome	Stretch injury, injection palsy
Multifocal mononeuropathy	Multiple entrapments	Vasculitis
Polyneuropathy	Guillain-Barré syndrome	Alcoholic neuropathy

Needle Electromyography

A needle electrode that is inserted into a muscle records the electrical activity generated by that muscle. Under normal circumstances with the muscle at rest, no electrical activity is recorded. With muscle contraction, the needle records the motor unit action potentials (MUAPs), which represent the summation of the electrical activity in all of the muscle fibers innervated by a specific motor unit. With increasing force of contraction, more and more MUAPs are recruited and more and more appear on the electromyograph screen. Normal motor units have a certain range of amplitude and duration, which varies slightly from muscle to muscle, with the age of the patient, and with other factors. Abnormalities on needle EMG take one of several forms: spontaneous activity (where there should be none), abnormal recruitment patterns, and abnormal motor units.

A normal muscle has no electrical activity at rest, and the recorded EMG activity is minimal. When a muscle demonstrates spontaneous activity, it usually takes the form of fibrillation potentials. This occurs when the axon supplying the muscle is damaged, or if the muscle is necrotic.

There are two types of recruitment abnormalities: increased recruitment and decreased recruitment. When the nerve supply to a muscle is impaired because of axon loss, there are fewer motor units available to sustain muscle contraction, and therefore a decreased number of motor unit potentials. Those present fire more rapidly than normal in an effort to generate force through an increased frequency of firing rather than through recruitment of additional units. This is a "neuropathic" pattern. When the muscle fibers themselves are diseased, as in myopathy, the number of muscle fibers in the motor unit is normal, and the number of motor units is normal. However, the diseased muscle fibers have difficulty generating force because of dysfunction related to the disease process. Since there is a normal number of motor units there is no difficulty in generating adequate numbers of MUAPs, but the motor units do not generate normal force. In the patient with myopathy, therefore, the muscle tries to generate force by firing an increased number of MUAPs for the level of contraction. This is increased recruitment, or a "myopathic" pattern.

When an axon dies, its muscle fibers send out trophic influences that attract reinnervating sprouts from other axons. The resultant "reinnervated" motor unit has an increased number of muscle fibers compared with a normal motor unit, and consequently an MUAP of larger amplitude and longer duration. Abnormally large motor units are therefore typically seen in a denervating process. In contrast, the muscle fibers involved by a myopathic process may be necrotic, atrophic, or otherwise diseased. These sick muscle fibers do not generate a normal amount of electrical current, and therefore the MUAPs seen in myopathic processes tend to be smaller than normal. Disorders involving the neuromuscular junction do not alter motor unit architecture. When myopathy is mild, the change in motor unit potential size may be so subtle as to escape detection. Myopathies characterized by muscle fiber necrosis (primarily inflammatory myopathies and dystrophies) may show increased spontaneous activity. These are termed "myonecrotic" myopathies. Other types of myopathies are not associated with muscle fiber necrosis and may produce motor unit potential abnormalities without any fibrillation activity. Table 9–7 summarizes the patterns of abnormality that may be seen on EMG in different types of disease processes. A myonecrotic myopathy is one with evidence of fiber necrosis on EMG and very high creatine kinase levels. A bland myopathy is one without much evidence of fiber necrosis on EMG and minimal or no elevation of creatine kinase.

Lumbar Puncture

Although not done as often as in the past, lumbar puncture (LP) remains an important part of the neurologic workup for many patients. There are two essential pieces of information obtained from the LP: the CSF pressure and the CSF composition. The opening pressure measurement is a vital part of the LP, and should never be omitted. The opening pressure is the most reliable indicator of the intracranial pressure. In some circumstances, the only abnormality seen on LP is an elevated opening pressure, as in pseudotumor cerebri. In other conditions, an elevation of the opening pressure may be an important clue to the presence of an intracranial pathological condition.

To obtain an accurate opening pressure, the physician must not al-

TABLE 9–7 PATTERNS OF NEEDLE ELECTROMYOGRAM ABNORMALITIES

Condition	Spontaneous Activity	Recruitment	MUAP Size
Normal	Absent	Normal	Normal
Denervation	Present	Decreased	Increased
Bland myopathy*	Absent	Increased	Decreased
Myonecrotic myopathy*	Present	Increased	Decreased

MUAP = motor unit action potential.
*See NEEDLE ELECTROMYOGRAPHY for more information on bland and myonecrotic myopathy.

low the patient to be tightly flexed into a ball. The increased intra-abdominal pressure with such positioning can lead to artifactual elevation of the opening pressure.

Once the opening pressure has been determined, fluid is usually withdrawn for analysis. Rarely, substances are injected into the CSF, such as an isotope for cisternography. Occasionally, CSF is simply withdrawn, as in the treatment of pseudotumor cerebri. The type of analyses done on the CSF varies depending on the clinical circumstances. A different set of studies is done on the patient with an acute infection than on the patient with suspected Guillain-Barré syndrome or the patient with suspected MS. An ever-increasing number of tests are possible on spinal fluid. Polymerase chain reaction testing is available for some organisms. It is not uncommon to request procedures such as antinuclear antibody, herpes simplex polymerase chain reaction, angiotensin-converting enzyme level, or Lyme titer.

In the majority of cases, the minimum amount of information requested includes cell count, differential, protein, and glucose. Several patterns of CSF are commonly encountered: "normal," acute bacterial infection, "aseptic meningeal pattern," and albuminocytologic dissociation pattern.

The pattern seen with acute bacterial infection is classically a markedly increased cell count, with the cells consisting primarily of polymorphonuclear lymphocytes, an elevated protein level, and a decreased sugar level. Protein elevation is nonspecific. Very low sugar levels usually indicate acute bacterial infection. Under these circumstances, the glucose is sometimes zero, and often less than 10 mg/dl. The "aseptic" pattern consists of an elevated cell count with predominantly mononuclear cells, elevated protein levels, and a normal sugar level. The term "aseptic" under these circumstances merely means the pattern is not that of acute bacterial infection. Viral infections, tuberculosis, and other chronic infections may well produce an aseptic pattern. Occasionally, an aseptic pattern with slightly to moderately decreased sugar levels occurs with viral infections, tuberculosis, and fungal or neoplastic meningitis. Common causes of an aseptic meningeal reaction are listed in Table 9–8.

The pattern of albuminocytologic dissociation is seen most often in Guillain-Barré syndrome and consists of an elevated protein level, sometimes an extremely elevated protein level, in the absence of an increased cell count or other abnormalities.

Sometimes, CSF that appears to be normal on routine studies proves to be abnormal when special studies are done. The most common of these special studies are done for the detection of evidence of demyelinating disease, primarily MS. When disimmune demyelination occurs in the nervous system, the CSF may reflect that process through the presence of an abnormal level of immunoglobulins. Synthesis of immunoglobulin within the nervous system causes an elevation of immunoglobulin G (IgG) in the spinal fluid. For accuracy, the IgG level must be compared with the albumin level, since the presence of protein from another process could cause the IgG level to be elevated on an absolute basis, but not in proportion to the albumin. The key abnormality is thus an increase in the IgG/albumin ratio or an abnormal IgG index [(CSF IgG/serum IgG)/(CSF albumin/serum albumin)]. It is also possible to calculate the IgG synthesis rate in the nervous system, which is also frequently abnormal in demyelinating disease. The immunoglobulins present are sometimes derived from limited clones of immunocompetent cells, and produce so-called oligoclonal bands on electrophoresis. When necrosis and inflammation are active in the nervous system, it is often possible to detect an elevation of myelin basic protein. The battery of tests often used to look for evidence of de-

TABLE 9–8 CAUSES OF ASEPTIC MENINGEAL REACTION

Viral infection

Tuberculosis

Fungal infection

Partially treated bacterial meningitis

Neoplastic meningitis

Parasitic infection

Parameningeal infection

myelinating disease thus consists of IgG/albumin ratio, IgG index, IgG synthesis rate, oligoclonal bands, and myelin basic protein.

An abnormal spinal fluid IgG/albumin ratio can sometimes be seen in conditions other than MS, such as neurosyphilis and subacute sclerosing panencephalitis. Systemic elevation of immunoglobulins, such as with multiple myeloma, can also alter the IgG/albumin ratio. It is therefore always necessary to have the results of serum protein electrophoresis to properly interpret abnormal CSF IgG studies.

Another common test done with CSF is cytology, which involves searching for tumor cells in patients suspected of having neoplastic meningitis.

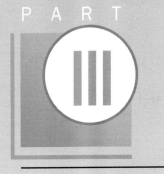

P A R T

III

Neurologic Disorders

10

Disorders Above the Foramen Magnum

Recall from Chapter 8 and Table 8–3 that conditions that affect the central nervous system (CNS) above the foramen magnum typically cause long-tract signs in a "hemi" distribution, and may demonstrate other localizing abnormalities, such as focal cortical signs, seizures, and cranial nerve dysfunction. This chapter discusses conditions in which the primary abnormalities occur above the foramen magnum, following the scheme of etiologic classification outlined in Chapter 8.

Tumor

Tumors may affect the nervous system directly or indirectly. Direct effects are due to the mass or infiltrative effects of the tumor. Indirect or remote or paraneoplastic effects can occur when the tumor is somewhere other than in the nervous system. Both direct and paraneoplastic effects may need to be considered in patients with a neurologic syndrome.

BRAIN TUMORS

With only rare exception, patients with CNS neoplasms present because of expanding mass effect, with the specific symptoms depending on the rate of expansion. Slowly growing tumors (meningiomas, low-grade astrocytomas, oligodendrogliomas) may well come to attention because of a seizure. Patients with more rapidly expanding tumors (high-grade anaplastic astrocytomas, glioblastomas, metastases) generally present because of a progressive neurologic deficit evolving over several weeks to several months. Although most patients with brain tumors mention the presence of headache if queried, they seldom present because of headache, nor do they describe the headache as severe.

Despite their relatively small size, some tumors cause prominent clinical symptoms because of their location or because of endocrinologic activity, such as acoustic neuromas presenting as hearing loss, pituitary adenomas presenting as acromegaly, pineal tumors presenting as precocious puberty, and optic nerve meningiomas presenting as visual loss. Many tumors occur characteristically in children and only rarely appear in adulthood, such as brainstem gliomas, medulloblastomas, craniopharyngiomas, and ependymomas. In adults, tumors are usually supratentorial; in children they are usually infratentorial. Intracranial tumors are second only to leukemia as a form of neoplasia in children.

Table 10–1 lists the more common types of primary brain tumors.

Gliomas

Gliomas include astrocytomas, oligodendrogliomas, and ependymomas, and range from relatively benign, "low-grade" gliomas that are slowly infiltrating lesions with an indolent course, to aggressive, malignant, "high-grade" lesions with a very short clinical course. The most malignant, virulent form of glioma is the glioblastoma multiforme (Figure 10–1). Gliomas can occur anywhere in the nervous system. The occipital lobes have a relatively low incidence of gliomas; lesions in that location are much more likely to be vascular. On occasion gliomas may present with a sudden deficit-simulating stroke, due to spontaneous necrosis or hemorrhage within the tumor. Gliomas can involve the spinal cord.

Meningiomas

Meningiomas arise from the meninges and can develop virtually anywhere in the nervous system, including the spinal meninges. They are

---

TABLE 10–1. COMMON TYPES OF PRIMARY BRAIN TUMOR

Glioma

Ependymoma

Medulloblastoma

Meningioma

Acoustic neuroma (schwannoma)

Pituitary adenoma

Craniopharyngioma

Pinealoma

Primary CNS lymphoma

CNS = central nervous system.

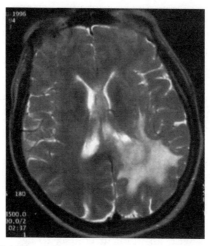

FIGURE 10–1. ■ Axial T2-weighted magnetic resonance image, demonstrating a large infiltrating glioblastoma multiforme in the deep white matter of the left parietal lobe. (Reprinted with permission from Brant-Zawadzki M, Bradley WG, Cambray-Forker J (eds): *MRI of the Brain I,* Philadelphia, Lippincott Williams & Wilkins, 2001.)

slow-growing, benign lesions by their inherent nature, but can sometimes act malignantly because of their location. Meningiomas over the convexity of the hemisphere are common and are usually easily resectable (Figure 10–2). Meningiomas arising from structures at the base of the brain or in other inaccessible locations are much more difficult, sometimes impossible, to remove surgically.

Metastatic lesions

The most common type of brain tumor is a metastatic deposit from a systemic neoplasm. Sometimes the brain metastasis is the presenting manifestation of the distant tumor. More often, brain metastases complicate the terminal course of patients with known primary tumors. Metastatic lesions can arise from almost any tumor, with the exception of prostate cancer, which rarely, if ever, metastasizes to the brain.

Metastases usually present as a seizure or progressive neurologic deficit. Like other aggressively malignant lesions, metastatic deposits sometimes spontaneously hemorrhage, causing a rapidly evolving neurologic deficit-simulating stroke (Figure 10–3A).

Meningeal neoplasia

Metastatic carcinoma, lymphoma, leukemia, and glioma can occasionally involve the meninges. Patients with these neoplasms usually

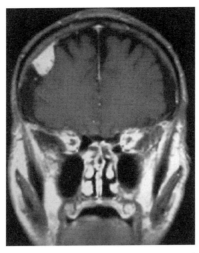

FIGURE 10–2. ■ Gadolinium-enhanced, T1-weighted magnetic resonance image, demonstrating a meningioma arising from the meninges over the cerebral convexity, a common location for such tumors. (Reprinted with permission from Brant-Zawadzki M, Bradley WG, Cambray-Forker J (eds): *MRI of the Brain II,* Philadelphia, Lippincott Williams & Wilkins, 2001.)

present with headache and multifocal neurologic deficits. Finding malignant cells in the cerebrospinal fluid (CSF) is the primary method of diagnosis. The clinical course is typically short and fulminant.

NERVE TUMORS

Neoplasms can occur on cranial and peripheral nerves. These may be gliomas, neurofibromas, schwannomas, or primitive malignant tumors. Virtually any peripheral nerve can be involved. The most common cranial nerve neoplasms are optic nerves gliomas, which typically present as progressive visual loss, and acoustic schwannomas, which typically cause progressive hearing loss.

PARANEOPLASTIC SYNDROMES

Malignancies can produce a host of nonmetastatic neurologic syndromes by various mechanisms, some that are fairly well understood, and others obscure. The neurologic syndrome may precede the malignancy by months or years, occur simultaneously with presentation of the tumor, or develop in patients with known cancer. Obviously, the first situation is clinically most problematic.

The paraneoplastic syndromes include but are not limited to the following: progressive cerebellar ataxia, peripheral neuropathy, Lambert-

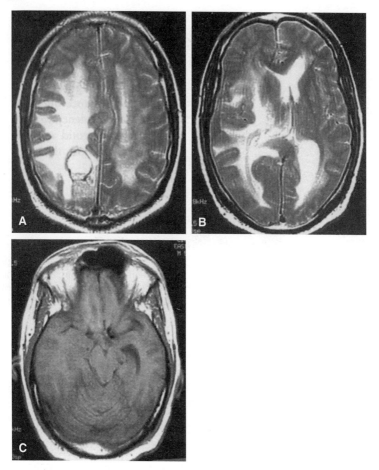

FIGURE 10–3. ■ (*A*) Axial T2-weighted magnetic resonance image, demonstrating a metastatic tumor deposit in the right parietal lobe. The slight low density in the posterior aspect of the discrete round lesion is due to acute hemorrhage within the metastasis. The bright white signal extending diffusely throughout the deep white matter of the right hemisphere is vasogenic cerebral edema caused by the metastasis. (*B*) A lower plane of section than in *A*, showing marked shift of the right hemisphere toward the left due to the mass effect and cerebral edema in the right hemisphere. The right lateral ventricle is markedly compressed and shifted. (*C*) Axial T1-weighted magnetic resonance image in the same case, demonstrating right uncal herniation with shift of the medial right temporal lobe into the tentorial hiatus, causing compression and shift of the upper brainstem to the left. (Reprinted with permission from Brant-Zawadzki M, Bradley WG, Cambray-Forker J (eds): *MRI of the Brain I.* Philadelphia, Lippincott Williams & Wilkins, 2001.)

Eaton syndrome, an opsoclonus-myoclonus syndrome, "limbic ence-phalitis" (memory and emotional disturbances), and sensory ataxia due to dorsal root ganglion cell degeneration. Tumors may also affect the nervous system by inducing coagulopathies and nonbacterial throm-botic endocarditis, not to mention dysproteinemias, alterations of serum viscosity, and abnormalities of the cellular constituents of the blood.

One of the most common remote effects of cancer on the nervous sys-tem is cerebellar degeneration. Patients typically have pancerebellar ataxia. Ovarian and small-cell lung carcinomas seem most prone to produce this syndrome. The development of a cerebellar syndrome in a middle-aged nonalcoholic patient should prompt an exhaustive evalu-ation for an underlying malignancy. In some cases, the presence of para-neoplastic, antineuronal antibodies in the blood confirms the diagnosis.

TREATMENT OF NERVOUS SYSTEM TUMORS

The treatment of most nervous system tumors is primarily surgical. Chemotherapy and radiation are used occasionally. Details of the ther-apy of neoplasia are beyond the scope of this discussion. For current information on the management of adult brain tumors, visit the Web site *www.cancerlinksusa.com/brain/txphysician.*

Neurologic Complications of the Use or Abuse of Drugs and Alcohol

Side effects and complications from the use and abuse of drugs and al-cohol account for some of the most common neurologic complaints seen in clinical practice. These complaints range from the relatively common and innocuous, such as dizziness due to drug-induced ortho-static hypotension or headaches due to a prescription medication, to the catastrophic, such as an intracerebral hemorrhage (ICH) due to co-caine. Table 10–2 summarizes many of the side effects and complica-tions associated with drug and alcohol use or abuse. These conditions can occur from the use or abuse of prescription drugs and from the abuse of illicit or recreational drugs and alcohol.

PRESCRIPTION DRUGS

A host of drugs can produce neurologic side effects and complications. Drowsiness is perhaps the most common drug side effect of all. The clue to the diagnosis of a drug-related neurologic syndrome is recognition of the possibility. The drug history from the patient may or may not be re-liable. Many patients cannot accurately relate which drugs they are tak-ing. Others deliberately deny or disguise their consumption or behave disingenuously regarding their drug history. Some patients think that

---

TABLE 10–2. NEUROLOGIC SYNDROMES ASSOCIATED WITH DRUG AND ALCOHOL USE OR ABUSE

Prescription and Other Legal Drugs

Headache

> Headache-remedy medications (analgesic rebound, especially codeine and ergots)
>
> Other drugs (e.g., proton pump inhibitors, histamine blockers, caffeine, calcium channel blockers, ACE inhibitors, nitrates, oral contraceptives, estrogens, vitamin A-containing compounds)

Excessive sleepiness (common drug side effect)

Insomnia (common drug side effect)

Other drug-induced sleep abnormalities (e.g., nightmares, parasomnias, sleep apnea)

Acute confusional state, delirium, toxic psychosis (many agents, such as anticholinergics, benzodiazepines, histamine-receptor antagonists, nonsteroid antiinflammatory drugs, and opioid analgesics)

Drug-induced seizures (AED withdrawal; phenothiazines; clozapine; cyclosporine; antimicrobial agents, such as penicillin and levofloxacin; CNS stimulants, such as theophylline, cocaine, and amphetamines; opiates, such as meperidine; radiologic contrast agents; lidocaine; aminophylline; others)

Drug-induced memory loss (anticholinergics, benzodiazepines)

Drug-induced myopathy (corticosteroids, paralytics, antimalarials, AZT, cholesterol-lowering agents, colchicine)

Rhabdomyolysis and myoglobinuria (numerous agents)

Generalized weakness due to electrolyte disturbances, such as hypokalemia or hypermagnesemia ($MgSO_4$, diuretics)

Peripheral neuropathy (numerous drugs, such as amiodarone)

Myelopathy (nitrous oxide, amphotericin B, radiologic contrast agents)

Drug-induced cerebrovascular disease (e.g., ischemic stroke, cerebral hemorrhage, cerebral vasculitis) [Many agents possible including anticoagulants, antineoplastic drugs, interleukin-2, interferons, ergot derivatives, oral contraceptives, IVIG, thrombolytics, and oral contraceptives.]

Syncope, with or without orthostatic hypotension (numerous agents)

Drug-induced aseptic meningitis (trimethoprim/sulfamethoxazole, ibuprofen, intravenous immunoglobulin, OKT-3)

Drug-induced parkinsonism (phenothiazines)

Tardive dyskinesias and dystonias (after antipsychotic exposure)

Drug-induced tremor (many agents such as lithium, sympathomimetics, and terfenadine)

Neuroleptic malignant syndrome

(continued)

TABLE 10–2. NEUROLOGIC SYNDROMES ASSOCIATED WITH DRUG AND ALCOHOL USE OR ABUSE (*CONTINUED*)

Serotonin syndrome

Drug-induced or exacerbated neuromuscular transmission disorders (many agents)

Complications of chemotherapy (many agents)

Drug-induced hepatic encephalopathy (valproic acid, benzodiazepines, narcotics, diuretics)

Drug-induced myoclonus (anticonvulsants, levodopa, lithium, MAO inhibitors, tricyclic antidepressants)

Pseudotumor cerebri (vitamin A, tetracycline, others)

Alcohol

Headache due to withdrawal (i.e., hangover headache)

Abstinence syndrome

Delirium tremens

Alcohol-related seizures (withdrawal and other)

Alcoholic blackouts (memory loss)

Alcoholic myopathy

Alcoholic rhabdomyolysis and myoglobinuria

Alcoholic peripheral neuropathy

Alcoholic cerebellar degeneration

Alcoholic myelopathy

Alcoholic psychosis

Alcohol-induced chronic auditory hallucinosis

Marchiafava-Bignami disease

Cortical atrophy

Alcoholic dementia

Wernicke encephalopathy

Korsakoff syndrome

Tremor

Acquired hepatolenticular degeneration

Central pontine myelinolysis

Illicit Drugs

Headache (cocaine, amphetamines, opiates, narcotic abstinence)

Acute confusional state, delirium, toxic psychosis (PCP, cocaine)

Drug-induced seizures (e.g., cocaine, heroin, amphetamines, PCP)

Coma

(*continued*)

TABLE 10–2. NEUROLOGIC SYNDROMES ASSOCIATED WITH DRUG AND ALCOHOL USE OR ABUSE (*CONTINUED*)

Myopathy

Rhabdomyolysis (i.e., drug-induced or due to prolonged immobility in overdose)

Drug-induced cerebrovascular disease (e.g., ischemic stroke, cerebral hemorrhage, cerebral vasculitis, complications of endocarditis) [Many agents possible including cocaine, amphetamines, ephedrine, and other sympathomimetics.]

Drug-induced movement disorders (e.g., parkinsonism, tremor, dystonia, chorea)

HIV and HTLV-I complications

Peripheral neuropathy (e.g., "huffer's neuropathy")

Cerebellar degeneration (inhalation of organic solvents, especially toluene)

Parkinsonism (analogue of meperidine)

Lead poisoning (due to inhalation of gasoline)

Dementia (chronic solvent vapor abuse)

Optic neuropathy (methyl alcohol, toluene)

Transverse myelitis (heroin)

ACE = angiotensin-converting enzyme; AED = antiepileptic drug; AZT = zidovudine; CNS = central nervous system; HIV = human immunodeficiency virus; HTLV-I = human T-cell lymphotrophic virus type I; IVIG = intravenous immunoglobulin; MAO = monoamine oxidase; $MgSO_4$ = magnesium sulfate; OKT-3 = anti-CD3 monoclonal antibody; PCP = phencyclidine.

the medication they are taking is actually something else, such as a patient taking diuretics, thinking they are taking "nerve pills," and developing hypokalemic paralysis. Blood and urine drug screens are often helpful in clarifying the patient's medication picture. There is a window in time, however, after which the drugs can no longer be detected.

In some instances, the clinical association between a clinical problem and known ingestion of a drug strongly suggests a causal link, as in the patient on cyclosporine having seizures, or the patient who develops aseptic meningitis while taking ibuprofen, or the patient who develops myopathy while on chloroquine. In other instances, the causal link may not be at all apparent, or the history of drug ingestion may be unknown. In some instances, the pathological or radiologic picture may be so characteristic that it suggests drug effects, even when ingestion is not known, as in the characteristic muscle histopathology of colchicine myopathy.

ALCOHOL

Alcohol can do many things to the nervous and neuromuscular systems. The most common complications of chronic alcoholism are seizures and peripheral neuropathy, but these symptoms are only the beginning. Alcoholics are infamous for attempting to conceal the amount of alcohol that they ingest. Some fervently deny drinking, even when repeatedly confronted with the possibility that their medical difficulties could be related to alcohol ingestion. A phone call to a family member or acquaintance is often edifying for revealing the patient's true level of alcohol consumption. It is a good rule of thumb to double the patient's admitted consumption level. There is also a maxim that the amount of alcohol the patient admits to drinking is actually what is spilled. Either saying makes the point: gross underreporting is the rule. Table 10–2 lists many of the complications of alcohol abuse. Some of the important conditions to recognize, either because they are common, or because they are treatable if recognized, include alcohol-related seizures, peripheral neuropathy, Wernicke-Korsakoff disease, and alcoholic cerebellar degeneration.

Wernicke Encephalopathy

Patients with thiamine deficiency, most often from alcoholic nutritional deficiency, may develop a syndrome consisting of impaired eye movements and altered mental status (AMS), frequently accompanied by other evidence of alcoholic nervous system damage such as cerebellar ataxia and peripheral neuropathy (Figure 10–4). The eye movement disorder may take virtually any form, from gaze-evoked nystagmus to

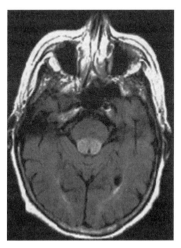

FIGURE 10–4. ■ Fluid-attenuated inversion recovery (FLAIR) magnetic resonance images, showing marked hyperintensity in the periaqueductal gray matter of the upper midbrain in a patient with acute Wernicke encephalopathy. (Reprinted with permission from Brant-Zawadzki M, Bradley WG, Cambray-Forker J (eds): *MRI of the Brain II.* Philadelphia, Lippincott Williams & Wilkins, 2001.)

global gaze palsy. If unrecognized and untreated, patients are left with a residual Korsakoff amnestic confabulatory psychosis.

Korsakoff Syndrome

Patients with Korsakoff syndrome typically have severe impairment of recent memory. To fill in the gaps in their memory, they often make up tales, referred to as confabulation. Wernicke encephalopathy is the acute manifestation, and Korsakoff amnestic confabulatory psychosis is the chronic sequela of thiamine deficiency. Korsakoff syndrome occurs most commonly in alcoholics as an aftermath of inadequately treated Wernicke encephalopathy. The two conditions are sometimes lumped together as Wernicke–Korsakoff disease. Although usually a complication of alcohol abuse, Wernicke-Korsakoff disease can occur in thiamine deficiency caused by other conditions.

Alcoholic Cerebellar Degeneration

Alcohol preferentially poisons the vermis, leading to a characteristic syndrome of gait ataxia with sparing of the limbs. Patients with this condition may have no demonstrable lower extremity, heel-to-shin ataxia while lying supine, yet be titubating and totally unable to walk. Unwary examiners may conclude such findings represent hysteria.

ILLICIT OR RECREATIONAL DRUGS

The most serious complications of illicit drug use are coma and death. Short of this, drugs can cause numerous neurologic complications, as summarized in Table 10–2. A negative serum or urine drug screen does not necessarily exclude drug use as the cause of a neurologic illness. In considering illicit substance abuse as a potential etiological factor, do not be fooled by demographics. Little old ladies and church deacons have been known to use illicit drugs. Grandmothers can have alcohol-withdrawal seizures. New substances, with previously unrecognized complications, continually appear. Old drugs regain favor. The drug-scape evolves. Clinicians must be ever vigilant.

Imbalances

Imbalances in key constituents, most notably gases, electrolytes, vitamins, and hormones can produce dramatic systemic and neurologic consequences. This section outlines imbalances in which the primary effects are on the nervous system.

With electrolytes and hormones, deleterious effects can be seen with either excess or deficiency. With vitamins, problems occur primarily because of deficiency, although excess vitamin intake of vitamin A and vitamin B_6 can cause neurologic complications (Table 10–3).

TABLE 10–3. NEUROLOGIC MANIFESTATIONS OF IMBALANCE IN KEY BODY CONSTITUENTS

Electrolytes

Hyponatremia: confusion, seizures

Hypernatremia: confusion

Rapid correction of hyponatremia: central pontine myelinolysis

Hypokalemia: weakness, cramps

Hypomagnesemia: seizures

Hypermagnesemia: neuromuscular transmission failure

Hypocalcemia: tetany, cramps

Hypercalcemia: altered mental status

Dehydration: syncope

Hormones

Addison disease: apathy, depression, confusion

Cushing disease: myopathy

Acromegaly: peripheral neuropathy, especially carpal tunnel syndrome

Hypothyroidism: cerebellar ataxia, peripheral neuropathy, dementia

Hyperthyroidism: myopathy, periodic paralysis, tremor

Antidiuretic hormone: diabetes insipidus or syndrome of inappropriate antidiuretic hormone

Vitamins

Vitamin B_{12} deficiency: dementia, optic neuropathy, peripheral neuropathy, subacute combined degeneration

Pyridoxine deficiency: neuropathy

Pyridoxine excess: neuropathy or neuronopathy

Vitamin A excess: pseudotumor cerebri

Vitamin E deficiency: spinocerebellar syndrome

Thiamine deficiency: Wernicke-Korsakoff disease

Gases

Hypoxia

Hypercarbia

Carbon monoxide toxicity

DEFICIENCY STATES

In addition to oxygen and glucose, the brain depends on numerous compounds to serve as enzymes and cofactors in its metabolic reactions. Deficiency of even minute amounts of some of these compounds can produce neurologic devastation.

Vitamin B$_{12}$ deficiency (pernicious anemia)

Patients with a deficiency of vitamin B$_{12}$ may develop several neurologic syndromes, including spinal cord disease (subacute combined degeneration), peripheral neuropathy, optic neuropathy, and dementia. Classic pernicious anemia is caused by a deficiency of gastric intrinsic factor due to an immunologic attack on parietal cells. There is an association with other organ-specific (e.g., myasthenia gravis, Hashimoto thyroiditis) and organ-nonspecific [e.g., systemic lupus erythematosus (SLE)] autoimmune disease, as well as an increased risk of developing carcinoma of the stomach. Since vitamin B$_{12}$ deficiency is easily treatable and can produce a spectrum of neurologic disease, a B$_{12}$ level is commonly included in neurologic workups, especially for neuropathy and dementia.

Other Deficiencies

Nutritional deficiency is also associated with optic neuropathy and peripheral neuropathy. Deficiency of vitamin E can cause a syndrome of spinocerebellar degeneration. Wernicke encephalopathy is due to thiamine deficiency.

Pyridoxine Imbalance

Most often a complication of isoniazid treatment of tuberculosis, lack of pyridoxine (vitamin B$_6$) produces an axonal polyneuropathy with distal weakness, sensory impairment, and reflex loss. Interestingly, an excess of pyridoxine can cause a severe, devastating sensory neuropathy. In neonates, pyridoxine deficiency is associated with seizures.

Mass Lesions

A mass lesion, also known as a space-occupying lesion, is any process that compresses neural tissue. A mass lesion can occur anywhere in the nervous system. Anything that has substance and volume can produce mass effect, including tumor, abscess, swollen brain due to infarction-induced necrosis, disc herniation, hematoma, and similar processes. Mass lesions commonly cause reactive (vasogenic) cerebral edema. This swelling of otherwise normal brain further exacerbates the effects of the mass (see Figure 10–3A). Steroids (dexamethasone is used most often) can sometimes dramatically alleviate the vasogenic edema induced by mass lesions.

Mass lesions can produce neurologic deficits because of direct and indirect effects. All mass lesions share in common the basic characteristic of dysfunction due to direct compression. These direct effects are primarily due to pressure-induced demyelination and necrosis of the compressed tissue. The indirect effects are due to any increase in pressure induced by a space-occupying lesion. Because the skull is a closed compartment with limited compliance, mass lesions within the skull can produce secondary effects due to increased intracranial pressure. With an intracranial mass lesion, the patient may therefore have both specific neurologic dysfunction due to direct tissue compression, and nonspecific neurologic dysfunction at a distance from the mass lesion itself due to the effects of a generalized increase in intracranial pressure.

The signs and symptoms due to the direct effects of an intracranial mass lesion depend on which part of the brain has been compressed. The signs and symptoms that result from a generalized increase in intracranial pressure include headache, nausea, vomiting, papilledema, third cranial nerve palsy, and herniation syndromes. Sixth cranial nerve palsy is common as a false localizing sign (Enrichment Box 10–1).

Intraspinal mass lesions, due to space-occupying lesions within the spinal canal, cause dysfunction due to direct pressure effects, but since the spinal canal is not a closed system, they do not cause indirect pressure effects such as those produced by intracranial mass lesions. Except for simple disc herniations, the signs and symptoms of an intraspinal mass lesion are usually transverse myelopathy, sometimes radiculopathy initially followed by the development of myelopathy, and rarely radiculopathy alone.

The signs and symptoms of an expanding mass lesion are characteristically progressive. The quintessential feature of the clinical syndrome due to an expanding mass is gradual worsening of the neurologic deficit. If the mass is expanding rapidly, such as might occur with a glioblastoma multiforme, the deficit may progress in a proportionately rapid fashion, typically over weeks or months.

Herniation syndromes are due to shifting of brain structures caused by increased intracranial pressure (see Figure 10–3B,C). They are evidence of severe involvement, and are life threatening. Several different herniation syndromes have been recognized. Three of the more important are central transtentorial, lateral transtentorial (uncal), and tonsillar herniation (see Enrichment Box 10–1) [Figure 10–5]. The clinical features of these herniation syndromes are summarized in Table 10–4.

Mass lesions

Small lesions compressing vital areas produce signs and symptoms early in the process. Lesions involving the motor cortex produce hemiparesis, lesions involving the occipital lobe produce hemianopia, and so forth. When mass lesions involve "silent" areas of the brain, such as the anterior frontal lobe, they can grow to remarkable size before the patient suffers any noticeable ill effects due to direct tissue compression.

False localizing signs are signs of dysfunction due to pressure-induced shifts that occur at a distance from the mass lesion itself. For instance, a sixth cranial nerve palsy, a classic false localizing sign, might occur on the side opposite the mass lesion.

Herniation syndromes

Central transtentorial herniation is due to symmetric downward displacement of the hemispheres, causing impaction of the diencephalon and midbrain into the tentorial notch. Pressure effects on the diencephalon and midbrain often cause small hemorrhages in the upper midbrain, referred to as Duret hemorrhages. Uncal herniation occurs when the temporal lobe and uncus shift medially into the tentorial notch, causing compression of the third cranial nerve and adjacent midbrain (see Figure 10–3C). Tentorial herniation, unless reversed, evolves into an orderly progression of neurologic dysfunction referred to as rostrocaudal deterioration. Herniation of the cerebellar tonsils downward into the foramen magnum compresses the medulla and upper spinal cord, and can result in rapid failure of vital functions. A dreaded complication of lumbar puncture (LP) is rapid worsening of an incipient herniation syndrome, especially cerebellar tonsillar herniation, due to removal of spinal fluid.

During rostrocaudal deterioration, neurologic dysfunction becomes progressively more dramatic. Clinical stages occur as if the brain had been transversely sectioned at a particular level (diencephalon, midbrain, pons, or medulla). Respirations become progressively more abnormal, evolving from a Cheyne-Stokes pattern early, to ataxic respirations, to eventual apnea. Pupils become progressively more abnormal and eventually become fixed and unreactive. Reflex eye movements are eventually lost. Motor responses evolve from localizing to nonlocalizing to decorticate to decerebrate to flaccid. The end result of unchecked rostrocaudal deterioration is death.

Seizure Disorders

Seizures are one of the most frequently encountered clinical problems in neurology, one in which the knowledgeable physician can have a great impact on the patient's quality of life. Seizures are prevalent;

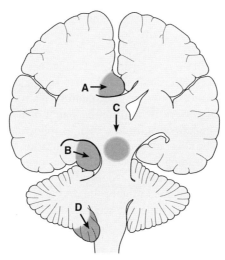

FIGURE 10–5. ▪Patterns of brain herniation. (*A*) Herniation of the cingulate gyrus under the falx cerebri. (*B*) Uncal (lateral transtentorial) herniation. (*C*) Central transtentorial herniation. (*D*) Herniation of the cerebellar tonsils through the foramen magnum. (Reprinted with permission from Wilkins RH, Rengachary SS: *Neurosurgery.* New York, McGraw-Hill, 1985.)

about 10% of the population suffers at least one seizure over an 80-year lifespan. In the past few years, several antiepileptic drugs (AEDs) have been added to the available treatment repertoire, which should permit even more effective therapeutic intervention.

TABLE 10–4. CLINICAL MANIFESTATIONS OF THE THREE CLASSICAL HERNIATION SYNDROMES

Herniation Syndrome	Clinical Manifestations
Central transtentorial	Impaired consciousness, abnormal respirations, symmetric small or midposition fixed or minimally reactive pupils, decorticate evolving to decerebrate posturing, rostrocaudal deterioration
Lateral transtentorial (uncal)	Impaired consciousness, abnormal respirations, third cranial nerve palsy (unilaterally dilated pupil), hemiparesis (may be false localizing), rostrocaudal deterioration
Cerebellar tonsillar	Impaired consciousness, neck rigidity, opisthotonos, decerebrate rigidity, vomiting, irregular respirations, apnea, bradycardia

Seizures result from "the excessive and disorderly discharge of neurons" [Hughlings Jackson, the original epileptologist, see JACKSONIAN (PARTIAL SIMPLE MOTOR) SEIZURES]. This disorderly discharge results from a disturbance in the normal delicate balance between excitatory and inhibitory influences. Recurrent seizures may be related to disturbances in the normal balance between the excitatory neurotransmitter glutamate and the inhibitory neurotransmitter γ-aminobutyric acid. In some of the secondary epilepsy syndromes, such as following a focal cerebral injury, there may be aberrant synaptic reorganization that facilitates excitatory functions, leading to hypersynchronous neuronal discharges.

The manifestations of a seizure depend on where this excessive and disorderly discharge begins in the brain, and how it spreads. Why the discharge begins matters little; the seizures due to a brain tumor or an old infarct, or for "idiopathic" reasons, look much the same.

Seizures can be divided into those that start in a specific part of one hemisphere, referred to as focal or partial seizures, and those that begin simultaneously in both hemispheres, referred to as generalized seizures. Simple partial seizures are focal or partial seizures that do not cause impairment of consciousness. Complex partial seizures are those that do impair consciousness or awareness.

Seizure discharges that begin focally may produce focal symptoms and signs. If the discharge remains focal, the clinical manifestations remain focal. For example, a focal motor seizure is the simplest form of seizure typically manifested as repetitive jerking of one body part, such as a hand or the corner of the mouth. If the discharge spreads along the cortex, a Jacksonian march is evident. If the discharge spreads down to deep midline structures, it is frequently then projected or propagated throughout the brain, resulting in loss of consciousness, a process referred to as secondary generalization.

Seizures that affect either the entire brain, or the deep midline structures that immediately project the discharge diffusely and bilaterally, are referred to as primary generalized seizures. Focal seizures that rapidly become secondarily generalized can be difficult to distinguish from primary generalized seizures. The importance of the distinction lies in the different likely causes of primary generalized seizures (idiopathic, familial, benign) as opposed to focal seizures with secondary generalization (focal cerebral lesions, e.g., tumor, abscess, or "scar" due to old stroke or trauma). Because of the importance of defining a focal origin for seizures, it is always critical to ask detailed questions about the prodrome, aura, and aftermath associated with any episode of loss or alteration of consciousness. A seizure is said to have a "focal signature" if there is an identifiable focal onset or a focal postictal deficit, either of which suggests a focal brain pathological condition (see TODD PARALYSIS). Patients with primary generalized seizures have a generally better prognosis and a greater likelihood of eventually discontinuing AEDs compared with patients with seizures due to a focal brain lesion.

The differential diagnosis of seizures is strikingly age dependent. The most likely etiological factors are different in an infant, a young child, an adolescent, a young adult, a middle-aged adult, and an elderly person (Table 10–5). The International Classification of the Epilepsies categorizes seizures by their neurophysiologic mechanism (Table 10–6).

Epilepsy is by definition characterized by recurrent seizures. Patients who have had an isolated seizure may or may not have epilepsy. The term "seizure disorder" is sometimes used to avoid the perjorative implications of the term "epilepsy," and sometimes because of uncertainty regarding the risk of having a recurrence of a seizure. The prognosis tends to be more favorable in the primary epileptic syndromes, which are generally age related and often remit in adolescence or early adulthood. The prognosis in secondary epilepsy syndromes depends on the underlying pathological condition. Some common causes of secondary epilepsy are tumor, cortical scar due to remote stroke or trauma, developmental defects, mesial temporal sclerosis, and infection.

The electroencephalogram (EEG) is the primary diagnostic test used for investigating patients with seizures. However, it is not a perfect tool. The interictal EEG, done between seizures, is normal in 10%–20% of patients with epilepsy. The likelihood of demonstrating an interictal

---

TABLE 10–5. LIKELY CAUSES OF RECURRENT SEIZURES IN VARIOUS AGE GROUPS

Age Group	Cause of Seizure
Neonatal and infancy	Birth injury or anoxia, metabolic disorders, congenital malformations, metabolic disorders, infantile spasms
Childhood	Febrile seizures, infantile spasms, perinatal anoxia or birth injury, idiopathic
Adolescence	Idiopathic, trauma
Early adulthood	Idiopathic, trauma, drug or alcohol use or withdrawal, neoplasm
Middle age	Neoplasm, alcohol or drug use or withdrawal, vascular disease, trauma
Elderly	Vascular disease, neoplasm, trauma, degenerative disease

TABLE 10–6. A CLASSIFICATION OF EPILEPTIC SEIZURES

Partial Seizures (Focal)

   Simple partial seizures with motor, autonomic, sensory, or psychic symptoms

   Complex partial seizures: simple onset followed by impairment of consciousness or with impairment of consciousness at onset

   Partial at onset, with evolution to generalized tonic clonic seizures

Generalized Seizures

   Nonconvulsive seizures (absence, myoclonic)

   Convulsive seizure: tonic clonic seizure, tonic seizure, clonic seizure

Unclassified Seizures

EEG abnormality depends on the type of epilepsy. Occasionally, a seizure may be fortuitously captured on EEG, permitting definitive diagnosis and characterization of the disorder both clinically and electrographically. EEG is discussed further in Chapter 9.

JACKSONIAN (PARTIAL SIMPLE MOTOR) SEIZURES

A neurologic classic: an electrical discharge "marches" across the motor cortex from one area of the homunculus to the next, causing the seizures to spread from one body part to another. The seizures might begin in the hand, spread to the arm, then to the face. As long as the seizures remain focal, the patient does not lose consciousness; with secondary generalization, loss or impairment of consciousness ensues.

GENERALIZED TONIC CLONIC (GRAND MAL, MAJOR MOTOR) SEIZURES

Generalized tonic clonic seizures involve a bilateral seizure discharge with loss of consciousness, bilaterally synchronous extremity movements, and often urinary and/or fecal incontinence and tongue biting. The extremity movements may consist of sustained tonic extension, repetitive clonic jerks, or (most commonly) a tonic phase followed by a clonic phase. The attacks are often heralded by a loud grunt (epileptic cry). During the attacks, the patient may become cyanotic during the tonic phase, then develop stertorous respirations. Following the seizure, patients typically go into a state of postictal lethargy and confusion, lasting from several minutes to half an hour or more. Grand mal attacks may occur because of a primary generalized seizure or during the secondarily generalized phase of a seizure that began focally.

GENERALIZED ABSENCE (PETIT MAL, MINOR MOTOR) SEIZURES

Absence seizures occur most often in children and produce transient staring spells with unresponsiveness, often mistaken for daydreaming. Sometimes minimal lip smacking or a few automatisms appear, but the motor manifestations are indeed "minor." These seizures are usually associated with a generalized 3-Hz spike and wave pattern on the EEG.

PARTIAL COMPLEX SEIZURES

Also known as temporal lobe or psychomotor seizures, these episodes are characterized by loss of awareness of the environment without actual loss of consciousness (i.e., a "dreamy state"), accompanied by various automatisms such as lip smacking, chewing, or idly picking at the clothing with one hand. Typical episodes last from about 2 to 15 minutes. If secondary generalization ensues, the patient may lose consciousness and have a generalized tonic clonic seizure. The seizure focus most often lies in the temporal lobe, occasionally in the frontal lobe. Uncinate fits are partial complex seizures with a prominent olfactory aura (Enrichment Box 10–2).

ALCOHOL WITHDRAWAL SEIZURES

The abstinence syndrome that results from abrupt discontinuation of heavy alcohol intake includes first "the shakes," beginning several hours after the last drink, then a tendency to have one (rarely several) generalized seizures within the first 24–48 hours, then the development of delirium tremens (DTs) at 48–72 hours. About 30%–40% of patients who have withdrawal seizures go on to develop DTs. Alcohol withdrawal seizures are nonfocal, usually self-limited, and associated with a normal interictal EEG. The neurologic examination is normal, as are imaging studies. Whether to treat the patient with AEDs is controversial; most neurologists do not. Extra caution should be used when any element of this syndrome is atypical; that is, the patient seizes while still drinking, the seizure follows rather than precedes DTs, the seizure has a focal signature, the neurologic examination is abnormal, or the EEG is abnormal. Patients who have just had a withdrawal seizure are at grave risk for DTs in the next 24–48 hours, and DTs carry a 50% mortality rate if left untreated (see Enrichment Box 10–2).

STATUS EPILEPTICUS

Prolonged seizures (> 15 minutes), or seizures occurring back to back without the patient regaining consciousness in between, constitute status epilepticus (SE). SE most often occurs in patients with known seizures who are noncompliant with their AEDs or in the setting of al-

ENRICHMENT BOX 10-2

Partial complex seizures

Because of the rich connections anatomically between the temporal lobe and the olfactory system, some patients with partial complex seizures have an olfactory or gustatory aura consisting of a strange, frequently indescribable, usually unpleasant smell or taste just before the seizure episode. These auras are referred to as "uncinate fits" because of the frequent location of the pathological condition in proximity to the uncus. Uncinate fits are classically associated with temporal lobe tumors.

Alcohol-related seizures

Alcoholics are not immune from other central nervous system (CNS) pathology (e.g., tumors), and they are more likely than nonalcoholics to have sustained head trauma with the formation of subdural hematoma (SDH) or encephalomalacia. To assume a withdrawal mechanism before adequate investigation is risky. However, after a workup has excluded other pathological conditions, it is generally superfluous and unnecessary to reinvestigate each time the patient has a seizure episode associated with drinking. Recent evidence suggests a more complicated situation, with the patient's likelihood to seize being correlated with total daily alcohol intake as well as with abstinence.

Pseudoseizures

Patients sometimes feign epileptic attacks for various reasons. Not infrequently, pseudoseizure patients also suffer from real seizures. They quickly learn the impact their seizures have on friends, family, teachers, and others and begin to manipulate others with feigned attacks, leading to a complex mixture of real seizures and pseudoseizures. Other patients develop pseudoseizures primarily. Pseudoseizure attacks are characterized by bizarre movements that lack the rhythmicity and symmetry of true seizures; patients tend to thrash and writhe about, have bicycling movements of the legs, struggle and lash out against assistance, and may have preservation of consciousness and recall the details of the "ictal" episode. Only rarely do they bite their tongue or have incontinence, but exceptionally determined and talented patients may manage to demonstrate these features. Some seizure foci in the brain, such as the frontal lobe, produce bizarre but very real seizures. Even experienced epileptologists may confuse such events with pseudoseizures.

cohol or drug withdrawal. SE is a neurologic emergency with a mortality rate in adults in the 10%–30% range, even with sophisticated management. Treatment regimens change over time, but often include intravenous (IV) fosphenytoin, phenobarbital, diazepam, or lorazepam. Some excellent AEDs have a limited role in SE because of the lack of an IV formulation. An IV preparation of valproic acid is now available, and is beginning to be used in SE. Intubation is frequently required because respiratory status may be compromised, especially when barbiturates and benzodiazepines have been used. Since altered metabolic states may cause SE, serum electrolytes, glucose, blood urea nitrogen, calcium, and magnesium levels need to be checked. In patients with no prior history of seizure disorder, a new intracranial lesion needs to be ruled out.

FEBRILE SEIZURES

A very common problem in children under 3 years of age, febrile seizures occur in about 5% of the "toddler" population. Typically, these seizures are brief, generalized, and occur with a rapidly rising fever that peaks at 103°F or higher. When the seizures occur in a child who was previously normal developmentally and neurologically, the events are usually benign and do not herald the later development of epilepsy.

NONEPILEPTIC SEIZURES (PSEUDOSEIZURES, HYSTERICAL SEIZURES)

[see Enrichment Box 10–2]

TODD PARALYSIS

Also known as postictal paralysis, Todd paralysis consists of a neurologic deficit that follows a seizure. The deficit usually lasts a few hours, rarely as long as 24 hours. Most often, the deficit is a hemiparesis, but hemianopia, aphasia, and other focal deficits occur as well. The occurrence of a postictal neurologic deficit suggests the possibility that the patient's seizure originated from a focal lesion in the brain, such as a tumor. Patients emerging from a seizure must be carefully examined for focal deficits, and this point must be assessed systematically in taking the history from any seizure patient, because postictal neurologic deficits provide a valuable clue to the cause of the seizure.

OTHER SEIZURE-RELATED ISSUES

Episodic loss of consciousness occurs for many reasons besides seizures, and distinguishing these other causes (e.g., vasovagal syncope, micturition syncope, Stokes-Adams attacks, drop attacks, cataplexy) is a regular clinical exercise. A complicating problem is the tendency of patients suffering sudden global cerebral hypoperfusion for any reason to have a few clonic jerks during the episode, referred to as "convulsive syncope." Even the occurrence of seizure activity does not necessarily indicate the primary event arose in the brain.

Patients are not easily rousable during the postictal state, which usually lasts about 30 minutes but may last longer; postictal coma must be considered in the differential diagnosis of patients who are "found down." In older patients, postictal focal deficits (Todd paralysis-type phenomena) are readily confused with cerebrovascular events.

TREATMENT OF EPILEPSY

AED treatment is justified for patients with epilepsy, that is, at risk of recurrent seizures. Single, isolated seizures are often not treated, especially when a likely explanation, such as alcohol abuse, is available. When AEDs are used, it is preferable to begin with monotherapy by using a single agent, and increasing the dose until the seizures are controlled or the treatment is limited by side effects. If the initial regimen is unsuccessful, a trial of monotherapy with a second agent is preferable to adding a second drug. Good control can be achieved in about 80% of patients. Those with difficult-to-control seizures often wind up on complicated, multiple drug regimens and are cared for by neurologists or even epileptologists.

The selection of an appropriate AED is based on its efficacy against the specific seizure type. For instance, phenytoin, carbamazepine, and valproic acid are effective against tonic clonic seizures. Valproic acid is particularly effective in absence seizures or seizures that have an absence component, such as juvenile myoclonic epilepsy. Careful attention must be given to the tendency of these drugs to cause specific serious adverse reactions and have interactions with other drugs. For current information on AEDs, including pharmacology and dosing information, visit the following Web sites: *elliott.hmc.washington.edu/education/drugs.html* or *www.mentalhealth.com/drug.*

The treatment of epilepsy during pregnancy is often particularly difficult, with problems of altered metabolism, complicating drug therapy, potential effects of the drug on the fetus, increased risk of bleeding, preeclampsia, eclampsia, and premature labor.

Craniocerebral Trauma

The clinical effects of trauma to the head involve complex dynamics, since one moving body, the brain, is traveling in relation to another moving body, the skull. With abrupt deceleration, the most frequent injury mechanism, the brain, suspended inside the skull, can rattle and bounce against the inner table and the rigid meningeal structures, causing coup and contrecoup injuries (Figure 10–6). Torsion vectors superimposed on acceleration changes further complicate matters.

Closed head injuries are those in which no fracture or only a simple linear fracture occurs. Open injuries are those with penetration or a depressed fracture. Fracture correlates only roughly with the force of injury. Severe brain damage can follow injuries in which no fracture oc-

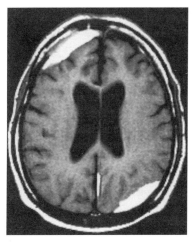

FIGURE 10–6. ■ Axial T1-weighted magnetic resonance image, showing bilateral subdural hematomas at opposite poles of the brain, right frontal and left occipital, due to a coup-contrecoup injury. (Reprinted with permission from Brant-Zawadzki M, Bradley WG, Cambray-Forker J (eds): *MRI of the Brain II*. Philadelphia, Lippincott Williams & Wilkins, 2001.) For an interactive example of a large subdural hematoma/hygroma, with mass effect and shift of midline structures, see *www.med.harvard.edu/AANLIB/cases/case10*.

curs, yet simple linear fractures of the cranial vault are often associated with only mild clinical effects. Concussion refers to an injury severe enough to cause loss of consciousness. Retrograde amnesia refers to loss of memory for events before injury; anterograde amnesia refers to events following the injury. Severity of injury correlates best with duration of loss of consciousness and length of anterograde amnesia. Following penetrating wounds or depressed fractures, there is a high incidence of posttraumatic seizures, which may not begin for months or years. Early seizures after injury have little implication for later epilepsy.

CLOSED HEAD INJURY

The most common type of closed head injury is simple concussion. These injuries produce brief loss of consciousness with no focal abnormalities on examination and normal imaging studies. The precise pathophysiologic mechanism underlying concussion remains unclear.

Loss of consciousness with concussion seldom lasts longer than minutes, although the antegrade and retrograde amnesia may be considerably longer. Prolonged unconsciousness, or a "lucid interval" of preserved function followed by deterioration after the injury should raise the question of an intracranial hematoma (see ACUTE SUBDURAL

HEMATOMA). Following concussion, some patients demonstrate an acute confusional state that lasts for a variable amount of time. Closed head injuries may also produce diffuse axonal damage, causing severe neurologic dysfunction.

The acute assessment should include a search for hemotympanum, Battle sign (discoloration over the mastoid), and raccoon eyes; these signs indicate probable basilar skull fracture, which may be difficult to demonstrate radiologically.

Cerebral contusion is a more severe form of closed head injury in which there is superficial hemorrhage over the cortex, which may be visible on imaging studies, and which may produce contamination of the subarachnoid space with blood. The most severe closed head injuries may produce ICH.

Postconcussion syndrome consists of a constellation of complaints following concussion, including headache, dizziness, lassitude, and difficulty with memory and concentration. Some individuals develop postconcussion syndrome after apparently minor closed head injuries. Symptoms resolve in most patients; the possibility of complicating depression or secondary gain arises with protracted recovery.

ACUTE SUBDURAL HEMATOMA

Subdural hematomas (SDHs) arise from torn veins bleeding into the subdural space, in contrast to epidural hematomas, which result from arterial bleeding. Acute SDHs most often follow obvious head trauma. The rapidly expanding intracranial mass produces impairment of consciousness and focal signs, and if untreated may progress to cause increased intracranial pressure, herniation, and death. Patients are most often young and multiply injured.

In infants and children, fragile bridging subdural veins can rupture during violent head movement, such as being shaken to and fro by an irate parent, and cause SDHs with no obvious external trauma (the shaken baby syndrome). A recent prominent legal case in the United States [*Commonwealth v. Woodward,* 427 Mass 659, 694 N.E.2d 1277 (1998)] may have involved such an injury.

CHRONIC SUBDURAL HEMATOMA

In contrast to the situation with acute SDHs, chronic SDHs develop more slowly and often follow minor head trauma, particularly in elderly patients (see Figure 10–6). Patients often give no history of head trauma, either because the head blow was so minor (e.g., bumping the head on a kitchen cabinet) or because the effects of the SDH impairs memory sufficiently that the patient fails to recall the traumatic episode. The intracranial mass effect develops slowly and typically produces impairment of consciousness with only minor focality on examination. Chronic SDHs develop osmotically active membranes of granulation tissue, which imbibe and release fluid, causing variations in the size of the SDH and a fluctuating clinical course. Chronic SDH figures prominently in the differential diagnosis of AMS and dementia, especially in elderly patients. Small chronic SDHs are sometimes managed with close observation; large SDHs require surgical drainage with or without excision of the membranes.

EPIDURAL HEMATOMA

Epidural hematomas most commonly follow fractures through the temporal squamosa that lacerate the middle meningeal artery. Patients may have a "lucid interval" following the injury, only to lapse into coma as the hematoma expands minutes to hours later.

TREATMENT OF CRANIOCEREBRAL TRAUMA

For current information on management of patients with traumatic brain injury, visit the following Web sites: *www.cdc.gov/ncipc/dacr-rdp/tbi.htm* or *www.braintrauma.org/pdflibrary.nsf/Main/Guidelines*. The latter site offers a large and very detailed monograph on the topic.

Degenerative Disease

Degenerative diseases are those for which no clear etiologic basis is known. The term is an admission of our lack of understanding. With advancing knowledge, some conditions are removed from this category as their etiologic basis is clarified. Conditions such as Creutzfeldt-Jakob disease, Huntington chorea, and Reye syndrome were often listed under this category until their cause was demonstrated. The clinical conditions now commonly included under the rubric of degenerative diseases include the dementias, amyotrophic lateral sclerosis (ALS), and Parkinson disease and related syndromes. ALS is discussed in Chapter 11, AMYOTROPHIC LATERAL SCLEROSIS.

DEMENTIA

Dementia refers to loss of mental capacity, and can occur either as a primary degenerative condition [e.g., Alzheimer disease (AD)] or as a secondary complication of another disease, such as hypothyroidism or CNS infection. The thrust of a dementia workup is exclusion of a "treatable dementia," in which an underlying condition has produced dementia as a complication. Treatable causes of dementia are listed in Table 10–7.

AD is the most common, but not the only, cause of dementia. Other neurologic conditions causing dementia are listed in Table 10–8. The

TABLE 10-7. TREATABLE CAUSES OF DEMENTIA

Depression ("depressive pseudodementia")

Hypothyroidism

Vitamin B_{12} deficiency

Normal pressure hydrocephalus

Cerebral vasculitis

Cerebrovascular disease

Neurosyphilis

HIV infection

Cerebral mass lesion (e.g., subdural hematoma, olfactory meningioma)

Chronic meningitis (e.g., tuberculosis, cryptococcosis)

Drug intoxication

HIV = human immunodeficiency virus.

incidence and prevalence of dementia are strikingly age dependent. The prevalence is approximately 1% at 60 years of age, but doubles every 5 years so that by 80 years of age 16% of the population is laboring under a degree of cognitive impairment. In the population 75–85 years of age, the prevalence may approach 30%–50%. AD, either in isolation or in combination with another process, accounts for about 50%–70% of the cases of dementia; some estimates are as high as 90%. Vascular, or multi-infarct, dementia can coexist with AD.

TABLE 10-8. NEUROLOGIC DISEASES IN WHICH DEMENTIA MAY BE A PROMINENT FEATURE

Alzheimer disease

Pick disease

Creutzfeldt-Jakob disease

Parkinson disease

Dementia with Lewy bodies

Corticobasal degeneration

Progressive supranuclear palsy

Paraneoplastic limbic encephalitis

A degree of cognitive impairment can be a component of many other neurologic conditions.

The core features of a dementing illness consist of progressive loss of memory, cognitive function, judgment, and social skills. Demented patients may sometimes exhibit clinical signs that provide a clue as to the cause, such as a prominent gait disturbance in normal pressure hydrocephalus (NPH), Argyll-Robertson pupils in neurosyphilis, or myoclonus in Creutzfeldt-Jakob disease. Aberrant behavior often becomes a major management problem. Sundowning refers to the common tendency of demented patients to become more confused and restless at night.

COMMON CLINICAL DEMENTIA SYNDROMES

The common dementia syndromes include AD and multi-infarct dementia (MID). The syndrome of NPH is frequently considered in the differential diagnosis of dementia. Loss of cognitive ability commonly complicates human immunodeficiency virus (HIV) infection.

Alzheimer Disease

AD is characterized by progressive cognitive deterioration and behavioral changes. AD was formerly referred to as senile dementia when it affected patients older than 65 years of age and presenile dementia when it affected patients younger than 65 years of age. These terms have fallen out of use and the condition is simply called AD or dementia of the Alzheimer type. It is by far the most common cause of dementia, and has become a major public health problem because of the aging population. Early memory loss progresses inexorably, leading to severe global cognitive dysfunction with eventual death due to inanition after a course of 5–7 years.

The pathological hallmark of AD is the presence of senile plaques and neurofibrillary tangles, along with synaptic and neuronal loss. Increasing evidence suggests that amyloid deposition plays a key role in the development of AD. Some of the genetic aspects of AD may be explicable through effects on amyloid deposition (Enrichment Box 10–3).

Loss of neurons and synaptic connections diffusely in the cortex likely underlies most of the manifestations of the disease. There is a predilection for involvement of certain neuronal groups, especially the nucleus basalis of Meynert in the basal forebrain. This nucleus is prominently involved in the cholinergic projections to the hemispheres. Abnormalities of acetylcholine metabolism are thought to be responsible for much of the cognitive and memory dysfunction in AD, and manipulation of acetylcholine forms the basis for the available pharmacotherapy.

Memory impairment is the clinical hallmark of AD. Progressive disruption of language functions usually accompanies the memory impairment. Behavioral aberrations are an integral part of AD, and can become as much or more of a management challenge as the cognitive

ENRICHMENT BOX 10-3

Alzheimer disease

The gene for apolipoprotein E is important in the genetics of Alzheimer disease (AD). It is located on chromosome 19, and has four alleles. The E4 allele is a marker that indicates increased risk of developing late-onset familial AD and sporadic AD. Apolipoprotein E influences the metabolism of amyloid, and the effects of the E4 allele may be mediated through amyloid deposition.

In the early stages of the disease, memory impairment is manifested primarily as difficulty in acquiring and retaining new information, with relative preservation of long-term memory. Remote events may be recalled with striking clarity, whereas recent events are muddled and unclear. With progression of the disease, remote memory is increasingly affected, and eventually the patient may be frankly disoriented and unable to recall even his or her own name.

With early involvement of language functions, difficulty with word finding and naming is usually apparent. With progression of the disease, there is impaired comprehension, and communication becomes increasingly problematic. Other evidence of cortical dysfunction eventually appears. Patients may develop various types of agnosias and apraxias, especially involving visual functions, along with impairment of judgment and abstraction ability.

The behavioral problems range from anxiety, agitation, sundowning, delusions, and frank psychosis to depression, extreme passivity, apathy, and a state approaching abulia. Personality change is common, and may even antedate the cognitive impairment. Delusions are commonly paranoid. Hallucinations, usually visual but occasionally auditory, are common.

These noncognitive manifestations of AD, especially the agitation, depression, and behavioral aberrations, are frequently a major management issue. It is important to recognize that some behavioral peculiarities, such as wandering, repetitive questioning, repetitive behaviors, and indecorous toilet behavior may simply be part of the disease and will not respond to medications.

Diagnostic criteria for AD may be helpful. There is an 85% confirmation at autopsy if patients have had a 1-year course of deterioration in two or more areas of cognitive functioning (memory, language, praxis, visual or spatial function), onset between 40 and 90 years of age, and preserved consciousness, and if treatable causes of dementia have been appropriately excluded.

(Continued)

ENRICHMENT BOX 10-3 (*CONTINUED*)

Alzheimer disease versus multi-infarct dementia and normal pressure hydrocephalus

In distinguishing between AD and multi-infarct dementia (MID), some features that favor MID as the cause of a dementing illness include abrupt onset, a stepwise or fluctuating course, relative preservation of personality, emotional incontinence, a history of hypertension, evidence of vascular disease elsewhere, ischemic white matter changes on imaging studies, and focal neurologic signs or symptoms. Although gait abnormality and dementia are classic for normal pressure hydrocephalus (NPH), most patients with a gait abnormality and dementia prove to have MID. In NPH, language functions tend to be preserved and there are no focal cortical signs.

Depression and pseudodementia

In addition to prominent complaints about memory loss, other features suggesting pseudodementia rather than AD include early solicitation of medical advice, a precise dating of the onset of symptoms, rapid progression of symptoms, and a history of past psychiatric problems. Patients with pseudodementia tend to describe their difficulties in detail, whereas patients with AD are vague about the problems they are experiencing. Pseudodementia patients emphasize their degree of disability, and exert poor effort in trying to perform even simple tasks. They often give "don't know" or near-miss responses to questions. Sundowning and personality changes are uncommon.

impairment. Diagnostic criteria for AD have been developed (see Enrichment Box 10–3).

Although there is considerable variability in disease severity and rate of progression, the typical patient with AD survives for about 8 years. Patients usually succumb to complications of immobility, urosepsis, or pneumonia, especially aspiration. The mental status may abruptly worsen when such complications supervene (so-called beclouded dementia).

In the workup of the patient with dementia, there is an emphasis on excluding treatable conditions. Patients with depression typically complain of problems with memory and seek medical attention directly, whereas those with AD are often less aware of their deficits and may be brought to medical attention by their families. Patients with nonneurodegenerative cognitive impairment often put forth poor effort during mental status testing, giving up readily, whereas those with AD make a good effort but cannot give right answers. After treatable causes of dementia have been excluded, there is little that can be done to confirm the diagnosis of AD.

Because of the disturbance in cholinergic metabolism, many attempts have been made to find a way to augment CNS cholinergic activity as a treatment for the disease. The centrally acting anticholinesterase agent tacrine was eventually proven to be of benefit, but tolerance was limited by side effects. Donepezil and rivastigmine are also effective and are better tolerated. Even when cognitive improvement with such agents is equivocal, patients may have improvement in functional abilities and an increased interest in the environment.

For current objective information on pharmacotherapy of AD, go to the Web site at *www.cochranelibrary.com/cochrane/cochrane-frame.html* and search the Cochrane abstracts for Alzheimer's.

Multi-infarct Dementia

MID is a dementing illness that results from multiple cerebral infarctions; it is also referred to as vascular dementia. Some of these infarctions may be quite small (lacunar) and silent, while others may be large and clinically obvious. MID is typically associated with diabetes, hypertension, and other causes of vascular disease. Most patients have a history of at least one clinical episode of stroke. Examination may show brainstem abnormalities, pyramidal signs, or other features not usually seen in AD. Magnetic resonance imaging (MRI) typically shows diffuse white matter disease, presumably due to vascular insufficiency, in addition to evidence of past focal vascular insults. Since both AD and vascular disease are common, MID and AD may occasionally coexist in the same patient (see Enrichment Box 10–3).

Communicating or Normal Pressure Hydrocephalus

In communicating hydrocephalus, there is either impairment of CSF reabsorption through the arachnoid villi into the venous sinuses, or obstruction to flow at a point in the CSF pathways beyond the outlet foramina of the fourth ventricle, most often at the base of the brain. Communicating hydrocephalus can occur after meningitis or intracranial hemorrhage because of scarring of the meninges, which impairs CSF circulation and/or causes dysfunction of the reabsorptive mechanisms.

NPH refers to a spontaneously occurring form of communicating hydrocephalus, featuring a clinical triad of dementia, gait difficulties, and urinary incontinence. Imaging studies show large ventricles, and lumbar puncture (LP) may result in temporary improvement. Since symptoms may improve after placement of a ventriculoperitoneal shunt, NPH represents one of the "treatable dementias" (see Enrichment Box 10–3).

Human Immunodeficiency Virus Dementia

HIV dementia is more likely to occur in a younger patient and present with memory loss that progresses over months. It may be the initial presentation of acquired immunodeficiency syndrome (AIDS), and affected patients may have other types of CNS infection or harbor a brain tumor. Frontal lobe dysfunction is usually prominent, especially personality changes.

Pseudodementia

Patients with depression frequently complain of memory loss and difficulty with thinking and concentrating, and depressive pseudodementia is another "treatable dementia." The patients, or their families, may think the patient has developed AD. Patients with AD usually do not complain of the memory loss, whereas those with depressive pseudodementia do so bitterly. (See Enrichment Box 10–3 for other features that may help distinguish pseudodementia from AD.)

PARKINSON DISEASE AND RELATED MOVEMENT DISORDERS

Movement disorders disrupt motor function not by causing weakness but by producing either abnormal, involuntary, or unwanted movements (hyperkinetic movement disorders), or by curtailing the amount of normal free-flowing, fluid movement by causing abnormal states of increased muscle tone (hypokinetic movement disorders). Pathological findings in these conditions primarily involve the basal ganglia: caudate, putamen, globus pallidus, substantia nigra, or subthalamic nucleus. The rich connections between the subcomponents of the basal ganglia and between the basal ganglia and other motor systems, as well as the numerous neurotransmitters involved, make the clinical manifestations of basal ganglia disease complex and varied. Depending on the precise location of the abnormality, the particular cell type involved, and the neurotransmitter affected, the clinical picture may range from abnormally decreased movement (the akinesia or bradykinesia of Parkinson disease) to abnormally increased movement (chorea, hemiballismus, dystonia).

Parkinson Disease

Parkinson disease is a very common disorder that is due to a degeneration of neurons in the dopaminergic nigrostriatal pathway. Pathologically, the disease is characterized by depigmentation and cell loss involving the substantia nigra with Lewy bodies in surviving neurons. The etiology remains unknown. Current thinking favors a multifactorial basis, possibly involving hereditary factors, environmental influences that may selectively affect dopaminergic nigral cells, and free radical toxicity.

Parkinson disease is the second most common movement disorder behind essential tremor, affecting about 1% of the population older than 50 years of age. Cardinal manifestations include tremor (a "pill rolling" tremor maximal at rest at a frequency of about 3 Hz), bradykinesia (slowness and poverty of movement), cogwheel rigidity (increased tone to passive movement, which has a rhythmic quality, presumably due to the superimposition of the tremor), and postural instability (poor balance with a tendency to fall).

Parkinsonism is a clinical diagnosis appropriate in the presence of resting tremor, bradykinesia, rigidity, and impaired postural reflexes. Parkinson disease is but one cause of parkinsonism, and must be differentiated from other conditions that may have some of its typical features as a component of another disorder. The terms parkinsonism, Parkinson syndrome, or Parkinson plus are sometimes used to designate such disorders (Table 10–9). Multisystem atrophy (MSA) produces degeneration in more than one system, and usually includes parkinsonian features. Shy-Drager syndrome is the most common type of MSA (Enrichment Box 10–4).

Clinical features that suggest Parkinson disease include prominent rest tremor, asymmetric signs, good preservation of balance and postural reflexes in the early stages of the disease, and a good response to levodopa replacement therapy. Asymmetry is characteristic. The disease often begins asymmetrically; the signs may be so lateralized as to warrant the designation of hemi-Parkinson, and some asymmetry usually persists even when the disease is well established.

TABLE 10–9. DIFFERENTIAL DIAGNOSIS OF PARKINSON DISEASE

Parkinson disease

Parkinsonian syndromes

   Progressive supranuclear palsy

   Multisystem atrophy

      Olivopontocerebellar degeneration

      Striatonigral degeneration

      Shy-Drager syndrome

   Diffuse Lewy body disease

   Drug-induced parkinsonism

Essential tremor

Depression

Wilson disease

Multisystem atrophy

Shy-Drager syndrome, one of the subtypes of multisystem atrophy (MSA), consists of a combination of parkinsonian signs and symptoms coupled with severe dysautonomia, most often manifest as orthostatic hypotension. The dysautonomia is due to degeneration of the neurons in the intermediolateral gray column of the thoracic and lumbar spinal cord. MSA can involve the basal ganglia, cerebellum, anterior horn cells, cerebral cortex, and brainstem in varying combinations. MSA patients may have elements of cerebellar ataxia, dementia, amyotrophy, parkinsonism, and dysautonomia. Shy-Drager specifically refers to that subset of patients with MSA who suffer primarily from the parkinsonian features associated with severe orthostatic hypotension. Dopaminergic agents help less than in Parkinson disease. The intermediolateral gray column degeneration can occur without any other abnormalities, in which case it produces a syndrome of idiopathic orthostatic hypotension. Dysautonomia can also occur in association with degeneration of other parts of the nervous system.

Parkinsonian versus essential tremor

The tremor of Parkinson disease is most prominent at rest, while that of essential tremor occurs with a sustained posture, such as with the hands outstretched, or on action. Parkinsonian tremor may persist with hands outstretched but damps with intention, whereas essential tremor usually worsens with intention. The head and voice are often involved with essential tremor, but only rarely with Parkinson disease. Alcohol and beta-blockers often improve essential tremor but have little effect on parkinsonian tremor.

Surgical treatment for Parkinson disease

New surgical approaches used for Parkinson disease include "brain transplants" with transplantation of adrenal medullary cells or fetal mesencephalic tissue into the striatum, thalamotomy, pallidotomy, and deep-brain stimulation. The pathophysiology of parkinsonism is complex, but dopamine deficiency ultimately results in an increased output from the internal segment of the globus pallidus and subthalamic nuclei, which results in excessive inhibition of the thalamus and suppression of the cortical motor system. Both pallidotomy and stimulation of the subthalamic nucleus reduce the excessive inhibitory output of the internal segment of the globus pallidus, restore more normal cortical motor activity, and can reduce the manifestations of parkinsonism. Thalamotomy is useful primarily for the control of tremor and may not result in significant improvement in disability, since tremor does not produce a great deal of functional limitation compared with akinesia and rigidity. Pallidotomy and deep-brain stimulation of either the internal pallidal segment or the subthalamic nucleus can ameliorate all features of parkinsonism.

In the early stages of Parkinson disease, typical signs are often subtle and patients may present complaining only of stiffness, impaired handwriting, or difficulty getting about. Stiffness and myalgic pains may suggest a diagnosis of arthritis, polymyalgia, or fibromyalgia. The facial masking and bradykinesia often lead to a misdiagnosis of depression. The gait abnormality in Parkinson disease is stereotypical. Patients walk with a stooped, flexed posture with a reduced stride length, sometimes markedly so, reduced arm swing, and a tendency to turn "en-bloc." Impaired postural reflexes lead to a tendency to fall forward, which the patient tries to avoid by walking with increasing speed but with very short steps, the festinating gait. Falls are common.

Advancing disease is characterized by increasing gait difficulty and worsening of tremor and bradykinesia. The tremor may begin to abate in the very late stages. Other major problems in advanced Parkinson disease include motor fluctuations related to levodopa therapy, behavioral changes, cognitive impairment, depression, hallucinations, impotence, dysphagia, speech difficulty, intractable drooling, and sleep impairment. Early or prominent hallucinations suggest the possibility of dementia with Lewy bodies.

The differential diagnosis of Parkinson disease is summarized in Table 10–9. One of the most common difficulties is differentiating early Parkinson disease from essential tremor (see Enrichment Box 10–4).

The other degenerative disorders with parkinsonian features typically produce other neurologic signs, such as gaze limitation, cerebellar signs, pyramidal signs, severe dementia, apraxia and other parietal lobe signs, or dysautonomia, although these other manifestations may not be very apparent early in the course. A suboptimal response to levodopa is often another important clue to the presence of a condition other than ordinary Parkinson disease.

Certain drugs can induce a reversible condition that mimics Parkinson disease. The most common agents that cause drug-induced parkinsonism are antipsychotics, especially the high-potency piperazine compounds such as haloperidol. The new class of atypical neuroleptics (e.g., clozapine, olanzapine, risperidone) are as potent in their antipsychotic effects as traditional compounds but less likely to induce parkinsonism. Drug-induced parkinsonism can mimic Parkinson disease closely, even to the point of causing asymmetric signs. Although dopamine receptor-blocking agents, especially those that block the D_2 receptor, are the most common offenders, other agents can induce parkinsonism. It is often not appreciated that metoclopramide, frequently given for gastrointestinal (GI) motility disorders, is a phenothiazine and can induce parkinsonism.

In the presence of typical clinical signs and symptoms and typical age of onset, no extensive workup is required. Imaging studies are usually normal. A thorough medication history, complete neurologic examination to look for nonextrapyramidal abnormalities, and screening for orthostatic hypotension are useful. Certain features suggest an alternative diagnosis, such as prominent dementia and hallucinations in the patient suffering from dementia with Lewy bodies, prominent dysautonomia in the patient with Shy-Drager syndrome, and dysarthria and early age of onset in Wilson disease.

Pharmacological treatment modalities include anticholinergic drugs, dopamine-releasing agents (amantadine), dopamine agonists that directly stimulate the dopamine receptor in the striatum (e.g., bromocriptine), and catechol-o-methyl transferase inhibitors and levodopa. The discovery of levodopa as a treatment for Parkinson disease was a major medical advance. The story of that discovery is told in British neurologist Oliver Sachs's book, *Awakenings* (Garden City, NY, Doubleday, 1974) and its movie adaptation. Some of the numerous drugs presently available for the treatment of Parkinson disease are listed in Table 10–10. Over 90% of patients with Parkinson disease respond very well to the initiation of levodopa replacement. The absence of a good initial response suggests the possibility of another diagnosis. Several surgical approaches seem to hold promise (see Enrichment Box 10–4).

For current information on the management of Parkinson disease, visit the following Web sites: *www.neuroland.com/move/index.htm, www.aafp.org/afp/990415ap/2155.html, www.postgradmed.com/issues/ 1999/08_99/conley2.htm,* or *www.parkinsons-information-exchange-*

TABLE 10–10. DRUGS USED IN THE TREATMENT OF PARKINSON DISEASE

Class	Drug
Anticholinergic	Trihexyphenidyl, benztropine, others
MAO-B inhibitor	Selegiline
Dopamine agonist	
Ergot derived	Bromocriptine, pergolide, lisuride, cabergoline
Non-ergot derived	Pramipexole, ropinirole
Dopamine precursor	Levodopa, carbidopa/levodopa
COMT inhibitor	Entacapone, tolcapone
Miscellaneous	Amantadine

COMT = catechol-O-methyltransferase; MAO-B = monoamine oxidase-B.

network-online.com/archive/ alg01.html (extensive discussion with an algorithm).

Essential Tremor

Although the etiology is unknown, essential tremor is mentioned here because of its frequent confusion with parkinsonian tremor. A form of enhanced physiologic tremor, essential tremor is higher in frequency and lower in amplitude than the tremor of Parkinson disease. It is the most common of all movement disorders. The prevalence of essential tremor increases with age, may first appear anywhere between the second and sixth decades of life, and tends to be slowly progressive. It is often familial. Essential tremor tends to affect the hands, head, and voice. It frequently abates with alcohol ingestion, an important historical point because this does not occur with the tremor of Parkinson disease. Essential tremor generally responds to beta-blockers. The etiology and pathophysiology remain obscure.

Migraine

Migraine is a multifaceted disorder. The headache is only one aspect, albeit the most common and familiar. Because the symptoms of neurologic dysfunction are sometimes more prominent than the headache, migraine enters the differential diagnosis of a number of clinical syndromes. Complicated migraine is often confused with cerebrovascular disease. Migraine, both "simple" headache and complicated migraine, is discussed further in the section on headache disorders in Chapter 12.

Multiple Sclerosis and Other Demyelinating Diseases

Demyelinating diseases primarily affect the myelin of the CNS. Disorders of peripheral myelin, such as Guillain-Barré syndrome (GBS), are not generally grouped under the rubric of demyelinating disease. Most demyelinating disease is immunologically mediated, multiple sclerosis (MS) being the most common example. More rarely, myelin is involved in infectious processes [e.g., progressive multifocal leukoencephalopathy (PML)] or fails to develop normally in the first place (e.g., leukodystrophy). Entities that are occasionally considered in the differential diagnosis of demyelinating diseases are listed in Table 10–11.

MULTIPLE SCLEROSIS

MS is a common disorder (400,000–500,000 affected individuals in the United States), caused by a presumably immunologic attack on CNS myelin, occurring for obscure reasons. It is more common in

TABLE 10–11. CONDITIONS TO CONSIDER IN THE DIFFERENTIAL DIAGNOSIS OF DEMYELINATING DISEASE

Multiple sclerosis

Acute disseminated encephalomyelitis

CNS vasculitis

Lyme disease

HTLV-I myelopathy

Tertiary syphilis

Progressive multifocal leukoencephalopathy

Connective tissue disorders, especially SLE and Sjögren syndrome

Behçet disease

Sarcoidosis

Vitamin B_{12} deficiency

Leukodystrophies

Degenerative disorders

CNS = central nervous system; HTLV-I = human T-cell lymphotrophic virus type I; SLE = systemic lupus erythematosus.

women by a ratio of 2:1, and more common in whites. There is some genetic influence, with an increased risk in first-degree relatives. The geographic distribution of MS is curious and possibly important. There is a significantly higher incidence in the more northern and southern latitudes, and a lower incidence in equatorial regions. Individuals escape the increased susceptibility only if they migrate from the high-risk environment before 15 years of age.

Pathologically, the disease creates "plaques" of obliterated myelin with spared axons. On palpation of the cut brain, these areas of demyelination feel hardened or "sclerotic." There tend to be many of them: hence the epithet. Demyelination impairs saltatory conduction and can slow conduction velocity along the involved fibers or cause conduction block at the site of the lesion. The effects of demyelination are more pronounced at higher temperatures, and increased temperature (e.g., fever or high ambient temperature) can temporarily cause increased neurologic dysfunction.

Clinical manifestations of MS are protean; among the most common are optic neuritis, transverse myelitis, cerebellar ataxia, and internuclear ophthalmoplegia. The disease generally begins in the "reproductive years" between 20 and 40 years of age with recurrent attacks followed by recovery, described as "relapsing and remitting."

Some patients with long-standing relapsing and remitting disease, and some older patients with the initial onset of MS, may follow a non-fluctuating inexorably downhill course referred to as chronic progressive MS. The disease sometimes runs a fairly benign course. The lack of major motor or cerebellar deficits after 5 years predicts relatively low disability after 15 years. MS patients often complain of intense fatigue, possibly due to the increased efforts necessary to compensate for their neurologic deficits, possibly of another origin.

A characteristic elevation of immunoglobulin G occurs in the CSF in addition to occasional oligoclonal bands of immunoglobulin. These immunoglobulin abnormalities originate in the CNS, remain isolated to the CSF, and do not appear in the serum. Oligoclonal bands are present in 90% of patients with definite MS. Some patients have a low-grade lymphocytic pleocytosis or mildly increased protein. The presence of myelin basic protein indicates myelin destruction and occurs in most patients after a significant exacerbation.

MRI shows multiple white matter lesions (Figure 10–7). Plaques of MS are often seen in a periventricular location. MRI findings suggestive of MS include four or more white matter lesions, periventricular lesions, ring enhancement with gadolinium, lesions perpendicular to the ventricles (Dawson fingers), and abnormalities in the corpus callosum or brainstem. Evoked potential studies may demonstrate lesions in white matter tracts that are not apparent clinically or radiologically.

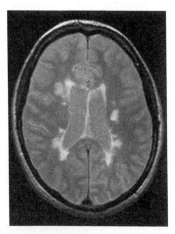

FIGURE 10–7. ■ T2-weighted magnetic resonance image, showing multiple, peri-ventricular white matter lesions in a patient with multiple sclerosis. (Reprinted with permission from Brant-Zawadzki M, Bradley WG, Cambray-Forker J (eds): *MRI of the Brain I*. Philadelphia, Lippincott Williams & Wilkins, 2001.) For an interactive example of a similar case, see *www.med.harvard.edu/AANLIB/cases/case38*.

MRI abnormalities and the presence of CSF oligoclonal bands aid most in buttressing clinical diagnosis.

Steroids, primarily IV methylprednisolone, are often given to patients during an MS exacerbation. Although steroids may shorten the duration of an acute exacerbation, it is not clear that they alter the long-term outcome of the disease. Recently, disease-modifying agents have been developed that alter the natural history of the disease toward fewer and milder attacks. These include interferon beta 1a, interferon beta 1b, glatiramer acetate, and mitoxantrone. Initiation of therapy with disease-modifying agents is advisable after a diagnosis of definite relapsing-remitting MS. For current information on MS treatment, visit the Web site *medstat.med.utah.edu/kw/ms/treat_options.html.*

ACUTE DISSEMINATED ENCEPHALOMYELITIS

Acute disseminated encephalomyelitis (ADEM), also referred to as postinfectious, parainfectious, or postvaccinial encephalomyelitis, is a dysimmune disorder affecting the white matter of the CNS, which typically follows a viral infection or immunization. The most common cause is a nonspecific upper respiratory infection. ADEM essentially constitutes the CNS analogue of GBS, and fortunately is much rarer. MRI typically demonstrates widespread, multifocal demyelinating lesions. Similar postinfectious or postvaccinial dysimmune attacks can involve the optic nerve (optic neuritis) and the spinal cord (transverse myelitis); in ADEM, the lesions are more widespread and the patients typically have multifocal deficits, often with alteration of consciousness and sometimes with seizures. The mortality rate is high and severe residua are common. There is no effective treatment, although high-dose steroids are usually given.

ACUTE TRANSVERSE MYELITIS OR MYELOPATHY

Patients with acute transverse myelitis typically present with a history of progressive numbness and weakness involving both legs, or more rarely, all four extremities, evolving over a period of hours or days. Bladder involvement is often early and prominent, and sometimes the patients present with urinary retention. At the height of the illness, the patient's clinical syndrome consists of weakness of all muscles below the level of the lesion; a sensory level that corresponds erratically with the actual site of abnormality; and varying degrees of bowel, bladder, and sexual dysfunction. The involvement is bilateral and symmetric with all functions below a certain "transverse" level of the spinal cord impaired. Acute transverse myelitis may occur after infection or immunization (see ACUTE DISSEMINATED ENCEPHALOMYELITIS), or as an attack of MS. Spinal fluid typically contains cells and an elevated level of protein. Devic disease (neuromyelitis optica) is a variant of MS in which the spinal cord and optic nerves are selectively involved.

In acute transverse myelopathy, a virtually identical clinical picture develops because of a mass lesion pressing on the spinal cord. Tumor (primary or metastatic), disc, and abscess can all produce an acute transverse myelopathy. A thorough workup to exclude compressive myelopathy is thus necessary before accepting a diagnosis of transverse myelitis.

OPTIC NEURITIS

Optic nerve dysfunction can occur for a number of reasons. One of the most common causes is demyelinating disease; conversely, optic neuritis is one of the most common manifestations of demyelinating disease. See Chapter 7 for further discussion of optic neuritis.

Congenital Disorders

Congenital disorders of the nervous system are ordinarily, and naturally, thought of as conditions that present in infancy or childhood. In fact, some congenital defects commonly present in the adult. Table 10–12 lists congenital defects that sometimes present in adulthood. The most common of these defects are probably Arnold-Chiari malformation (Enrichment Box 10–5) and spinal dysraphism syndromes. Spinal dysraphism syndromes are discussed in Chapter 11.

TABLE 10–12. DEVELOPMENTAL DEFECTS THAT SOMETIMES PRESENT IN ADOLESCENCE OR ADULTHOOD
Hydrocephalus syndromes (e.g., aqueductal stenosis)
Arnold-Chiari malformation type I
Occult spinal dysraphism
Porencephaly
Arachnoid cyst
Klippel-Feil syndrome
Platybasia
Basilar impression
Congenital myasthenic syndromes
Congenital myopathies

ENRICHMENT BOX 10–5

Arnold-Chiari malformation refers to a congenital defect that involves the brainstem and cerebellar tonsils. The cerebellar tonsils are herniated or displaced down into the upper cervical spinal cord. Patients have clinical manifestations such as headaches, cerebellar ataxia, nystagmus, and other brainstem deficits. Three varieties of Arnold-Chiari commonly occur. Type 1 involves the hindbrain malformation only, and can present in adulthood. Mild type 1 Arnold-Chiari malformations are not uncommonly found on magnetic resonance imaging (MRI) done for other reasons, and may be totally asymptomatic. Type 2 Arnold-Chiari is the hindbrain defect associated with a lumbar meningomyelocele. This congenital syndrome is always distressingly obvious at the time of birth. Type 3 Arnold-Chiari is the same as type 2 except that the meningomyelocele or encephalocele occurs in the occipitocervical region.

Hemorrhagic Disorders

In contrast to ischemic cerebrovascular disease, intracranial hemorrhage characteristically produces either severe headache, early impairment of consciousness, or both. Intracranial hemorrhage may occur in the parenchyma or in one of the spaces that surround the brain. Intra-parenchymal bleeding may occur in the supratentorial compartment (intracerebral), the cerebellum, or the brainstem. Supratentorial hemorrhage is often further divided into basal ganglia (usually putaminal) hemorrhage, thalamic hemorrhage, and so-called lobar or subcortical hemorrhage, which involves the deep white matter in the corona radiata.

Extraparenchymal hemorrhage may involve the subarachnoid, subdural, or epidural spaces. Most extraparenchymal hemorrhage is due to head trauma. Spontaneous intracranial, extraparenchymal hemorrhage is usually in the subarachnoid space. Occasionally, patients, usually the elderly or infants, may develop SDH without an obvious history of head trauma.

INTRACEREBRAL HEMORRHAGE

Hemorrhages can occur anywhere in the brain. Those due to hypertension usually involve the basal ganglia, subcortical white matter, thalamus, pons, or cerebellum, with basal ganglia and thalamic bleeds accounting for the vast majority (Figure 10–8). Hypertensive hemorrhages are usually related to fibrinoid necrosis and microaneurysm formation, involving the deep penetrating vessels such as the lenticulostriate arteries, and thus occur in the same distribution as lacunar infarction. Patients

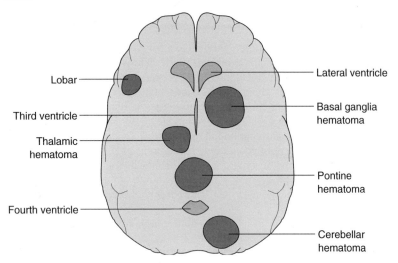

Lobar

Lateral ventricle

Third ventricle

Basal ganglia hematoma

Thalamic hematoma

Pontine hematoma

Fourth ventricle

Cerebellar hematoma

FIGURE 10-8. ■ Typical locations of intracerebral hemorrhage: basal ganglia, thalamus, pons, cerebellum, and lobar (subcortical).

with hypertensive ICH typically have apocalyptic events with dense deficits and rapid impairment of consciousness. Large bleeds, especially with intraventricular extension, have a very poor prognosis, but smaller hemorrhages often have a surprisingly good outcome. Rarely, other conditions produce ICH, such as arteriovenous malformations (AVMs), amyloid angiopathy, drug abuse (especially cocaine and amphetamines), coagulopathy (especially the use of coumadin), pregnancy (especially with eclampsia), and trauma.

Computed tomography (CT) scanning is very valuable in the diagnosis and management of ICH. The ICH is typically very obvious, as is the presence of any shift or intraventricular extension. When the ICH occurs in a location typical for hypertension in a patient with known hypertension, little in the way of further workup is usually necessary. When the ICH is not in a typical location, hypertension is absent, or the demographics are not typical, then further workup may be necessary to exclude one of the more unusual causes of hemorrhage.

CEREBELLAR HEMORRHAGE

Ten percent of hypertensive hemorrhages occur in the cerebellum. The patient usually presents with acute loss of balance and vertigo, which rapidly progresses to coma. The mortality rate without treatment is extremely high. The most common misdiagnosis in one study was "labyrinthitis." This condition is extremely important to recognize, since with surgical evacuation there is usually a decent outcome, and without it morbidity and mortality rates are very high.

SUBARACHNOID HEMORRHAGE

Trauma is the most frequent cause of subarachnoid hemorrhage (SAH). Nontraumatic SAH is most often due to ruptured aneurysm, occasionally to AVM, and in 10%–15% of cases to no identifiable cause.

The major types of aneurysms are congenital, atherosclerotic, mycotic, and dissecting. Most congenital berry aneurysms occur at branching sites of the major arteries of the circle of Willis. Mycotic aneurysms, due to infected emboli from endocarditis, are typically located more peripherally. Fusiform atherosclerotic aneurysms usually involve the large proximal vessels, especially the carotid siphon. Dissecting aneurysms usually involve the carotid or vertebral arteries in the neck and are not often associated with intracranial hemorrhage. The most common sites of intracranial berry aneurysms are the distal internal carotid artery, posterior communicating artery, anterior communicating artery, tip of the basilar artery, middle cerebral bifurcation, and the posterior inferior cerebellar artery.

AVMs are the second most common cause of nontraumatic SAH.

Bleeding from an AVM often has both intraparenchymal and subarachnoid elements, and is usually less severe than with aneurysmal SAH. Less common causes of spontaneous SAH include bleeding diatheses, amyloid angiopathy, and the use of drugs such as cocaine.

The archetypical history of SAH is sudden onset of severe headache. Depending on the extent of bleeding, neurologic deficits and impairment of consciousness may occur. Nuchal rigidity is commonly present within a short time. Focal findings may occur related to the location of the responsible aneurysm, such as a third cranial nerve palsy in the internal carotid–posterior communicating artery aneurysm. The initial diagnostic procedure is usually CT (Figure 10–9). However, CT scanning misses 5%–20% of SAHs, depending on the quality of the scanner, the quality of the interpretation, and the time elapsed since the event. The gold standard for diagnosis is an LP showing bloody CSF, which does not clear from tubes 1 to 4, and which has a xanthochromic supernatant. Because of the possibility of SAH, the physician must always take very seriously a patient with a history of headache of sudden onset or unusual intensity. The conditions most often causing difficulty in the differential diagnosis of SAH are severe migraine and meningitis.

Once the diagnosis of SAH has been made, angiography is usually performed to identify the responsible lesion, although some patients with severe deficits are managed expectantly. If feasible, aneurysms are treated surgically. Early clipping of the aneurysm is the preferred ap-

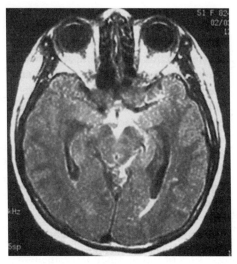

FIGURE 10–9. ■Unenhanced computed tomography scan, demonstrating high-density signal in the prepontine cisterns just anterior to the brainstem. This area should normally be of cerebrospinal fluid intensity (black). The high density is due to blood in the subarachnoid space. (Reprinted with permission from Brant-Za-wadzki M, Bradley WG, Cambray-Forker J (eds): *MRI of the Brain I*. Philadelphia, Lippincott Williams & Wilkins, 2001.)

proach, but interventional neuroradiologic treatment is increasingly available.

Common problems in the management of patients with SAH include cerebral vasospasm, hydrocephalus, hyponatremia, and seizures. There is a significant risk of rebleeding, and rebleeding significantly increases the morbidity and mortality rates. Vasospasm typically begins 3–5 days after the event and can lead to major clinical worsening. Transcranial Doppler has become the standard method to follow patients for vasospasm.

Intracranial extracerebral hematomas are another variety of hemorrhagic disease (see CRANIOCEREBRAL TRAUMA).

TREATMENT OF INTRACRANIAL HEMORRHAGE

For further information on the management of intracranial hemorrhage, visit the Web sites *www.neuroland.com/cvd* and *www.americanheart.org/Scientific/statements/1994/119403.html*.

Stroke (Ischemic Cerebrovascular Disease)

Stroke is one of the most common problems encountered in neurology; it is a maxim that trainees learn neurology "stroke by stroke." The term "cerebrovascular accident," or CVA, is used mostly by nonneurologists and is, thankfully, falling out of favor. Cerebrovascular disease can be classified in a number of ways: ischemic versus hemorrhagic, anterior circulation (carotid) versus posterior circulation (vertebrobasilar), large vessel (atherosclerotic) versus small vessel (hypertensive, diabetic), and thrombotic versus embolic. Table 10–13 shows a classification scheme for stroke.

Patients may present with many varieties of stroke that are related to these variables, as well as to the particular location of the event in the brain. About 70%–80% of strokes are ischemic; of these, cardiac embolism produces about 15%–30% of cases, small vessel lacunar disease causes about 15%–30%, and the remainder are due primarily to thrombotic infarction. About 10%–30% of strokes are due to ICH.

Some of the major risk factors for stroke include increasing age, hypertension, diabetes mellitus, dyslipidemia, history of transient ischemic attacks (TIAs), cigarette smoking, carotid artery stenosis, and atrial fibrillation. The hypertensive, diabetic smoker is at grave risk. Heart disease significantly increases the risk of stroke, especially atrial fibrillation, valvular disease, myocardial infarction, congestive heart failure, and mitral valve prolapse.

There are significant sex and racial variations in the propensity to develop different types of occlusive cerebrovascular disease. Extracranial occlusive disease most commonly occurs in white males and is as-

---

TABLE 10–13. A CLASSIFICATION SCHEME FOR STROKE

Ischemic stroke

  Thrombotic

    Occlusion of large extracranial or intracranial artery

    Occlusion of small penetrating artery (lacunar syndrome)

  Embolic

    Central embolic source (heart or aortic arch)

    Carotid bifurcation

    Paradoxical embolism

  Watershed stroke related to global hypoperfusion

Hemorrhagic stroke (hemorrhagic conversion of an ischemic infarct)

Spontaneous intracranial hemorrhage

  Intracerebral hemorrhage

  Subarachnoid hemorrhage

sociated with coronary artery disease, peripheral vascular disease, and dyslipidemia. In contrast, blacks and women of both races are more prone to develop intracranial occlusive disease involving the proximal major arteries and the small penetrating branches.

Ischemic disease tends to present with an acute focal deficit in an alert patient. Intracranial hemorrhage is more likely to have an apocalyptic onset with coma and a poor outcome. It is not rare for an event that is primarily ischemic to have a hemorrhagic component due to extravasation of blood into the infarcted tissue. This is referred to as a hemorrhagic stroke, and is different from primary ICH. The term "bland infarct" refers to an ischemic infarct with no hemorrhagic component. Hemorrhagic conversion of an infarct occurs most often in large infarcts, in cardiogenic embolism, and in patients who have received anticoagulants or thrombolytics.

Certain clinical accompaniments may help determine the subtype of stroke (Enrichment Box 10–6). Large-vessel disease involves the major extracranial and large named intracranial vessels, is usually related to atherosclerosis, is more common in whites, and is more likely to be treated with antiplatelet agents and anticoagulants. Small-vessel disease involves deep, penetrating small arteries and arterioles, is frequently related to hypertension, is more common in blacks, and is less likely to be treated aggressively with anticoagulants. Large-vessel disease tends to present as TIA or cortical stroke and small-vessel disease as a subcortical "lacunar" syndrome. Anterior circulation events typically produce hemispheric infarction, causing hemiparesis and higher cortical function defects such as aphasia, whereas posterior circulation events cause brainstem ischemia and produce "crossed" syndromes involving dysfunction of one or more cranial nerves and the opposite side of the body, often accompanied by vertigo. Thrombotic events tend to have onset during sleep and cause less severe, more restricted deficits. Embolic events classically occur during activity, are more devastating, and more likely to have associated cardiac disease. Strokes sometimes occur because of globally decreased perfusion producing watershed infarction (see Enrichment Box 10–6).

CLINICAL CEREBROVASCULAR SYNDROMES

The following sections provide brief summaries of some of the more important clinical entities.

Transient Ischemic Attack

Patients with TIAs experience brief episodes of neurologic dysfunction, by traditional definition lasting less than 24 hours but in fact usually lasting only 10–30 minutes. Three basic forms are recognized: carotid dis-

Clinical differentiation of stroke subtypes

Early loss of consciousness is much more common in patients with intracranial hemorrhage. Headache at onset is more common in patients with intracerebral hemorrhage (ICH) and those with large infarcts. Severe headache is virtually always present in SAH. In contrast, headache is unusual in patients with lacunar events. Vomiting is more common with intracerebral and subarachnoid hemorrhage (SAH) than with ischemic infarcts. Seizures at or shortly after the onset of the stroke suggests an embolic event. The pattern of neurologic deficit helps to distinguish cortical from subcortical events.

Watershed infarcts

The cortical areas that lie between the principal fields of perfusion of the major cerebral arteries have a precarious blood supply, which is dependent on the terminal ramifications of the major vessels. Under ordinary circumstances perfusion is adequate, but when systemic pressure falls below the critical levels at which cerebral autoregulation can compensate, as in hypovolemic shock, the first zones where circulation fails are these "watershed" areas. The arm area of the homunculus is a region often falling in the watershed territory between the perfusion fields of the anterior and middle cerebral arteries, so that the classical neurologic picture in watershed infarction following shock is bilateral arm weakness with relative preservation of face and leg function (man-in-the-barrel syndrome).

Drop attacks

Drop attacks are attributed to transient ischemia of the medullary pyramids. Patients with drop attacks have spells where they abruptly and without warning drop to the ground without loss of consciousness, then promptly recover. Such attacks are uncommon, but their occurrence should prompt a search for evidence of vertebrobasilar insufficiency (VBI).

Embolic stroke

In embolic strokes, the development of transesophageal echocardiography (TEE) has made it less difficult to detect embolic sources. TEE has shown that atheromas in the aortic arch are a much more common source of embolism than previously recognized. Transcranial Doppler can also help to establish embolism as the cause of a stroke. Paradoxical embolism occurs when clots from the peripheral venous system gain access to the arterial circulation through a right-to-left shunt, such as a patent foramen ovale or pulmonary arteriovenous fistula.

Anterior cerebral artery stroke

The anterior cerebral artery is one of the terminal divisions of the internal carotid. It arches forward and upward, then loops backward in

(Continued)

the interhemispheric fissure. It perfuses the medial frontal lobe in its initial portions and the medial aspect of the frontal and parietal lobes in the latter part of its course. Since the cortical area subserving lower extremity functions lies on the medial aspect of the hemisphere, occlusion of the anterior cerebral artery is characterized by leg weakness and numbness. The classic patient with an anterior cerebral stroke has a monoparesis with impaired sensation involving the contralateral lower extremity.

Posterior cerebral artery stroke

The posterior cerebral artery is a terminal division of the basilar artery. It courses posteriorly and perfuses the visual cortex. Patients with posterior cerebral artery strokes typically have visual field cuts, but no significant weakness or sensory loss. Depending on whether the dominant or nondominant side is involved, there may be various combinations of alexia and agraphia. Patients occasionally have bilateral posterior cerebral artery stroke, causing the classical neurologic syndrome of "cortical blindness," visual impairment of which the patient is unaware (Anton syndrome).

Lacunar syndromes

The other lacunar syndromes are much less common than pure motor stroke. Pure sensory stroke is due to infarction of the thalamus, and produces an isolated hemisensory deficit. The syndrome of ataxic hemiparesis originally had the cumbersome but descriptive name of "homolateral ataxia with crural paresis." Patients have weakness that is much more severe in the leg than in the arm, in addition to ataxia of the arm out of proportion to the mild weakness. Uncertainty persists regarding the location of the lacunar infarction in this syndrome, but it may involve the basis pontis, including the corticospinal tract and cerebellar peduncle, or the posterior limb of the internal capsule. Patients with dysarthria clumsy hand syndrome have dysarthria along with a curious clumsiness of one hand without significant weakness, spasticity, or ataxia. The responsible lacunar infarction may be in the anterior limb of the internal capsule or in the pons.

---

tribution TIA (brief hemispheric spells), vertebrobasilar TIA (brainstem ischemia or visual field deficits), and amaurosis fugax (AF; transient monocular visual disturbances due to ischemia in the ophthalmic artery distribution). Anterior circulation TIAs are usually attributed to small fibrin-platelet or cholesterol emboli, and generally indicate carotid bifurcation atherosclerosis with stenosis. TIAs presage major stroke in about 25%–30% of patients; the stroke risk is about 5%–6% per year for the first 5 years and is greatest in the first year after a TIA. TIAs are usually treated initially with aspirin for its antiplatelet effects. With acceptably low surgical morbidity and mortality rates, carotid endarterectomy benefits symptomatic patients with greater than 70% stenosis.

Amaurosis Fugax

AF is a common type of TIA that is most often caused by a retinal embolus. Amaurosis means blindness; fugax means fleeting. The currently popular term is "transient monocular blindness." AF causes fleeting visual disturbances that may range from complete blindness (embolus to the central retinal artery) to partial field defects (embolus to a retinal branch artery). These branch emboli often produce so-called shade or curtain effects, wherein the patient loses the upper or lower half of the field (also called "altitudinal" field loss; see Chapter 7), or the right or left half of the field. AF typically lasts only 5–10 minutes; most patients have atheromatous disease of the ipsilateral carotid bifurcation. So-called Hollenhorst plaques are white or grayish material seen in retinal vessels, especially at bifurcations, which are probably fibrin-platelet emboli. These are very suggestive of ipsilateral carotid bifurcation atheromatous disease.

Hemispheric Transient Ischemic Attack

The symptoms of carotid TIA vary with the hemisphere involved. Attacks involving either hemisphere usually produce contralateral body numbness and weakness and may cause a visual disturbance ipsilateral to the other symptoms due to visual cortex involvement or contralateral to the other symptoms due to ophthalmic artery involvement. Attacks affecting the dominant hemisphere may cause transient aphasia or dysnomia. A carotid bifurcation bruit or Hollenhorst plaques in the retina contralateral to the extremity symptoms are useful confirmatory signs.

Vertebrobasilar Transient Ischemic Attack

Common symptoms of vertebrobasilar TIA, or vertebrobasilar insufficiency (VBI), include weakness of the extremities, in either a hemi distribution or involving all four limbs, accompanied by numbness or paresthesias of the extremities or face. Circumoral paresthesias are particularly characteristic. Patients may develop visual field disturbance, decreased balance, incoordination, diplopia, dysarthria, or dysphagia. Vertigo is common but vertigo alone is seldom due to a vertebrobasilar TIA. Drop attacks are a classic manifestation of VBI (see Enrichment Box 10–6).

Stroke In Evolution

Patients with stroke in evolution, or progressive stroke, either experience a progressive onset, or show stepwise progression occurring in fits and starts. Carotid distribution events seldom show progression after 24 hours except for worsening due to cerebral edema. Vertebrobasilar events occasionally stutter for up to 72 hours. Some patients with anterior circulation stroke in evolution harbor high-grade, critical carotid stenotic lesions; they are at risk for total occlusion and a devastating infarction.

Completed Stroke

Patients with completed stroke have stable or improving neurologic deficits, reflecting a fixed anatomic lesion, in contrast to patients with evolving stroke. Many patients thought to have had TIAs, especially those with duration of symptoms longer than a few minutes, prove with modern imaging techniques to have had small completed strokes. If the deficit remains subtotal, such as hemiparesis rather than hemiplegia or anomia rather than global aphasia, the event is referred to as a partial completed stroke. The trick lies in distinguishing a partial completed stroke from an intermediate stage of stroke in evolution. After a completed stroke there is a risk of a recurrent event of about 6%–10% per year.

Embolic Stroke

In embolic stroke, there is sudden occlusion of a brain artery by an embolus. Some potential sources of embolism include the heart, aortic arch, and carotid arteries. Paradoxical embolism may sometimes arise from the venous system and reach the arterial side via a patent foramen ovale. Most cardiac emboli are thrombus material and most artery-to-artery emboli are platelet-fibrin. Table 10–14 lists important cardiac diseases associated with cerebral embolism. Rarely, other types of embolic material may reach the brain, such as air or fat.

An embolic infarct is often hemorrhagic, in part because the fragmentation and distal migration of the embolus allows for the reperfusion of infarcted tissue. Another characteristic clinical feature of major embolic infarction, particularly cardiogenic embolism, is that seizures occur at the onset much more often than with other types of infarcts.

The greatest embolic threat is posed by atrial fibrillation, especially when associated with mitral valvular disease; intracardiac thrombi due to recent myocardial infarction, ventricular aneurysms, or cardiomyopathy; prosthetic valves; and endocarditis. Evolving technology has demonstrated that more ischemic strokes are embolic than previously thought (see Enrichment Box 10–6).

Embolic stroke usually presents apocalyptically, during activity. Such strokes are usually large, with severe deficits, often associated with seizures and with a tendency to hemorrhagic conversion of the in-

TABLE 10–14. CAUSES OF CARDIOGENIC CEREBRAL EMBOLISM

Cardiac arrhythmias, especially atrial fibrillation, atrial flutter, and sick sinus syndrome

Recent myocardial infarction

Valvular disease

   Rheumatic mitral stenosis

   Rheumatic aortic stenosis

   Calcific aortic stenosis

   Congenital bicuspid aortic valve

   Mitral annulus calcification

   Mitral valve prolapse

Ventricular aneurysm

Ventricular hypokinesia (segmental or global)

Atrial or ventricular thrombi

Cardiomyopathy

Prosthetic valves

Endocarditis, bacterial or nonbacterial (marantic)

Atrial myxoma

Atrial septal aneurysm

Patent foramen ovale

farct. Embolic infarcts may be difficult to distinguish clinically from ICH because of the abrupt onset and severe deficit.

The definitive management of an embolic stroke may involve thrombolytic treatment acutely and anticoagulation to prevent recurrence. Intracranial hemorrhage as a complication of thrombolytic treatment is especially worrisome because of the underlying tendency of embolic strokes to undergo hemorrhagic transformation. Also, the timing of anticoagulation to prevent recurrence without causing hemorrhagic transformation is delicate.

Sleepy Stroke

Since bilateral hemispheric or brainstem reticular pathology is necessary to impair consciousness, cerebral infarctions and bleeds do not cause drowsiness, lethargy, or coma unless there has been damage to the brainstem reticular-activating system. When a patient with a stroke who has been alert initially becomes drowsy, or is drowsy at the time of presentation, this generally reflects cerebral edema with shifting of intracranial contents, incipient herniation with impairment of deep midline structures subserving consciousness, or secondary impairment of the uninfarcted hemisphere due to increased intracranial pressure. Such patients have usually either had very large infarcts or hemorrhages, are at risk of herniation and death, and generally fare badly (Figure 10–10). Impairment of consciousness ("sleepiness") in a stroke patient is a poor prognostic sign; such patients must be monitored very closely.

Patients who worsen are sometimes said to have had "extension of the infarct." This is, in fact, uncommon, and more likely causes for worsening in a previously stable stroke patient include recurrent embolism, hemorrhagic transformation of the infarct (see Figure 10–10), cerebral edema, systemic hypotension (especially from overzealous treatment of hypertension), seizures, medication effects, or the development of a medical complication such as aspiration, pneumonia, myocardial infarction, or urosepsis.

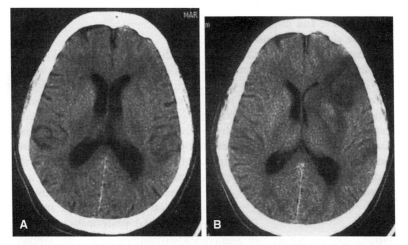

FIGURE 10–10. ■ (A) Unenhanced computed tomography (CT) scan performed on the first day after sudden hemiparesis in a 64-year-old woman. The study shows no clear abnormality, which is typical for CT in the first 24 hours after cerebral infarction. (B) Unenhanced CT performed 2 days later, demonstrating a large left middle cerebral infarct with a small area of high density within the infarct due to hemorrhagic transformation. Note the wedge shape of the infarct and the mass effect with compression of the left lateral ventricle. (Reprinted with permission from Brant-Zawadzki M, Bradley WG, Cambray-Forker J (eds): *MRI of the Brain I.* Philadelphia, Lippincott Williams & Wilkins, 2001.) For an interactive example of a large infarct, see *www.med.harvard.edu/AANLIB/cases/case37.*

Middle Cerebral Artery Stroke

The middle cerebral artery is a terminal branch of the internal carotid. It courses laterally and posteriorly in the Sylvian fissure to supply the lateral aspect of the cerebral hemisphere. Areas of particular clinical importance perfused by the middle cerebral artery include the frontal eyefields, Broca area, Wernicke area, and the cortical areas subserving motor and sensory function for the arm and face (Figure 10–11). Patients with a complete middle cerebral artery stroke involving the dominant hemisphere typically have aphasia and contralateral hemiplegia along with hemisensory loss. They may or may not have a visual field cut. Middle cerebral distribution lesions in the nondominant hemisphere produce hemiplegia, various forms of apraxia, sometimes a visual field deficit, and various combinations of a peculiar syndrome involving neglect of the left side of space, denial of disability, and sometimes total failure to recognize the paralyzed extremities as part of the body (anosagnosia). The middle cerebral artery distribution is the most commonly involved in ischemic large vessel infarction. Anterior and posterior cerebral artery strokes occur less commonly and are often more difficult to recognize (see Enrichment Box 10–6).

Brainstem Stroke

In the brainstem, descending corticospinal and corticobulbar fibers before decussation, as well as ascending sensory pathways that have already crossed, lie in intimate relation to the lower motor neurons of the cranial nerve nuclei. For this reason, brainstem strokes are charac-

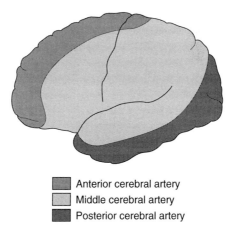

■ Anterior cerebral artery
▢ Middle cerebral artery
■ Posterior cerebral artery

FIGURE 10–11. ■ The territories of perfusion of the major cerebral arteries. ACA = anterior cerebral artery; MCA = middle cerebral artery; PCA = posterior cerebral artery.

terized by "crossed" syndromes of cranial nerve dysfunction ipsilateral to the stroke and long motor or sensory tract dysfunction contralateral to the stroke (Figure 10–12). For instance, a lower motor neuron facial palsy on the right with hemiparesis of the left side of the body would indicate a lesion involving the right pons. In addition, because of the rich vestibular and cerebellar connections, patients with brainstem strokes often have accompanying vertigo, nausea, vomiting, and cerebellar ataxia. The syndrome seen depends on whether the occlusive process has involved the paramedian perforating, short circumferential, or long circumferential branches of the basilar artery.

Wallenberg (Lateral Medullary) Syndrome

Wallenberg initially described the syndrome of lateral medullary infarction, the most common form of brainstem stroke, which is most often due to ischemia in the distribution of the posterior inferior cerebellar artery, usually because of occlusion of a vertebral artery. Typical findings include impaired sensation to pin and temperature involving the ipsilateral face and contralateral body, dysphagia with paralysis of the ipsilateral palate, an ipsilateral Horner syndrome, ataxia of the ipsilateral arm and leg, vertigo, and nystagmus.

Lacunar Infarction

Hypertension produces fibrinoid necrosis, or lipohyalinosis, of small arterioles throughout the body. In the brain, this process is most promi-

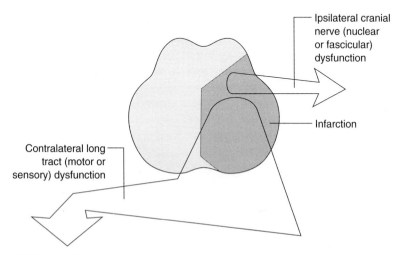

FIGURE 10–12. ■ Schematic of a brainstem stroke, illustrating the pattern of a cranial nerve defect on one side and long-tract motor or sensory dysfunction on the opposite side, typical of a brainstem stroke.

nent in the distribution of the short penetrating endarteries, such as the lenticulostriate vessels off the middle cerebral, the thalamoperforators off the posterior cerebral and posterior communicating arteries, and the paramedian perforators that come off the basilar in the midline to supply the deep structures of the brainstem. Lacunar infarcts affect subcortical structures such as the basal ganglia, thalamus, internal capsule, subcortical white matter, cerebellum, and brainstem (Figure 10–13). They do not involve the cerebral cortex. Occlusion of these small endarteries produces infarction, and the small infarctions result in cavitation. When the brain is cut at autopsy, the small cavities filled with fluid resemble tiny lakes. The French neurologists who first described this condition used the term "lacune," which is French for lake. When the small infarcts are multiple, as they often are, the term "etat lacunaire" (lacunar state), is applied. Such patients have had recurrent lacunar infarcts and deep white matter ischemic changes that result in a syndrome of dementia, pseudobulbar palsy, and gait abnormalities.

Hypertension is responsible for about 80%–90% of lacunar infarctions. Diabetes mellitus is another important predisposing condition. Smoking may play a role in some patients. There are important gender and ethnic influences, as mentioned earlier.

There are four classical lacunar strokes: pure motor stroke, pure sensory stroke, dysarthria-clumsy hand syndrome, and ataxic hemi-

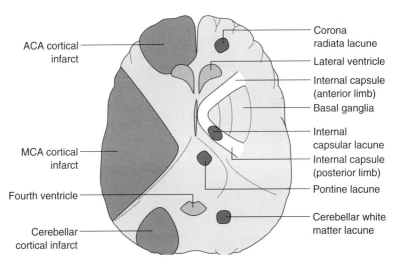

FIGURE 10–13. ■ Illustration of the typical areas and size of cortical infarctions on the left side (of the figure), and typical areas and size of lacunar infarctions on the right side (of the figure). ACA = anterior cerebral artery; MCA = middle cerebral artery.

paresis (see Enrichment Box 10–6). Of these, pure motor stroke is by far the most common. Other lacunar syndromes have been described in recent years. The importance of recognizing a lacunar syndrome is its indication that the patient has likely had an infarct related to hypertension and small-vessel disease, and not large-vessel atherosclerosis. The patient's long-term management is oriented more toward scrupulous control of hypertension than toward antiplatelet agents.

Because fibrinoid necrosis is also the basic pathological substrate of hypertensive hemorrhage, lacunar infarction and hypertensive hemorrhage tend to occur in the same general distribution (basal ganglia, thalamus, pons, and cerebellum).

Helpful in the diagnosis of lacunar stroke are the presence of risk factors, primarily hypertension and/or diabetes, a clinical syndrome typical of a lacunar stroke, a normal EEG, and imaging studies showing a lacunar infarct, or at least no cortical infarct. The neurologic recovery from a lacunar stroke is often better than from a cortical infarction.

Internal Capsular, or Pure Motor Stroke

The corticospinal fibers descending from the motor cortex occupy a compact bundle in the posterior limb of the internal capsule. Lacunar strokes commonly involve the posterior limb of the internal capsule, in which case they tend to damage the corticospinal tract fibers in isolation. The patients thus have a dense hemiparesis but no sensory loss, visual field deficits, speech disturbance, eye movement disorder, or other evidence of dysfunction of the cerebral cortex. This syndrome is thus referred to as a "pure motor stroke" because the only deficit is motor weakness. The corticospinal tract fibers to the arm, leg, and face are closely grouped in the internal capsule, and the infarction typically involves the entire bundle, producing weakness that is symmetrically severe in the arm, leg, and face. This pattern contrasts with that of a cortical stroke, where arm, leg, and face functions are spread over a wide area, and where infarctions usually produce different degrees of weakness of the arm, leg, and face.

Dissecting Aneurysms

Dissecting aneurysms are an unusual cause of stroke. They most often involve the carotid or vertebral artery in the neck, sometimes caused by trauma (often surprisingly trivial), related to underlying fibromuscular dysplasia, or for no apparent reason. Dissections occur more commonly in young patients. Patients with carotid dissection typically develop a progressive hemispheric stroke, often with an accompanying ipsilateral Horner syndrome and a headache.

STROKE IN THE YOUNG ADULT

In young people, those not in the stroke-prone age group, cerebrovascular disease carries a somewhat different differential diagnosis. Although premature atherosclerosis, especially in patients with diabetes and hypertension, remains a prominent possibility, other conditions merit consideration. These conditions include cardiac disease (mitral valve prolapse, atrial myxoma, congenital or acquired valvular disease, septal defects, patent foramen ovale with paradoxical embolism, and cardiomyopathy), cerebral vasculitis, complications of drug abuse (especially cocaine and heroin), oral contraceptives, arterial dissection, fibromuscular dysplasia, antiphospholipid syndrome, protein C and protein S deficiency, antithrombin III deficiency, inborn metabolic errors (Fabry disease, homocystinuria), and complicated migraine. While far from inclusive, this list should serve to convey the flavor of the differences in the approach to the workup of younger patients compared with the approach in patients in the usual vascular-disease age group.

VASCULITIS

Vasculitis may occur as a primary disorder of the nervous system, or as a complication of systemic vasculitis or connective tissue disorder. Some patients develop vasculitis from the use of drugs. Vasculitis is primarily of concern in patients with stroke, but it can involve other parts of the nervous system, including the peripheral nerves. The primary symptoms of CNS vasculitis are stroke-like episodes, but it may present with headache, confusion, dementia, chronic meningitis, or a syndrome resembling MS. Angiography typically shows segmental zones of alternating arterial constriction and dilatation, referred to as beading and ectasias. Initial treatment is usually with corticosteroids.

TREATMENT OF ISCHEMIC CEREBROVASCULAR DISEASE

The treatment of ischemic cerebrovascular disease has evolved a great deal in recent decades. Potential therapeutic agents now include anticoagulants, heparin substitutes, antiplatelet agents, antifibrinolytic agents, lipid-lowering agents, surgery, and interventional neuroradiologic procedures including angioplasty and stenting. Long-term management of hypertension, diabetes, hypercholesterolemia, and other stroke risk factors can have a major impact on the likelihood of stroke.

For detailed information on current concepts in the management of ischemic cerebrovascular disease, visit the following Web sites: *www.stroke-site.org, www.strokecenter.org/prof,* or *www.americanheart.org/Scientific/statements.*

Heredofamilial Disorders

Many neurologic syndromes of formerly obscure pathogenesis have proven to be familial. Recent genetic advances have clarified the modes of inheritance and chromosomes involved in many of these syndromes. In a few, investigators have identified the abnormal gene and the protein or enzyme defect. Some of these disorders are discussed elsewhere (see Chapter 11, DUCHENNE MUSCULAR DYSTROPHY and MYOTONIC MUSCULAR DYSTROPHY).

HUNTINGTON DISEASE (HUNTINGTON CHOREA)

The cardinal features of Huntington disease are chorea and dementia, with a typical onset in the late thirties or early forties. It is an autosomal dominant condition with variable penetrance. The folk singer Woody Guthrie ("This land is your land, this land is my land") died of Huntington disease. It is to be hoped that his son Arlo Guthrie ("Alice's Restaurant," "City of New Orleans") has escaped the disease.

Chorea (from the Greek "dance") consists of quick, fleeting involuntary movements, which patients often try to disguise by pretending they were intentional. Imaging studies may show atrophy of the caudate. The condition is inexorably progressive and ultimately fatal. The typical course is from 15 to 20 years. Some symptomatic treatments are available, but nothing that arrests the progression. The specific gene defect is an expanded and unstable CAG trinucleotide repeat on chromosome 4, which produces a protein called huntingtin. How this leads to the progressive degeneration, which primarily affects the caudate and putamen, is unclear.

DNA diagnostic testing can now confirm the diagnosis, even in presymptomatic individuals. Genetic testing is a process with major potential medical, psychological, and ethical considerations, and is not to be undertaken lightly.

Other conditions associated with chorea include Sydenham chorea, chorea gravidarum (occurs during pregnancy), SLE, and the effects of certain drugs.

SPINOCEREBELLAR DEGENERATION

Most often familial, occasionally sporadic, the different spinocerebellar syndromes result from degeneration of the cerebellum, the spinocerebellar tracts, or the corticospinal tracts in various combinations. Patients may have a purely cerebellar syndrome, or various mixtures of cerebellar and corticospinal dysfunction. The most common example is Friedreich ataxia (Enrichment Box 10–7).

Friedreich ataxia

Friedreich ataxia is an autosomal recessive form of spinocerebellar degeneration with prominent evidence of spinal cord involvement. In childhood or adolescence, patients develop both cerebellar ataxia as well as spasticity. Involvement of posterior roots produces loss of deep tendon reflexes. Friedreich ataxia is one of the causes (along with pernicious anemia) of the unusual combination of absent ankle jerks with upgoing toes.

Tuberous sclerosis

Tuberous sclerosis is an autosomal dominant condition that causes seizures, mental retardation, and various characteristic skin lesions, including adenoma sebaceum on the face (easily mistaken for acne), café-au-lait spots, and hypomelanotic macules (ash leaf spots).

Sturge-Weber disease

Also known as encephalotrigeminal angiomatosis, Sturge-Weber disease describes the association between a vascular nevus of the face (port wine stain) and a vascular malformation involving the ipsilateral cerebral cortex. Affected patients are prone to seizures and mental retardation. Unlike most other neurocutaneous syndromes, Sturge-Weber is sporadic. Not all individuals with facial port wine stains have Sturge-Weber; some physicians claim that hemangioma involving the medial canthus of the eye reliably marks those patients who do.

von Hippel-Lindau disease

von Hippel-Lindau disease is characterized by the association of vascular tumors (hemangioblastomas) involving the retina and various portions of the central nervous system (CNS), especially the cerebellum.

Ataxia-telangiectasia (Louis-Bar syndrome)

Ataxia-telangiectasia is an autosomal recessive condition in which there is early childhood onset of cerebellar ataxia associated with telangiectasias that characteristically involve the conjunctiva. There are many other features of this disease. The essential feature is a failure of DNA repair mechanisms, which also leads to an increased risk of malignancy.

NEUROCUTANEOUS SYNDROMES (PHACOMATOSES)

Portions of the nervous system share a common ectodermal embryological origin with the skin. As a result, some conditions produce abnormalities of both skin and nervous system. The recognition of the skin lesions permits prediction of the neuropathology and in turn the prognosis and the pattern of inheritance. The term "phako" is Greek for "mother-spot," referring to the skin (or eye) lesions that are the usual initial clue to the presence of a neurocutaneous syndrome. The usual neurologic accompaniments are seizures and mental retardation, but other abnormalities can occur as well. The most common neurocutaneous syndrome is neurofibromatosis.

Neurofibromatosis

Von Recklinghausen disease (neurofibromatosis type I) is an autosomal dominant disorder characterized by multiple neurofibromas involving nerves throughout the body. Involvement of small cutaneous nerve twigs produces pedunculated skin tumors that sometimes cover the patient from head to toe. Café-au-lait spots are also characteristic. Other nerve tumors (e.g., plexiform neuromas, acoustic neuromas) also occur. John Merrick, the main character in the movie *The Elephant Man,* suffered from neurofibromatosis with multiple plexiform neuromas. The neurofibromatosis I gene is on chromosome 17. Neurofibromatosis type II, also autosomal dominant, with the gene located on chromosome 22, is a milder form of the disease, lacking the cutaneous features but associated with bilateral acoustic neuromas.

Other Neurocutaneous Syndromes

Other common neurocutaneous syndromes include tuberous sclerosis, Sturge-Weber disease, von Hippel-Lindau disease, and ataxia-telangiectasia (see Enrichment Box 10–7).

Psychiatric Disorders

Psychiatric disease is extremely common and complicated. The psychiatric disorders most often of neurologic concern are depression, hysteria, malingering, and hypochondriasis, the same conditions that are a concern for any physician. These disorders are also frequently referred to as "functional" or "nonorganic." Depression tends to exaggerate any symptomatology, neurologic or otherwise. See Chapter 8, PSYCHIATRIC DISEASE, for further discussion of hysteria and malingering, and Chapter 4 for a discussion of depression. It is worth reemphasizing that the diagnosis of nonorganic disease can be treacherous. So-called "hysterical signs" on physical examination are often extremely misleading. Except for blatantly obvious things like "Hollywood amnesia" or hysterical coma, it is wise to tread carefully.

In addition to depression, hysteria, malingering, and hypochondriasis, certain other neurologic conditions and psychiatric conditions may be confused with each other, and there may be overlap. Some physicians concentrate their clinical practice on the borderland between neurology and psychiatry. The topic can become complex. For example, patients with degenerative diseases such as diffuse Lewy body disease, AD, and end-stage Parkinson disease may develop prominent hallucinations. Determining whether the elderly patient with new onset hallucinations suffers from a neurologic disorder or a psychiatric disorder is often difficult. Patients with disease in certain brain regions, notably the frontal and temporal lobes, may have symptoms resembling those seen in patients with primary psychiatric disease, including obsessiveness, compulsiveness, strange personalities, hallucinations, and so forth. Does the physician consider the difficult headache patient who develops chronic daily headache and abuses analgesics a neurologic patient or a psychiatric patient?

Systemic Disease

Neurologic complications of systemic disease are common. Patients frequently present with neurologic signs and symptoms because of an underlying medical or surgical disorder, and the underlying disorder may not be at all apparent. The possibility that the patient's neurologic syndrome may not represent a primary neurologic disorder must always be borne in mind, particularly in older patients. The systemic disorders relevant to disease at each neurologic level are included in the tables in Chapter 8.

Central Nervous System Infections

Numerous pathogenic microorganisms can infect the CNS. These range from ordinary bacteria to unconventional "slow" viruses or novel infectious particles known as prions. Clinical manifestations depend on the nature of the infecting organism, adequacy of host defenses, and the CNS area predominately involved. The clinical course may range from hyperacute (meningococcal meningitis), to chronic (tuberculous meningitis), and extremely chronic (prion infection). Many infections that were once rare have become commonplace since the advent of AIDS.

Postinfectious or parainfectious neurologic syndromes are those that follow infections, usually viral. The predominant pathophysiology in such cases is demyelination, in the CNS producing ADEM and related syndromes, and in the peripheral nervous system producing Guillain-Barré and related syndromes. Such postinfectious syndromes can sometimes follow infection with other agents. For example, Sydenham chorea follows streptococcal infection (Enrichment Box 10–8).

ACUTE BACTERIAL MENINGITIS

In acute bacterial meningitis, the patient typically appears acutely ill and toxic with fever, headache, altered sensorium, and stiff neck. Low sugar

Sydenham chorea

Sydenham chorea follows infection with Group A beta hemolytic streptococcus, essentially the CNS counterpart of rheumatic fever and poststreptococcal glomerulonephritis. It is usually a self-limited disorder that most often affects children. In Sydenham chorea, antibodies to neurons in the striatum, particularly the caudate and subthalamic nuclei, likely develop because of cross-reactivity with streptococcal antigens. How these antistriatal antibodies cause the clinical manifestations of the disease remains unclear. A similar pathogenesis may be at work in other postinfectious chorea syndromes.

Herpes simplex encephalitis

Because herpes simplex encephalitis (HSE) can have a terrible neurologic aftermath, acyclovir is usually begun empirically when there is reasonable suspicion about possibility of the diagnosis. Brain biopsy, formerly done routinely, is now generally reserved for atypical cases or patients who do not respond to acyclovir. HSE is caused by type 1 herpes simplex virus. No association whatsoever exists between the occurrence of herpes labialis and the risk of HSE.

Herpes zoster

Herpes zoster can produce radicular pain for days or weeks before vesicles appear (zoster sine zoster, a diagnosis usually made in retrospect). Some patients continue to have severe pain long afterward (postherpetic neuralgia). Zoster is usually treated with acyclovir. Steroids may decrease the incidence and severity of postherpetic neuralgia, but their role in the acyclovir era is unclear. Postherpetic neuralgia sometimes responds well to topical capsaicin. For recent information on the therapy of zoster, see the Web site *www.aafp.org/afp/20000415/2437.html*.

Creutzfeldt-Jakob disease

Creutzfeldt-Jakob disease is a rapidly progressive dementing illness typically associated with prominent myoclonus and sometimes with a variety of other neurologic features. The disease, formerly attributed to a "slow virus," follows infection with a "prion" (proteinaceous infectious particle). These infections were termed "slow" because of the very long incubation periods; once symptoms appear, the disease progresses swiftly. The EEG shows characteristic periodic discharges, and spongiform changes are present pathologically. Cases of "new variant" Creutzfeldt-Jakob are occurring, primarily in England, due to transmission of the agent from "mad cows" to humans.

Subacute sclerosing panencephalitis

Subacute sclerosing panencephalitis (SSPE) has fortunately become

(Continued)

ENRICHMENT BOX 10-8 (*CONTINUED*)

rare, but was a significant clinical problem not many years ago. SSPE produces progressive neurologic deterioration in children, has characteristic periodic EEG discharges, and is due to infection by an atypical form of measles virus.

Rabies

Fortunately rare in this country, human rabies virus infection follows the bite of an infected animal and produces devastating and uniformly fatal viral encephalitis with massive spasms and myoclonic jerks following sensory stimuli. Rabies virus is strongly neurotropic and migrates along nerve trunks from the bite site to the CNS.

Poliomyelitis

The term poliomyelitis connotes inflammation of the gray matter. The spinal cord is chiefly affected. During the rampant polio epidemics that preceded the Salk and Sabin vaccines, the causative organism was polio virus. The disease still occurs rarely in a sporadic fashion and may be caused by other viruses, such as ECHO, coxsackie, or enteroviral infection.

and polymorphonuclear leukocytosis characterize the CSF. Partial treatment, usually inadvertent, can cloud the clinical picture and make separation from viral, tuberculous, and fungal meningitis much more difficult. Also, meningitis in the very young, the very old, the chronically ill, and the immunocompromised may not present with the usual clinical features. Microorganisms may gain access to the CNS through hematogenous spread or direct extension from adjacent focal infection.

The differential diagnosis depends greatly on age and circumstances. For instance, *Escherichia coli* commonly infects neonates but rarely adults. Young children most often suffer infection with *Haemophilus influenzae*. An adolescent or young adult from a dormitory or barracks setting most likely has meningococcal meningitis. Pneumococcal meningitis typically attacks chronic alcoholics. Although the brain is not directly involved, the spread of bacterial toxins to the CNS commonly produces coma, seizures, and increased intracranial pressure.

Suspect the possibility of bacterial meningitis and expeditiously perform an LP on any patient with headache or AMS accompanied by fever. See Enrichment Box 10–9 for a discussion of meningitis treatment.

ASEPTIC (VIRAL) MENINGITIS

Patients with aseptic meningitis present in much the same way as do patients with bacterial meningitis, except they generally appear less sick. In addition, the CSF in aseptic meningitis contains a predomi-

Treatment should begin promptly on suspicion of the diagnosis of bacterial meningitis, without awaiting bacteriologic confirmation. High-dose intravenous (IV) antibiotics remain standard. The most appropriate antibiotic varies with the age of the patient and the presence of specific epidemiological factors. The most common causative agent in young adults is meningococcus. In patients older than 45 years of age, pneumococcus and *Listeria* become more likely.

The optimal treatment regimens tend to evolve with the development of new antibiotics. A currently favored empiric treatment in adults is a third-generation cephalosporin, such as cefotaxime sodium or ceftriaxone sodium, with ampicillin if listerial meningitis cannot be ruled out. Vancomycin is added in some instances. In patients with obvious meningococcal disease, penicillin remains the drug of choice. The initial choice of antibiotics may be modified when culture and sensitivity information is available.

Management of the complications of meningitis, which can include seizures, stroke, hydrocephalus, cerebral edema, and many others, is a major challenge. With current therapeutic regimens, the mortality rate remains at about 20% for adults.

The Web site *gold.aecom.yu.edu/id/eaa-bm.htm* (developed by the Infectious Disease division at Albert Einstein College of Medicine) contains an algorithm for the management of meningitis in various situations. See *www.telco.es/braincenter/Meningitis.htm* for a brief discussion.

nance of mononuclear cells, a normal sugar level, and variable protein elevation. Patients with bacterial meningitis have a predominance of polymorphonuclear cells, and the sugar level is typically decreased. CSF protein elevations occur in both conditions and do not help in distinguishing between them. Many different viruses, including HIV, can produce aseptic meningitis. Enteroviruses are a common cause.

Patients with typical aseptic meningitis do not require antibiotics. Parameningeal bacterial infection and partially treated bacterial meningitis can closely mimic viral meningitis. Treatment of viral meningitis is generally supportive. Effective antiviral treatment is not yet available in most instances.

CHRONIC MENINGITIS

Some organisms produce an indolent form of meningitis with a mononuclear CSF pleocytosis. Chronic meningitis carries a broad differential diagnosis; major considerations include tuberculosis, cryptococcosis and other fungi, Lyme disease, syphilis, lymphoma or carcinoma, and sarcoidosis. The CSF sugar level is frequently low, but rarely as low as in bacterial meningitis. Protein elevations, sometimes striking, are the rule. Patients present with a history going back weeks to months of headache, confusion, dementia, or cranial nerve palsies. Overt evidence of systemic infection is often scant. Some apply the term "aseptic" to these forms of meningitis, since routine bacteriologic cultures prove sterile. Most clinicians apply the term aseptic to viral meningitis.

Treatment of the various forms of chronic meningitis is beyond the scope of this discussion. The Web sites *www.kcom.edu/faculty/ chamberlain/Website/tritzid/chronmen.htm* and *www.sums.ac.ir/~semj/ sept2000/meningitis.htm* have good brief discussions of chronic meningitis. The site *www.idsociety. org/pg/toc.htm* has practice guidelines for the management of various infectious diseases, including some of the agents that cause chronic meningitis.

BRAIN ABSCESS

Brain abscesses can arise either because of direct spread from a contiguous infected source, such as a mastoid, or because of hematogenous spread, such as in subacute bacterial endocarditis. Patients typically present with varying combinations of headache, progressive neurologic deficits, seizures, and evidence of infection. However, fever and leukocytosis are absent in about half of the patients harboring a brain abscess; therefore, the absence of these signs does not exclude the possibility of an abscess in a patient with a mass lesion.

Imaging studies classically show a "ring-enhancing lesion" on both CT and MRI with a central area of fluid (necrosis) that is low density on CT and is CSF fluid-signal intensity on MRI. The ring-enhancing appearance is not specific for abscess, and can also occur with infarct, tumor, and demyelinating disease.

Management of brain abscess is complex and is usually done in conjunction with a neurosurgeon. For an illustrative case discussion, visit the Web site *www.hopkins-id.edu/education/caserounds/caserounds9.html*.

VIRAL ENCEPHALITIS

Viral encephalitis differs from viral meningitis by virtue of the involvement of the brain parenchyma, which may produce altered consciousness progressing to coma, seizures, or focal signs such as hemiparesis, visual field deficits, and aphasia. Herpes simplex encephalitis (HSE) is the most common type of sporadic viral encephalitis. Most of the other forms of viral encephalitis are seasonal and frequently occur in epidemics.

The epidemic forms of viral encephalitis most often follow an arbovirus infection. Arthropods (mosquitoes) carry arboviruses from a natural host (such as horses) to man. The arboviral encephalitides include eastern equine encephalitis, western equine encephalitis, St. Louis encephalitis, Japanese B encephalitis, and California encephalitis. Further varieties exist elsewhere in the world (e.g., Russian spring/summer encephalitis). Encephalitis due to West Nile fever virus is now being seen in the United States. Viral encephalitis can vary from a relatively mild disorder with a reasonably good prognosis (California encephalitis) to an extremely severe, neurologically devastating condition with a high mortality rate (eastern equine encephalitis). Treatment remains supportive; no specific antiviral agents exist for these infections.

HERPES SIMPLEX ENCEPHALITIS

While arboviral encephalitis emerges most commonly during the times of the year (summer and early fall) that mosquitoes are abundant, HSE occurs sporadically at all times of the year. The typical patient is a young and previously healthy adult who suddenly develops alteration of consciousness, followed rapidly by the onset of seizures and a focal neurologic deficit. Imaging studies frequently show abnormalities in one temporal lobe (Figure 10–14). MRI may show high signal intensity lesions in the medial and inferior temporal lobe on the T2-weighted images. The EEG pattern is frequently characteristic, and

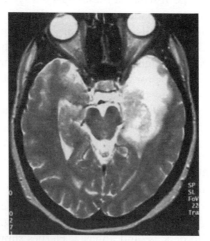

FIGURE 10–14. ▪ Axial T2-weighted magnetic resonance image in a case of herpes simplex encephalitis, demonstrating diffuse abnormal high-intensity signal involving the anterior and medial left temporal lobe. (Reprinted with permission from Brant-Zawadzki M, Bradley WG, Cambray-Forker J (eds): *MRI of the Brain I*. Philadelphia, Lippincott Williams & Wilkins, 2001.)

EEG may have higher sensitivity than imaging studies early in the disease. The CSF may show red cells and xanthochromia, unusual in other CNS infections. The CSF polymerase chain reaction, while highly specific and sensitive for herpes simplex virus encephalitis, may be negative in the first 24–48 hours of infection. CSF and serum should also be sent for herpes simplex virus antibody assay. HSE may respond to treatment with acyclovir (see Enrichment Box 10–8).

HERPES ZOSTER

Reactivation of a latent varicella-zoster virus resident in dorsal root ganglion cells triggers a herpes zoster outbreak ("shingles"). Affected patients develop an extremely painful rash in the distribution of the involved dorsal root ganglia, usually a single dermatome. Although thoracic segments are involved most often, zoster can strike anywhere. Involvement of the ophthalmic division of the trigeminal nerve is relatively common and can have serious ophthalmologic and neurologic complications (encephalitis, aseptic meningitis, and cranial neuropathy). The rash consists of vesicles on an erythematous base, which may coalesce into bullae as the disease develops (see Enrichment Box 10–8).

NEUROSYPHILIS

Neurosyphilis is a specific subtype of tertiary syphilis and occurs after a long latent period following the primary and secondary stages. Once rare, neurosyphilis is on the rise in association with HIV infection. Although the manifestations are protean, several specific syndromes are recognized. Tabes dorsalis follows syphilitic involvement of the posterior roots of the spinal cord and produces degeneration of the posterior columns. Tabetic patients have sensory ataxia, absence of deep pain, spontaneous "lightning" pains in the extremities, and Argyll-Robertson pupils (small, asymmetric, reactive to near but not to light stimulation). General paresis refers to neurosyphilis involving the brain, rarely with gumma formation. Patients with general paresis are demented and may have psychotic features (delusions of grandeur are classic). Meningovascular syphilis refers to syphilitic involvement of blood vessels, mostly at the base of the brain related to a presumed low-grade chronic inflammation. These patients present with stroke, either large or small vessel, and often with a history of multiple strokes. Serologic testing for syphilis is frequently done as part of a stroke workup to exclude this possibility.

The treatment of neurosyphilis is penicillin. For periodically updated guidelines on therapy, see the Web site *www.cdc.gov/nchstp/dstd/1998_STD_Guidelines/1998_guidelines_for_the_treatment.htm*.

LYME DISEASE

Lyme disease, caused by the spirochete *Borrelia burgdorferi,* is transmitted to humans by a tick bite. The nervous system manifestations of this disease consist of early and late phases. The early phase may present as meningitis, cranial nerve palsies, and radiculoneuritis. The late phase may consist of encephalopathy, encephalomyelitis, and polyradiculoneuropathies. Lyme disease can cause intermittent neurologic events confused with cerebrovascular disease. The diagnosis is suggested by a history of tick bite or the characteristic skin rash, or involvement of other organs such as the heart or the joints. Lyme titers, especially paired serum and CSF antibody titers or a Lyme polymerase chain reaction in the CSF or blood are very helpful in diagnosis. The CSF may show a lymphocytic pleocytosis; some of the CSF abnormalities may resemble those seen in MS. MRI may also show white matter changes, which can resemble those seen in MS. Treatment of neurologic Lyme disease (except for facial nerve palsy) consists of IV antibiotics for at least 2 weeks. The facial nerve palsy may be treated with oral doxycycline. For a practice guideline on the treatment of Lyme disease, visit the Web site *www.idsociety.org/pg/toc.htm.*

HUMAN IMMUNODEFICIENCY VIRUS INFECTION

In addition to predisposing to a variety of other infections or conditions (e.g., cerebral toxoplasmosis, cytomegalovirus encephalitis, cryptococcal meningitis, tuberculous meningitis, neurosyphilis, CNS lymphoma) the HIV virus can itself directly infect the CNS, producing meningitis or encephalitis. These direct infections generally occur early in the course of the disease, when the virus first invades the body. They do not differ substantively from the usual pictures of viral meningitis and viral encephalitis discussed earlier.

With well-established disease, AIDS patients may develop a number of different neurologic syndromes, including dementia, myelopathy or myelitis, polyradiculopathy, neuropathy, and inflammatory myopathy. Toxoplasma gondii so frequently attacks AIDS patients that many physicians empirically treat for toxoplasmosis when evidence of diffuse, focal, or multifocal CNS infection appears. Mycobacterial and spirochetal infections tend to run atypical and aggressive courses in AIDS patients. PML occurs frequently, as does CNS lymphoma. The antiviral drugs used to treat HIV infection can cause neurologic complications (polyneuropathy, myopathy).

The treatment of HIV/AIDS is very complex and beyond the scope of this discussion. For periodically updated treatment guidelines, visit the Web sites *www.hivatis.org/trtgdlns.html* and *www.ama- assn.org/special/hiv/treatmnt/treatmnt.htm.*

PROGRESSIVE MULTIFOCAL LEUKOENCEPHALOPATHY

Rarely occurring in normal individuals, PML has always been recognized as a complication of immunosuppression, and now is most often seen in AIDS patients. CNS infection by papovavirus produces a characteristic pattern of white matter lesions, most prominent in the parieto-occipital regions, along with rapidly progressive dementia (see Figures 9–2 and 9–3). Lesions seen on MRI may resemble MS. None of the various therapeutic agents tried have had notable success with PML.

OTHER INFECTIONS

Other important but uncommon neurologic infections include Creutzfeldt-Jakob disease, subacute sclerosing panencephalitis, rabies, and poliomyelitis (see Enrichment Box 10–8). Some infections, and even infestations, cause their neurologic complications by the elaboration of a toxin, which then affects the nervous system. Such infections include botulism, tetanus, and diphtheria, all of which are rare. Tick paralysis is due to infestation by a tick that elaborates a toxin that interferes with nerve transmission and causes generalized weakness and areflexia.

Toxins

Neurologic disease due to toxin exposure occurs rarely, although the possibility is considered often, particularly in peripheral neuropathy patients. Toxins are generally separated from drugs in that drugs have some medicinal or quasi medicinal intent. Occasionally, the distinction is blurred, such as when a toxin is used as a drug. This was done often in the early days of medicine, but is done much less so now. A current example is the use of botulinum toxin to treat movement disorders.

Environmental toxins include heavy metals (e.g., lead); industrial agents used in the manufacture of goods (e.g., n-hexane); pesticides (e.g., organophosphates); gases to which a patient might be accidentally or deliberately exposed (e.g., carbon monoxide); and biologic toxins derived from plants (e.g., chickpeas), fish (e.g., ciguatera), or bacteria (e.g., diphtheria). Sometimes people play with toxins. Adventurous diners in Japan sometimes toy with tetrodotoxin, ingesting contaminated puffer fish and titrating themselves to the brink of paralysis. The upside is usually unclear to people who have not tried it. Occasional miscalculations occur.

The diagnosis of a neurotoxicologic syndrome is usually difficult. The patient must have a known exposure, a compatible clinical syndrome, and other likely responsible conditions must be rigorously excluded. A history of exposure in the isolated case is often difficult or impossible to obtain. There is frequently disagreement among the various parties regarding the level of exposure. The systemic manifestations may provide a clue to the cause of the neurologic syndrome, such as anemia and basophilic stippling of lead intoxication, which raise the possibility of a toxic cause. Sometimes toxin exposure occurs in the course of an illegal activity, such as moonshine ingestion or taking illicit drugs. The exposure history under these circumstances is even more difficult to obtain than usual. It is a good general rule that when exposure is eliminated, the neurotoxicologic syndrome should stabilize or regress. Patients who continue to progress in the absence of continued exposure usually have another condition.

Most neurotoxicologic syndromes are not treatable except by eliminating exposure. Some toxins, for example, heavy metals, can be treated by using chelating agents that bind the metal and allow it to be excreted in the urine. The following paragraphs summarize heavy metal intoxications; Table 10–15 summarizes other more common or important chronic neurotoxicologic syndromes. Acute intoxications are usually encountered in the emergency room setting. Biologic toxins primarily occur in the setting of infection or infestation (see CENTRAL NERVOUS SYSTEM INFECTIONS).

LEAD INTOXICATION

Lead intoxication may occur in an industrial setting or by accidental exposure through the ingestion of contaminated material. A common mode of accidental exposure is moonshine ingestion. Lead intoxication has many effects. In adults, the primary neurologic complication is a peripheral neuropathy. Heavy metal screens are often done in peripheral neuropathy patients to search for evidence of exposure, but are rarely helpful. Lead exposure has diverse purported consequences in children that are quite different from adults; the details are beyond the scope of this discussion.

TABLE 10–15. CHRONIC NEUROLOGIC EFFECTS OF VARIOUS TOXINS

Toxin	Major Clinical Manifestations of Chronic Neurologic Toxicity
Organic solvents	Numerous effects, such as cognitive impairment, ataxia, parkinsonism, optic atrophy, seizures, peripheral neuropathy, myopathy
Carbon monoxide	Parkinsonism, degeneration of the globus pallidus
Organophosphate insecticides	Peripheral neuropathy

ARSENIC

Patients are usually exposed to arsenic by homicidal or suicidal intent. Arsenic exposure is much more common in certain regions of the United States (e.g., North Carolina) than elsewhere. The primary neurologic manifestation in the chronic phase is peripheral neuropathy. In the acute phases patients are extremely ill with systemic effects, particularly GI effects, and may also develop encephalopathy, seizures, and other complications. Acute arsenical peripheral neuropathy can closely simulate GBS. Severely intoxicated patients seldom survive. Arsenic intoxication has been suspected in the deaths of such historical figures as Napoleon and Andrew Jackson.

Inflammatory Disorders

This section describes noninfectious disorders characterized by a pathological picture of inflammation. Most of these disorders are of obscure etiology. Some of them are probably autoimmune, such as the inflammatory myopathies. In other instances, the etiopathogenesis remains obscure, and a reaction to an exogenous agent cannot be excluded. The inflammatory reaction in such instances may be a misdirected host defense mechanism against an infectious agent. Examples of similar nonneurologic inflammatory disorders of obscure etiology include such conditions as the connective tissue disorders, inflammatory bowel disease, Reiter syndrome, and systemic vasculitis. Table 10–16 lists neurologic conditions of an inflammatory but presumably noninfectious etiology.

There is some overlap with other etiologic categories. Some demyelinating diseases have associated inflammation, such as ADEM and similar postinfectious syndromes. However, the predominant pathological change is the demyelination, and these disorders are discussed with the demyelinating diseases. Likewise, the inflammatory myopathies are discussed with the other muscle diseases, and the inflammatory neuropathies with the other peripheral neuropathies. This section is devoted to inflammatory disorders that tend to be diffuse or multifocal.

NEUROSARCOIDOSIS

Sarcoidosis is a systemic disease. The lung, skin, and eye are most commonly affected, but any organ system may be involved. Clinically obvious neurologic involvement occurs in 5%–10% of patients. Subclinical involvement may be even more common. Granulomas in skeletal muscle may be seen in as many as 50% of sarcoid patients, even in the absence of symptoms, making muscle biopsy a useful diagnostic tool. Patients occasionally present with neurologic symptoms; careful workup reveals evidence of systemic sarcoidosis in the majority of

TABLE 10–16. DISORDERS CHARACTERIZED BY INFLAMMATION OF PRESUMABLY NONINFECTIOUS ORIGIN

Neurosarcoidosis

Acute inflammatory demyelinating polyradiculoneuropathy, Guillain-Barré syndrome

Chronic inflammatory demyelinating polyradiculoneuropathy

Acute disseminated encephalomyelitis

Transverse myelitis

Orbital pseudotumor

Tolosa-Hunt syndrome

Polymyositis, dermatomyositis, inclusion body myositis

Aseptic meningitis due to drugs

Recurrent meningitis and meningoencephalitis (Mollaret meningitis, Vogt-Koyanagi-Harada disease, and like entities)

Vasculitis (temporal arteritis, granulomatous arteritis of the brain, systemic vasculitis)

Neurologic complications of systemic connective tissue disorders

Rasmussen encephalitis

Paraneoplastic limbic encephalitis

Some disorders can occur as a postinfectious syndrome; others arise for no clear reason.

them, but the diagnosis is frequently difficult. Truly isolated neurosarcoidosis is uncommon. Because of its immunologically privileged status, the nervous system may be involved less often than might otherwise be expected. Sarcoidosis is far more common in blacks than in whites, and it appears likely that neurologic complications are more common in blacks as well.

Any part of the nervous or neuromuscular systems can be involved (Enrichment Box 10–10). Table 10–17 lists some of the neurologic complications. The most common neurologic complication of sarcoidosis is facial nerve palsy, which may be bilateral. The treatment of neurosarcoidosis is primarily with corticosteroids and other immunosuppressants.

BEHÇET DISEASE

Behçet disease is a rare inflammatory condition that may involve the nervous system. It is primarily relevant in the differential diagnosis of MS (see Enrichment Box 10–10).

Sarcoidosis

The etiology of sarcoidosis remains unknown. Interestingly, cell-mediated immunity is impaired, producing anergy, in the face of an ongoing inflammatory response. Various antigenic stimuli have been suspected, particularly mycobacteria, but no definite associations have been proven.

Neurosarcoidosis is sometimes multifocal, with disease present in more than one location simultaneously. The most common neurologic complications are due to infiltration of the basal meninges with sarcoid granulomas, producing cranial neuropathies and pituitary and hypothalamic dysfunction. For unknown reasons, sarcoidosis characteristically varies in its clinical activity, waxing and waning spontaneously, causing relapses and remissions similar to those that occur with multiple sclerosis (MS). Sarcoid can also involve the white matter on imaging studies. Neurosarcoidosis is therefore often included in the differential diagnosis of demyelinating diseases.

The cerebrospinal fluid (CSF) in active neurosarcoidosis frequently demonstrates a mild mononuclear pleocytosis and elevated protein, and may show oligoclonal bands and immunoglobulin G elevation.

Behçet disease

Behçet disease is a disorder of obscure pathogenesis characterized pathologically by inflammation involving multiple organ systems and clinically by chronic relapsing multisystem involvement with complete or incomplete remissions between attacks, although sometimes by a chronic progressive course. The primary manifestations are recurrent oral or genital ulcerations, ocular disease, primarily uveitis, and involvement of other organ systems including the skin, joints, gastrointestinal (GI) tract, lungs, urinary tract, and cardiovascular system.

Central nervous system (CNS) involvement occurs in as many as half of the cases, and the condition may present with neurologic manifestations. The most common neurologic complication is recurrent meningoencephalitis. Other common neurologic features are headache, confusion, increased intracranial pressure, and brainstem or corticospinal tract dysfunction. The CSF is often abnormal. Behçet disease can produce a magnetic resonance image resembling that seen in MS, and the disease is often considered in the differential diagnosis of both MS and sarcoidosis.

Treatment is primarily with corticosteroids and other immunosuppressants.

TABLE 10–17. NEUROLOGIC COMPLICATIONS OF SARCOIDOSIS

Basilar meningeal infiltration

Recurrent meningitis

Cranial neuropathies

    Facial nerve

    Optic nerve

Neuroendocrine dysfunction

    Panhypopituitarism

    Hyperprolactinemia

    Diabetes insipidus

    Hypothalamic dysfunction

Neuropsychiatric symptoms

    Psychosis

    Bipolar disorder

    Amnesic syndromes

    Schizophrenic-like states

Hydrocephalus

    Communicating

    Obstructive

Pseudotumor cerebri

Headaches

Seizures

Intracranial mass lesion

Cerebrovascular syndromes

    Ischemic stroke

    Subarachnoid hemorrhage

    Intraparenchymal hemorrhage

    Central nervous system vasculitis

Spinal cord disease

    Myelopathy

    Radiculopathy

    Polyradiculopathy

Peripheral neuropathy

Myopathy

Complications of immunosuppressant treatment

Antibody-Mediated or Autoimmune Disorders

Autoimmune disorders may be either cell mediated, with a pathological picture demonstrating inflammation, or antibody mediated, where inflammation is not prominent. The nervous system may be secondarily involved in systemic autoimmune disorders such as SLE and related conditions or when the autoimmune process is directed against blood vessels. The CNS may suffer the primary insult in other autoimmune conditions, such as MS and stiff man syndrome. Many of the conditions in Table 10–16 are likely autoimmune. They are discussed earlier (see inflammatory disorders). The autoimmune neuropathies, myopathies, and neuromuscular transmission disorders are discussed in Chapter 11. Examples of humorally mediated disorders, definite or probable, include myasthenia gravis, Lambert-Eaton syndrome, Sydenham chorea, some channelopathies, some paraneoplastic syndromes, autoimmune hearing loss, and stiff man syndrome. An autoimmune etiology has been postulated for ALS. In several conditions, antibodies have been demonstrated against nerve or muscle tissue, as in the inflammatory neuropathies and myopathies. The pathogenetic role of such antibodies remains uncertain, because they might develop secondarily due to exposure of previously sequestered antigens by a destructive process of another origin. Thus the demonstration of an autoantibody does not conclusively prove that the disease process is mediated by that antibody.

Disorders Below the Foramen Magnum

This chapter focuses on the more common disorders that involve structures below the foramen magnum and the peripheral neuromuscular system. See Table 8–3 for a summary of the characteristics of disease affecting these parts of the nervous system. The key feature is bilaterality of abnormalities, compared with the unilaterality often seen in processes involving structures above the foramen magnum. There are exceptions; for example, plexopathy, radiculopathy, and mononeuropathy may cause symptoms and signs involving only one extremity.

DISORDERS OF THE SPINE AND SPINAL CORD

Conditions affecting the spine and spinal cord are common, especially if the physician considers the numerous patients with back and neck pain of soft tissue origin in whom spine disease warrants differential diagnostic consideration. Diseases of the spinal column and diseases of the spinal cord are closely related, and therefore are discussed together. The most common spinal cord disorders are degenerative spine disease, which produces radiculopathy or myelopathy, acute spinal cord injury (SCI), demyelinating disease, acute transverse myelopathy due to cord compression or transverse myelitis, subacute combined degeneration, and tumor, most often metastatic.

Disease of the spinal cord can be clinically confusing, mistaken by novice and experienced clinicians alike for other conditions. Many patients who were thought to have hysteria and conversion syndromes actually suffered from spinal cord disease. The misdiagnosis resulted in clinical mismanagement, significant morbidity, occasional mortality, and litigation.

TUMORS

Primary tumors, such as glioma, schwannoma, or neurofibroma, can involve the spinal cord and spinal roots, but the most common tumor to involve the spinal cord is metastatic cancer. Metastases to the cord parenchyma are rare, but metastatic disease in the epidural space, producing cord compression, is very common. Almost any systemic cancer can metastasize and cause cord compression. Breast and lung tumors are most common. Prostate cancer, which only rarely metastasizes to the brain, frequently metastasizes to the spinal column and can cause spinal cord compression. Epidural metastases usually present with back or neck pain and a progressive neurologic deficit, primarily weakness and bladder impairment. Spinal cord involvement with other types of tumors is rare.

Aggressive management with steroids, surgery, and radiation is necessary to preserve function. For further information on management of spinal cord compression, see the Web site *cancer.med.upenn.edu/support/tips/tip38.html*. If patients have already become nonambulatory, they are not likely to regain walking ability, despite optimal treatment (Enrichment Box 11–1).

DRUGS AND ALCOHOL

See Table 10–2 for mention of agents that may cause myelopathy.

IMBALANCES

The primary imbalance likely to cause spinal cord dysfunction is vitamin B_{12} deficiency, which causes subacute combined degeneration. Other imbalances affecting the spinal cord are rare.

The term subacute combined degeneration describes the pathological appearance of the spinal cord in vitamin B_{12} deficiency, with demyelination and gliosis of the posterior columns combined with the lateral columns. Clinically, affected patients have weakness, spasticity, and prominent loss of vibratory and position sense with relative preservation of pain and temperature. These clinical deficits reflect the structures in the spinal cord that are primarily damaged by B_{12} deficiency. Hematologic evidence of B_{12} deficiency is often lacking. A simple serum vitamin B_{12} level is not an adequate screening test in patients with suspicious neurologic findings. Subacute combined degeneration of the spinal cord may coexist with B_{12}-induced peripheral neuropathy, producing the unusual combination of absent ankle jerks with upgoing toes (also seen in Friedreich ataxia). Vitamin B_{12} deficiency is discussed further in Chapter 10.

Spinal cord compression

In suspected cord compression, finding a discrete sensory level on examination is very helpful. When symptoms of cord compression occur in a patient with known systemic cancer, the diagnosis is readily suspected. In some patients, epidural metastasis that causes spinal cord compression is the presenting manifestation of the cancer. In such instances the diagnosis may be considerably more difficult. Patients present with acute transverse myelopathy if the compression involves the spinal cord proper. When metastatic deposits involve the cauda equina, the patient presents with a cauda equina syndrome rather than a transverse myelopathy. Distinguishing acute compressive transverse myelopathy from acute transverse myelitis is critical. A diagnosis of transverse myelitis is only acceptable after cord compression has been excluded.

Central cord syndrome

Central cord syndrome is one of the regularly recurrent variants seen with incomplete cervical spinal cord injury (SCI). It involves necrosis with softening of the central aspect of the spinal cord and relative sparing of the periphery. Patients with central cord syndrome thus have segmental weakness at the involved level due to anterior horn gray matter necrosis, with only minor long tract findings; they are not paraplegic or quadriplegic. The segmental weakness typically involves the hands and distal upper extremities.

Brown-Sequard syndrome

Brown-Sequard described the clinical picture that follows functional hemisection of the spinal cord. It is actually more often seen with extramedullary tumor compression than it is with trauma. Patients with Brown-Sequard syndrome have corticospinal tract and posterior column dysfunction ipsilateral to the lesion and spinothalamic tract–mediated pain and temperature loss contralateral to the lesion. There may be evidence of root dysfunction at the level of the lesion.

Neurogenic versus vascular claudication

Some features of the history can sometimes help to distinguish neurogenic from vascular claudication. With neurogenic claudication, symptoms decrease with sitting or bending forward, the pain occurs in a wider distribution, and there may be neurologic accompaniments such as lower extremity weakness or numbness. Patients usually have to sit down for relief, and the symptoms subside slowly. Vascular claudication tends to produce focal, intense, crampy pain in one or both calves and the pain subsides quickly if the patient just stops and stands. Patients with vascular claudication have more symptoms walking uphill because of the increased leg work. Neurogenic claudication may decrease when

(Continued)

walking uphill because of the increased spinal flexion in forward leaning. Patients with vascular claudication have as much trouble riding a bicycle as they do walking because of the leg work involved, whereas forward flexion on the bicycle opens up the spinal canal, allowing patients with neurogenic claudication to ride a bike with greater ease than they can walk.

Spinal dysraphism

Patients with congenital malformations of the lumbosacral spine related to occult dysraphism often present with dysfunction of the cauda equina, producing combinations of weakness and sensory loss of the lower extremities with variable bowel and bladder dysfunction. Foot deformities due to long-standing denervation and impaired trophic influences such as pes cavus or pes equinovarus, or a dimple, sinus tract, or lipoma over the sacral region, may be clues to the presence of a congenital anomaly. Such anomalies of the spinal cord included tethered cord syndrome, diastematomyelia, arteriovenous malformation, and various tumors such as dermoid, epidermoid, and lipoma.

Anterior spinal artery syndrome

Anterior spinal artery syndrome is due to ischemia in the distribution of the anterior spinal artery, which perfuses the anterior two-thirds of the spinal cord, all except the posterior columns. Ischemia of the anterior spinal artery produces dysfunction that involves the entire spinal cord except posterior column function. Patients are typically paraplegic or quadriplegic with loss of pain and temperature sensation below the level of the lesion, but with retained sensation to light touch, position, and vibration.

MASS LESIONS

Spinal cord mass lesions are most commonly due to tumor (often metastatic), abscess, or disc herniation. These lesions all behave in a similar fashion neurologically. See the previous discussion on tumor for details. The Web site *medweb.bham.ac.uk/neurosurgery/cord.html* discusses mass lesions from a neurosurgical perspective.

TRAUMA

Acute SCI occurs most often after motor vehicle accidents. Young males are predominantly affected. Although more indolent processes, such as cervical spondylosis, mechanically damage the spinal cord, the term SCI is generally used only to refer to acute events. Patients with complete injuries lose all function below the level of the injury, and those with incomplete injuries have variable preservation of function. The American

Spinal Injury Association has published a scale, the ASIA scale, for rating the severity of an SCI. An ASIA grade A injury is complete, and grades B-E injuries are variably incomplete. SCI may be associated with different types of vertebral injury, ranging from fracture dislocation lesions to no detectable bony abnormality. Spinal shock refers to the flaccidity that occurs acutely, producing hyporeflexia or areflexia. As the spinal shock stage resolves, spasticity develops. Multiple complications may occur in the SCI patient, most commonly urinary tract infection and decubitus ulcers. The strength in a series of "key muscles" is used to establish the level of the lesion; the key muscles range from the elbow flexors to the ankle plantar fractures. There are, in addition, key sensory levels to further aid in localization. The acute management of SCI includes immobilization pending orthopedic and neurosurgical evaluation and management. High-dose intravenous (IV) steroids, the "Bracken regimen," are given if the injury occurred less than 8 hours previously. For further information, see the Web site *www.cochrane.de/cochrane/revabstr/ab001046.htm.*

Most SCI patients have a transverse myelopathy; central cord and hemicord syndromes occur occasionally (see Enrichment Box 11–1).

DEGENERATIVE DISEASES

The intervertebral disc is the largest avascular structure in the body. It begins to desiccate and lose elasticity in the fifth to sixth decade; individuals in this age group are prone to intervertebral disc rupture. In the seventh to ninth decade, the tendency is to hardening and calcification, resulting in spondylosis and spinal stenosis.

The annulus fibrosus provides circumferential reinforcement for the disc; the spherical nucleus pulposus allows the vertebral bodies above and below to glide and slip across it, like a ball bearing. The nucleus pulposus is eccentrically placed, closer to the posterior aspect of the disc.

With aging and recurrent micro and macro trauma, degenerative spine disease develops. This involves both the disc [degenerative disc disease (DDD)] and the bony structures and joints [degenerative joint disease (DJD)]. These processes are separate but related. Together, DDD and DJD are referred to as spondylosis. Several different clinical syndromes may ensue from degenerative spine disease. Common problems include simple, single-level radiculopathy; multilevel radiculopathy; cauda equina syndrome; cervical myelopathy; cervical radiculomyelopathy; and neurogenic claudication. Arthritic, degenerative, and inflammatory disease of the spine may cause local pain plus referred pain to an extremity, even without neurologic pathology. Separating patients with such referred nonradicular pain from those with true radiculopathy is a common clinical exercise.

Herniated Intervertebral Disc

Disc herniations can theoretically occur at any level of the vertebral column, but the clinically significant and most common herniations involve the C5, C6, C7, C8, L5, and S1 roots. The clinical syndrome includes pain that may be localized over the spine and/or referred along the distribution of the involved root. There may or may not be associated weakness, sensory loss, or reflex depression, depending on the severity of the root compression. Some patients have signs of radicular inflammation on examination, so that stretching of the involved root increases the pain in the distribution of the root, producing a positive straight-leg raising sign.

Small tears in the annulus may cause nonspecific, nonradiating pain. More extensive tears lead to disc bulging, protrusion, or ruptures. Disc herniations tend to occur posterolaterally, especially in the lumbosacral region, in part because of lateral incompleteness of the posterior longitudinal ligament and the relative thinness of the annulus posteriorly; occasionally herniations are directly lateral or central. Which nerve roots are damaged depends largely on the direction of the herniation. A central herniated nucleus pulposus (HNP) may compress the spinal cord or cauda equina. The root level involved in a radiculopathy may or may not correspond with the vertebral level of the pathological process (Figure 11–1 and Enrichment Box 11–2).

Cervical Radiculopathy

The incidence of cervical radiculopathy is highest in men 50–54 years of age. A history of physical injury or exertion is present in only 15% of patients. The onset is acute in half, subacute in one-fourth, and insidious in one-fourth of patients, with the majority of them symptomatic for about 2 weeks before diagnosis.

A number of clinical conditions can be confused with cervical radiculopathy. These conditions primarily include brachial plexopathy, entrapment neuropathy, and musculoskeletal conditions such as cervical myofascial pain and shoulder pathology (bursitis, tendinitis, impingement syndrome).

Physical examination in patients with suspected cervical radiculopathy should include an assessment of the range of motion of the neck, shoulder, and arm; a search for root compression signs; detailed examination of strength and reflexes; a screening sensory examination; and probing for areas of muscle spasm or trigger points. Pain or limitation of motion of any upper extremity joint should signal the possibility of nonradicular pathology. Reflex examination should include not only the upper extremity reflexes, but also the knee and ankle jerks and the plantar reflexes. Increased lower extremity reflexes and extensor plantar responses suggest myelopathy, complicating the radiculopathy.

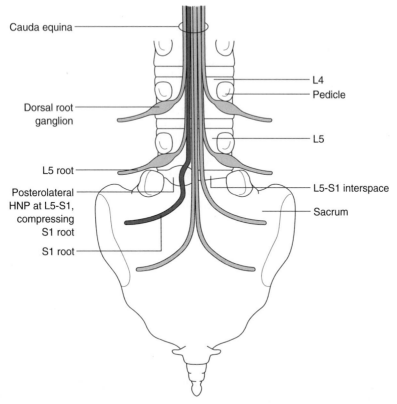

Cauda equina

L4
Pedicle

Dorsal root
ganglion

L5

L5 root

Posterolateral
HNP at L5-S1,
compressing
S1 root

L5-S1 interspace

Sacrum

S1 root

FIGURE 11–1. ■ Posterior view of the cauda equina with exiting nerve roots. A posterolateral herniated nucleus pulposus (*HNP*) is compressing the S1 root as it passes by the L5-S1 interspace. (From Campbell WW: *Essentials of Electrodiagnostic Medicine.* Baltimore, Williams & Wilkins, 1999, p 186.)

Lumbosacral Radiculopathy and Low Back Pain

Low back pain (LBP) has numerous potential origins. Most benign self-limited episodes of LBP arise from musculoligamentous structures, and discomfort is localized to the low back region. However, numerous pain-sensitive structures can underlie a clinical episode of back pain: the intervertebral disc, especially the outer fibers of the annulus; the facet joints; other bony structures; and spinal nerve roots. In addition, pain can be referred to the lower back from visceral structures in the abdomen and pelvis. With true HNP, leg pain usually predominates over back pain. With HNP the pain is typically worse when sitting, better when standing, better still when lying down, and generally worse in flexed compared with extended postures, all of which reflect the known changes in intradiscal pressure that occur in these positions.

In the cervical spine, the nerve root exits over the vertebral body of like number; for example, the C6 root exits at C5–6. The C8 root exits beneath C7 and all subsequent roots exit beneath the vertebral body of like number; for example, the L5 root exits at L5-S1. The roots exit more or less horizontally in the cervical spine. Downward slant increases more caudally. When the cord terminates at the level of L1–2, the remaining roots drop vertically downward in the cauda equina to their exit foramina.

In the cervical region, there is about a one-segment discrepancy between the cord level and the spinous process, in the thoracic region, about a two-segment discrepancy, and in the lumbosacral region, a three-to-four segment discrepancy. Therefore the L5 nerve root exiting at the L5-S1 interspace arises as a discrete structure at L1-L2 and traverses the interspaces at L2–3, L3–4, and L4–5 before exiting at L5-S1, sliding laterally all the while. This means that the L5 root could be injured by a central disc at L2–3 or L3–4, a posterolateral disc at L4–5, or a far lateral disc at L5-S1. A posterolateral disc at L4–5 is the most likely culprit, but not the sole suspect.

Pain radiating down the back of the leg is termed sciatica, and is an important clue to the presence of radiculopathy. Involvement of other pain-sensitive structures can produce referred pain that radiates to the extremity (buttock, hip, or thigh), and which can simulate the radiating pain of nerve root origin. Referred pain to the leg occurs nearly twice as often as true radicular pain, and can closely mimic the clinical presentation of radiculopathy. Considerable pain can be referred to the buttock and thigh with disease limited to the disc, the facet joint, or the sacroiliac joint. Sciatica may occur from either L5 or S1 radiculopathy, but the pain of L5 origin tends to involve the dorsum of the foot, whereas the pain of S1 origin tends to involve the heel.

The straight-leg raising test is one of the mainstays in detecting radicular compression. The test is performed by slowly raising the symptomatic leg with the knee extended. Tension is transmitted to the nerve roots between about 30° and 70°, and pain increases. Pain at less than 30° raises the question of nonorganicity, and discomfort and tightness beyond 70° is routine and insignificant.

The neurologic examination should include assessment of power in the major lower extremity muscle groups, but especially the dorsiflexors of the foot and toes, and the evertors and invertors of the foot. Sensation should be tested in the signature zones of the major roots. The status of knee and ankle reflexes reflects the integrity of the L3–4 and S1 roots. There is no good reflex for the L5 root.

Cervical Spondylosis

As patients mature into the seventh decade and beyond, the liability to disc rupture decreases, but degenerative spine disease attacks in a different form. Osteophytic spurs and bars; bulging discs; thickened laminae and pedicles; arthritic, hypertrophied facets; and thickened spinal ligaments all combine to narrow the spinal canal and foramina and produce the syndrome of spinal stenosis. Cervical spondylosis is a common condition. Progressive DDD and DJD may produce pressure on exiting nerve roots and cause clinical radiculopathy. Midline bulging discs with variable degrees of calcification, sometimes with hypertrophy of the ligamentum flavum, and with the superimposition of acute "soft disc" herniations into the spinal canal can compress the cord and produce long tract signs such as spasticity and bladder incontinence. Cervical spondylosis may thus be associated with radiculopathy, myelopathy, or a combination of the two. The latter condition is the most common and is referred to as spondylotic radiculomyelopathy. Patients with this condition may have upper motor neuron weakness in the lower extremities with accompanying lower motor neuron weakness in the upper extremities. This clinical picture can mimic amyotrophic lateral sclerosis (ALS).

Lumbar Spondylosis

Although analogous to cervical spondylosis in basic pathophysiology, the clinical manifestations of lumbar spondylosis are different. Patients may or may not complain of LBP. Because of the diffuse involvement, they commonly have evidence of a multilevel lumbosacral radiculopathy. One unique feature of lumbar spondylosis is so-called claudication of the cauda equina, also known as neurogenic claudication or pseudoclaudication. Patients with spinal stenosis and neurogenic claudication experience pain, weakness, numbness, and paresthesias or dysesthesias when standing or walking; these symptoms are generally attributed to mechanical pressure on the nerve roots and blood vessels of the cauda equina. Such pain in the legs on walking can obviously be easily confused with vascular claudication. See Enrichment Box 11–1 for distinguishing features.

DEMYELINATING DISEASE

The most common demyelinating disease to involve the spinal cord is transverse myelitis, which may occur as an independent, often postinfectious, disorder, or as a manifestation of multiple sclerosis. See Chapter 10 for further details.

CONGENITAL DISEASES

It is not rare for congenital malformations of the spinal cord and spinal column to present well after childhood. These malformations are most often instances of occult spinal dysraphism due to abnormalities of neural tube closure (see Enrichment Box 11–1).

Syringomyelia is difficult to classify. Most cases are probably congenital, although they may not present until later in life. Syringomyelia can develop after spinal cord trauma (posttraumatic syringomyelia) or in association with a spinal cord tumor. There is cavitation within the central portion of the spinal cord. The first anatomic structure disrupted by such cavity formation is the anterior white commissure, which lies just anterior to the central canal. Because the second-order neurons of the lateral spinothalamic tract cross in the anterior white commissure, the earliest clinical manifestation is loss of pain and temperature sensation corresponding to the earliest clinical segmental level involved.

Patients with syringomyelia typically display "suspended" [involving a certain segmental level (e.g., C6–8 bilaterally, with normal function above and below that level)], "dissociated" (involving pain and temperature sensation but sparing light touch, pressure, position, and vibration) sensory loss. When syringomyelia involves the cervical segments, a syrinx thus produces the classical suspended, dissociated, cape or shawl-like sensory loss to pain and temperature. Most patients with a syrinx also harbor a type I Arnold-Chiari malformation.

HEMORRHAGIC DISEASE

Spinal hematomas are rare but important to recognize because they are eminently treatable, and the untreated consequences can be neurologically devastating. Spinal epidural hematoma is more common than spinal subdural hematoma. Either can occur in the setting of obvious trauma with spinal fracture, or may follow lumbar puncture or other needling of the spinal column. The patient typically presents with severe local pain in the neck or back, followed by a rapidly evolving transverse myelopathy following the inciting event. Coagulopathies raise the risk of either form of spinal hematoma. With hematomas below the L2 vertebral level, the patient may instead present with a rapidly evolving cauda equina syndrome (asymmetric pain, weakness, sensory loss, and reflex loss in both lower extremities with variable bowel and bladder involvement).

Arteriovenous malformations are not rare, and can be extremely difficult to diagnose. Although bleeding can occur from these lesions, they more often present with mass effect due to spinal cord compression or with a progressive myelopathy due to ischemic changes as the malformation "steals" blood from the normal spinal cord.

Hematomyelia refers to hemorrhage into the substance of the spinal cord. It is a rare but neurologically devastating condition.

STROKE

Ischemic disease of the spinal cord is rare. The most common ischemic spinal cord syndrome is anterior spinal artery syndrome, which occurs most often after aortic surgery (see Enrichment Box 11–1).

HEREDOFAMILIAL DISORDERS

Except for the rare syndrome of hereditary spastic paraparesis, the spinal cord is rarely involved in isolation in hereditary diseases, although myelopathy may occur as part of the clinical picture in a number of genetic conditions (Table 11–1).

TABLE 11–1. SYSTEMIC DISEASES AND OTHER CONDITIONS THAT MAY BE COMPLICATED BY MYELOPATHY

Retroviral infection (HIV and HTLV-1)

Cytomegalovirus infection

Lyme disease

Varicella-zoster virus infection

Schistosomiasis

Remote neoplasm (carcinomatous myelopathy)

Leukemia or lymphoma

Connective tissue disorders

Wegener granulomatosis

Hyperparathyroidism

Achondroplasia

Mucopolysaccharidosis

Adrenomyeloneuropathy

Neurosarcoidosis

Chronic alcoholism

Extramedullary hematopoiesis

Epidural lipomatosis

Chiropractic manipulation

Radiation therapy

Thyrotoxicosis

Celiac disease

HIV = human immunodeficiency virus; HTLV-I = human T-cell lymphotrophic virus type I.

PSYCHIATRIC DISEASE

Paraparesis with inability to walk is one of the classic presentations of hysterical conversion disorder or malingering. Accept such a diagnosis only after rigorous exclusion of organic disease and confirmation of a psychiatric disorder. See Chapter 8 for a discussion of the pitfalls of diagnosing conversion disorder.

COMPLICATIONS OF SYSTEMIC DISEASE

Myelopathy may complicate numerous systemic diseases. Table 11–1 lists some of the diseases that are not discussed elsewhere.

One of the most common spinal cord conditions complicating systemic disease is radiation myelopathy. Therapeutic antitumor radiation can damage the nervous system in a variety of ways. One of the more common of these unfortunate side effects is the development of a myelopathy months to years following the radiation, most often affecting the cervical cord. Recurrence of the original tumor is always a major consideration in the differential diagnosis.

INFECTIONS

Because of the therapeutic implications, the most important infectious disorder affecting the spinal cord is spinal epidural abscess. The possible consequences of an untreated spinal epidural abscess are the same as for spinal epidural or subdural hematoma: paraplegia or quadriplegia. Spinal epidural abscess may be acute or chronic, and arises from direct extension of infection from an adjacent vertebral source (in which case plain films of the spine may show osteomyelitis), or through hematogenous spread. The patient presents with a combination of evidence of infection (fever, leukocytosis) and severe back pain, followed by radicular pain and a rapidly progressive transverse myelopathy. A characteristic clinical feature is severe back pain with exquisite tenderness localized over the area of the spine corresponding to the location of the abscess. With antibiotics and surgical drainage, there is reasonable expectation of recovery. In patients with chronic epidural abscess, the evolution of the disease may be insidious and evidence of systemic infection lacking, causing confusion with other processes, including spinal cord neoplasm. The organism most often associated with spinal epidural abscess is *Staphylococcus aureus*. A patient with an untreated spinal epidural abscess usually winds up paraplegic or quadriplegic.

A vacuolar myelopathy frequently complicates acquired immunodeficiency syndrome (AIDS). Tropical spastic paraparesis is caused by the human T-cell lymphotrophic virus type I, which produces a chronic progressive myelopathy. It is seen primarily in patients from the Caribbean, but also occurs occasionally in the United States. Syphilitic infection may cause tabes (Latin, "wasting away") dorsalis, which preferentially affects the posterior columns. See Table 11–1 for mention of other spinal cord disorders related to infection.

TOXINS

Only rarely do toxins cause isolated myelopathy.

INFLAMMATORY AND AUTOIMMUNE-MEDIATED DISORDERS

Except for complications of systemic disease and for neurosarcoidosis, only rarely do inflammatory or autoimmune-mediated conditions affect the spinal cord (see Table 11–1).

Disorders of the Motor Unit

A motor unit consists of an individual anterior horn motor neuron, its axon, and all of the muscle fibers it innervates. Disease can strike anywhere along this pathway, producing motor neuron disease, radiculopathy, plexopathy, peripheral neuropathy, neuromuscular junction (NMJ) disorder, or myopathy. The discipline of neuromuscular disease addresses conditions affecting all of these different components of the motor unit; some "motor unit" disorders may have sensory dysfunction as well, primarily radiculopathies and peripheral neuropathies.

Patients with suspected neuromuscular disorders are often subjected to all or part of a battery of tests. These tests are done to help localize and characterize a neuromuscular disorder, and from most simple to most complex include creatine kinase (CK) determination, electromyogram (EMG), and muscle biopsy. CK is an enzyme involved in muscle energy metabolism, and is present in great quantities in muscle tissue. Under certain circumstances, CK is released into the serum, and when present in large quantities indicates muscle fiber necrosis. The situation is not so simple that an elevation of CK indicates muscle disease and the lack of elevation of CK indicates no muscle disease. Some muscle diseases, such as steroid myopathy, produce little or no CK elevation. Some nonmuscle neuromuscular diseases, such as ALS, often produce mild elevation of CK.

EMG is an electrophysiologic test done to help distinguish neuromuscular from nonneuromuscular problems, and to help localize and characterize a neuromuscular disorder. It is described further in Chapter 9.

When the diagnosis remains uncertain or when further information is required, muscle biopsy is often performed. Thin sections are stained in various ways, then examined by light microscopy or electron microscopy. For light microscopy, two sorts of staining procedures are used, routine H and E stains, and histochemical stains. Sometimes routine H and E staining is adequate, as in polymyositis (PM). However, routine H and E appears normal in many muscle diseases, and histochemical stains show marked abnormalities. Under most circumstances, the full battery of stains, including histochemistries, should be performed if muscle tissue is to be removed from the patient. Other tests sometimes used in the evaluation of the patient with neuromuscular disease are listed in Table 11–2.

MOTOR NEURON DISEASE (MOTOR NEURONOPATHY OR ANTERIOR HORN CELL DISEASE)

The most common disorders affecting motor neurons are the acquired degenerative disease ALS and the hereditary spinal muscular atrophy (SMA) syndromes.

Amyotrophic Lateral Sclerosis

ALS, also known as Lou Gehrig's disease, is a progressive degenerative disorder of unknown etiology involving motor neurons of the brain and spinal cord. Current thinking favors a multifactorial basis, at least in part related to excitotoxicity. About 10% of the cases are familial, and some have a mutation involving the superoxide dismutase gene.

Patients typically present with painless, progressive, asymmetric muscle weakness and wasting, typically involving the distal part of one extremity. A weak, wasted, yet hyperreflexic extremity is virtually pathognomonic of ALS (Enrichment Box 11–3). As the disease progresses, it tends to lay waste to one extremity, then move on to another. Degeneration of cortical motoneurons produces associated

TABLE 11–2. TESTS OFTEN USED IN THE EVALUATION OF PATIENTS WITH NEUROMUSCULAR DISORDERS

Acetylcholine receptor antibody

Nerve antibody panel

Carbohydrate-deficient transferrin

Ischemic lactate test

Muscle metabolic analysis

Paraneoplastic antibody panel

Muscle dystrophin analysis

Genetic testing

ACE level

ACE = angiotensin-converting enzyme.

Cervical spondylosis often arises as part of the differential diagnosis of amyotrophic lateral sclerosis (ALS), producing lower motoneuron abnormalities of the upper extremities because of radiculopathy, and upper motoneuron abnormalities in the lower extremities because of compressive radiculomyelopathy. An important distinguishing feature is that patients with cervical spondylosis tend to have decreased reflexes in their upper extremities (due to the radiculopathy component), whereas ALS patients have increased reflexes in the upper extremities (because of degeneration of cortical motor neurons). Fasciculations are common in both conditions.

spasticity, hyperreflexia, and upgoing toes. Classical ALS thus has a mixture of upper and lower motor neuron signs in the same patient at the same time. Involvement of bulbar muscles leads to progressive dysphagia and dysarthria. The tongue typically becomes weak and wasted with prominent fasciculations. Without extreme measures of support, such as a ventilator or artificial feeding, death from inanition, aspiration, or infection generally ensues after a course of 3–5 years. ALS patients usually have prominent fasciculations. These fleeting muscle twitches, of which the patient is usually unaware, also commonly appear in tense, cold, or hypercaffeinemic individuals, especially medical personnel. In the absence of weakness, these twitches do not indicate disease.

There is no effective treatment for ALS, although there has been intense clinical trial activity pursuing various promising areas. Riluzole may help selected patients. For recent information on ALS treatment, see *www.wfnals.org* or *www.neuro.wustl.edu/neuromuscular/motor.html*.

Werdnig-Hoffman Disease

Werdnig-Hoffman disease, or SMA type I, is the most severe form of hereditary SMA. Inherited as an autosomal recessive trait, infants are born weak and floppy due to diffuse degeneration of motor neurons in the anterior horn of the spinal cord. Werdnig-Hoffman disease is always a prominent consideration in the differential diagnosis of the floppy baby syndrome. Survival is rarely past 2 years of age. More benign forms of SMA (types II and III) represent allelic variations of the Werdnig-Hoffman syndrome.

RADICULOPATHY

See DISORDERS OF THE SPINE AND SPINAL CORD.

PLEXOPATHY

Numerous pathological processes may affect either the brachial or lumbosacral plexus. The most common and clinically important brachial plexopathy is the syndrome of neuralgic amyotrophy. Other plexopathies involving the brachial plexus include acute trauma due to traction, laceration, missile wounds, neoplasms, radiation, obstetric palsies, and postsurgical plexopathy (Enrichment Box 11–4). Lumbosacral plexopathy is usually a complication of diabetes mellitus. Other plexopathies affecting the lumbosacral plexus include diabetes, neoplasms, retroperitoneal hematoma, and radiation (see Enrichment Box 11–4). Either plexus may rarely be involved in systemic processes, such as systemic lupus erythematosus or sarcoidosis.

Neuralgic Amyotrophy

Neuralgic amyotrophy has gone by a number of names, most frequently brachial plexitis, Parsonage-Turner syndrome, and acute brachial plexus neuropathy. Neuralgic amyotrophy is a stereotyped clinical syndrome characterized by the acute onset of very severe pain in the shoulder and upper arm, followed by weakness of variable severity, primarily affecting upper arm and shoulder muscles. It runs a protracted course of slow, sometimes incomplete recovery, and sometimes as one arm is recovering the other is stricken. Recurrence is not rare. Many patients have had an antecedent event triggering an immune reaction, such as viral infection, immunization, or surgery.

Diabetic Amyotrophy

Like neuralgic amyotrophy, diabetic amyotrophy has a stereotyped clinical presentation. The typical patient is older, with type 2 diabetes that is usually mild and occasionally not previously diagnosed. Symptoms begin subacutely with pain in one hip or thigh that becomes severe. Weakness of the hip flexors, gluteal muscles, and quadriceps ensues and the patient begins to lose weight, often 20 lb or more. Pain continues, the quadriceps atrophies, and the knee jerk disappears. Similar but milder pain, weakness, and atrophy occur on the opposite side. At its zenith, the patient has painful, bilateral but asymmetric weakness and wasting of the thighs along with substantial weight loss. The process eventually stabilizes and a slow and occasionally incomplete recovery follows over months to a couple of years.

PERIPHERAL NEUROPATHY

Current custom divides neuropathies into generalized versus focal and demyelinating versus axonal. Generalized neuropathies, or polyneuropathies, affect all of the nerves, although the tendency of axonopathies to

Radiation plexopathy

Radiation brachial plexopathy appears after a delay of months to years, and a common and often difficult problem is to distinguish recurrent tumor, usually breast or lung, from radiation plexopathy. Pain can occur with either condition, but is more likely to be an early and dominant symptom in neoplastic plexopathy.

Traumatic plexopathy

Iatrogenic postoperative brachial plexopathy primarily occurs during coronary artery bypass graft surgery. The injury usually involves the lower elements of the plexus; a number of mechanisms have been postulated. Traumatic brachial plexopathies are most often due to stretch, especially in motorcycle accidents. Stretch injuries also occur during childbirth. These injuries most often involve the upper plexus (Erb palsy), and less often the lower plexus (Klumpke palsy).

Thoracic outlet syndrome

Thoracic outlet syndrome (TOS), entrapment of the lower elements of the brachial plexus and vascular structures of the thoracic outlet by cervical ribs and bands, can cause various symptoms related to ischemia, venous stasis, or nerve dysfunction. TOS has a long and controversial history. Many neurologists believe this syndrome is vastly overdiagnosed. Most patients thought to have TOS suffer from carpal tunnel syndrome, cervical radiculopathy, or droopy shoulder syndrome. Although convincing cases of TOS are rare in neurologic practice, first-rib resections for TOS are commonly performed in the United States, occasionally with disastrous results.

Lumbosacral plexopathy

Except for diabetic amyotrophy, lumbosacral plexopathies are uncommon. Neoplasms, especially colorectal, breast, and cervical, may metastasize to or directly invade the plexus; distinguishing neoplastic from radiation lumbosacral plexopathy is usually a conundrum. Retroperitoneal hematoma in the region of the psoas muscle, usually in a patient on anticoagulants, can damage the plexus and cause severe leg pain and weakness. Whether there is a primary, spontaneous "plexitis" affecting the lumbosacral plexus analogous to the entity of neuralgic amyotrophy of the brachial plexus has been a matter of conjecture. If so, it occurs at only a fraction of the incidence of the upper extremity condition.

produce maximal dysfunction of the longest fibers often produces clinical symptoms having distal predominance. At the least, generalized neuropathies have symmetric symptoms and signs. Focal neuropathies, or mononeuropathies, affect only one nerve, such as from local trauma or isolated nerve infarction. When several, but not all, nerves are affected by a disease process, the condition is termed a multiple mononeuropathy. Bilateral carpal tunnel syndrome is a multiple mononeuropathy.

Demyelinating neuropathies result from a pathological process directed largely, if not exclusively, at the myelin sheath or Schwann cell. Pressure-induced focal neuropathies are typically demyelinating. Acute and chronic inflammatory demyelinating polyradiculoneuropathies are the most common example of generalized demyelinating neuropathies. Myelin can repair itself rapidly, and patients with demyelinating neuropathies may recover quickly; they have characteristic earmarks during clinical examination and electrodiagnostic testing. Axonopathies result when the pathological process involves primarily the axon. These neuropathies are typically toxic or metabolic, have a distal "dying back" pattern on examination, and tend to resolve slowly and incompletely.

Generalized Neuropathies

For a good brief review of the diagnosis and treatment of generalized neuropathies, see *www.dcmsonline.org/jax- medicine/august2000/ neuropathies.htm.*

Alcoholic neuropathy. The neuropathy of alcoholism is typically a generalized sensorimotor axonopathy, frequently with painful paresthesias and dysesthesias. The debate over whether the neuropathy results from malnutrition or a direct toxic effect of alcohol remains unsettled; most evidence favors the former mechanism. Treatment involves abstinence, multivitamin use [being careful not to give too much pyridoxine (B_6), which can itself cause a neuropathy in doses as low as 100 mg per day], and symptomatic remedies for the pain.

Diabetic neuropathy. Diabetes mellitus affects the peripheral nervous system in a variety of ways, and is one of the most common causes of neuropathy in the United States. Typically, patients with long-standing diabetes develop an insidious sensorimotor axonopathy, often with painful distal paresthesias (burning feet syndrome). Dysautonomia often accompanies neuropathies that are due to diabetes. Diabetic patients are also much more likely than normal individuals to develop compression or entrapment neuropathies such as carpal tunnel syndrome, even at a time when their generalized neuropathy remains subclinical. The microvasculopathy of diabetes also makes patients prone to nerve infarction, most commonly involving the oculomotor nerve.

Human immunodeficiency virus-associated neuropathies. AIDS patients may develop neuropathy early or late in the disease. Demyelinating neuropathies tend to occur early, and human immunodeficiency virus (HIV) infection warrants consideration in any patient presenting with Guillain-Barré syndrome (GBS) or chronic inflammatory demyelinating polyradiculoneuropathy (CIDP). A nondescript, axonal, sensorimotor neuropathy affects many AIDS patients with long-standing disease.

Guillain Barré syndrome. GBS, also known as acute inflammatory demyelinating polyradiculoneuropathy, is the most common cause of acute generalized weakness requiring ventilatory support. In about half of the cases, a prior event (e.g., viral infection, immunization, parturition, surgery) has seemingly primed the immune system. Onset is typically with numbness and paresthesias in the feet, followed by progressive weakness, leading in a substantial number of patients to respiratory failure. Examination may show distal, proximal, or generalized weakness. Hyporeflexia or areflexia occurs early. Sensory complaints usually overshadow demonstrable sensory loss. Facial weakness ensues in at least half of the patients, probably more. There is no sphincter dysfunction except at the height of the illness in severely affected patients; it never appears as a presenting complaint. Clinical indicators favoring GBS over transverse myelitis or myelopathy are the presence of facial weakness and the absence of sphincter dysfunction. Cerebrospinal fluid classically displays albuminocytologic dissociation with elevated protein but no cells. GBS has been described as "subacute ascending paralysis with variable sensory loss and retained sphincteric function," and it is difficult to provide a better definition.

Most patients with GBS present to physicians several times before the diagnosis is made, often being sent home from the emergency room on multiple occasions. This mistake happens three times more frequently when the disease attacks a young woman than when it affects a man or an older woman. The peripheral paresthesias and subjective dyspnea can easily lead to a misdiagnosis of hyperventilation syndrome.

GBS patients must be watched carefully, their respiratory functions monitored closely, and treatment instituted with signs of significant progression. Patients who are already nonambulatory, or seem to be rapidly progressing in that direction, are typically treated with either plasmapheresis or IV immunoglobulin; both have been proven effective in controlled trials. Most authorities consider steroids ineffective and possibly detrimental. For further information and a discussion of treatment, see *www.neuro.wustl.edu/neuromuscular/antibody/gbs.htm* or *www.neuroland.com/nm/guillain.htm*.

Good to excellent recovery occurs in 85%–90% of patients; the remainder has residual disability ranging from minor to severe.

Chronic inflammatory demyelinating polyradiculoneuropathy. GBS and CIDP are probably variants of the same disease process, which develops over different time courses. CIDP is common, and represents a significant proportion of all initially undiagnosed acquired chronic neuropathies, perhaps as many as 10%–20%, and is important to recognize because of the likelihood that it may respond to therapeutic intervention. To distinguish CIDP from GBS, which is fully developed in 90% of patients by 4 weeks, the condition must evolve over a period of at least 8 weeks. CIDP is primarily a motor neuropathy. Depression of reflexes is typically global and profound. The cerebrospinal fluid protein is often elevated. The electrodiagnostic features of CIDP are an important clue to the diagnosis. Potential treatments include administration of prednisone, azathioprine, cyclophosphamide, IV immunoglobulin, and plasma exchange.

Focal Neuropathies

The vast majority of focal neuropathies are due to trauma, either acute, or more often, chronic and repetitive.

Carpal tunnel syndrome. A very common malady, carpal tunnel syndrome results from compression of the median nerve beneath the transverse carpal ligament, producing complaints of hand pain and numbness. Symptoms are typically intermittent and worse at night or on first awakening in the morning. Proximal referral of pain to the forearm or shoulder is not uncommon. Advanced cases develop weakness and sometimes atrophy of the thenar muscles. Diagnosis is based on the clinical features, often supplemented by EMG. Conservative treatment consists of splinting and administration of nonsteroidal anti-inflammatory drugs; definitive treatment is surgical division of the transverse carpal ligament.

Other common focal neuropathies due to peripheral nerve compression include ulnar neuropathy at the elbow and peroneal neuropathy at the fibular head (Enrichment Box 11–5).

Bell palsy. Like GBS, Bell palsy frequently follows a viral infection or an immunization, with involvement limited to one facial nerve, producing a peripheral seventh cranial nerve palsy with weakness of both upper and lower face. Symptoms often begin with pain behind the ear, followed within a day or two by facial weakness with variable degrees of drooling and difficulty speaking due to the slack facial muscles. Lesions proximal to the take-off of the chorda tympani cause difficulty with the sense of taste; lesions proximal to the branch to the stapedius may cause hyperacusis. Most cases of Bell palsy are idiopathic. Recent evidence suggests that herpes simplex type 1 may be responsible for many of the

ENRICHMENT BOX 11–5

Ulnar neuropathy

Ulnar neuropathies at the elbow typically present with complaints of numbness and tingling of the fourth and fifth fingers of one hand. Weakness and atrophy of ulnar innervated intrinsic hand muscles occur in more severe cases. Pain is seldom a significant clinical feature. Such neuropathies are often blamed on excessive leaning on the elbows. Ulnar neuropathy can also result from entrapment of the nerve beneath the aponeurosis joining the two heads of the flexor carpi ulnaris muscle. When ulnar neuropathy at the elbow follows remote fracture or dislocation of the elbow, the condition is termed tardy ulnar palsy.

Peroneal neuropathy

Another common mononeuropathy follows compression or stretch of the peroneal nerve in the region of the fibular head, producing a foot drop. External compression may result, for example, from habitual leg crossing, tight casts, or prolonged bed rest. Stretch injuries may follow prolonged squatting or forceful ankle inversion.

cases. Initial treatment is generally with prednisone, possibly combined with acyclovir. Both HIV infection and Lyme disease can occasionally present with facial neuropathy. For an extensive discussion of the facial nerve and conditions that affect it, see *www.bcm.tmc.edu/oto/studs/face.html* or *icarus.med.utoronto.ca/carr/manual/afnp2.html*.

NEUROMUSCULAR JUNCTION DISORDERS

Diseases involving the NMJ cause weakness due to impaired neuromuscular transmission. Acquired myasthenia gravis (MG), an autoimmune disorder, is by far the most common of these syndromes. Other NMJ disorders include Lambert-Eaton syndrome and botulism (Enrichment Box 11–6).

MG develops following an autoimmune attack on the acetylcholine receptors lying along the postsynaptic membrane. Classical symptoms include ptosis, diplopia, dysarthria, dysphagia, and proximal muscle weakness. Weakness increases with use and recovery follows rest of the body part. The disease is frequently associated with simple hyperplasia of the thymus gland, particularly in younger patients; frank thymoma occurs in 10% of patients, mostly older men. Diagnosis rests on the clinical features, certain characteristic electrodiagnostic abnormalities, alleviation of weakness following the administration of anti-acetylcholinesterase agents, and the presence of the autoantibody in the serum. Symptomatic treatment is with anti-acetylcholinesterase agents; more definitive treatment involves aggressive immunosuppression by using a variety of measures.

Lambert-Eaton syndrome

The Lambert-Eaton myasthenic syndrome (LEMS) results from impaired release of acetylcholine at the presynaptic nerve terminal. Because the clinical features of LEMS differ considerably from those of myasthenia gravis (MG), the appellation "myasthenic syndrome," which was applied early and stuck, remains an unfortunate point of confusion. It is a presynaptic disorder, whereas MG is a postsynaptic disorder. Ptosis and diplopia, classic in MG, are relatively uncommon in LEMS; most patients suffer primarily with proximal muscle weakness, particularly in the lower extremities. Depression of reflexes is common, as is autonomic dysfunction, producing dry mouth, constipation, and impotence. About half of the patients harbor an occult neoplasm, usually a small cell carcinoma of the lung.

An autoantibody attack sabotages the function of the voltage-gated calcium channel on the presynaptic nerve terminal and impairs transmitter discharge because calcium is a required element in the release mechanism. In patients with tumor, the neoplasm presumably shares an antigenic determinant with the calcium channel. In patients, mostly women, who have the syndrome without an associated neoplasm, the reason for the presence of the autoantibody remains unknown. Therapeutic efforts are directed toward controlling the tumor, if present, and/or aggressive immunosuppression.

Botulism

Botulism is caused by the toxin produced by *Clostridium botulinum*, which blocks the release of acetylcholine from the presynaptic nerve terminal, impairing neuromuscular transmission and causing generalized weakness and respiratory failure. Abnormal pupils are a classical accompaniment, but are certainly not present in every case. The toxin is most often ingested from contaminated food. In some cases the bacterium releases the toxin while living in the body (infantile botulism and wound botulism).

Because of the subjective nature of the complaints of fatigue and "blurry vision," along with a mild fluctuating weakness and the frequent presentation in young women, it is not uncommon for patients with MG to suffer for long periods of time before diagnosis. Patients are frequently labeled as either hysterical or depressed. The average patient with MG has seen several physicians before the diagnosis is finally made.

MYOPATHIES

There are many possible causes for muscle disease. Table 11–3 lists some of the more common or important etiological factors, and Table 11–4 provides details of some of the entities. The most common cause of an

TABLE 11-3. COMMON PRIMARY MUSCLE DISEASES

Inherited diseases

Dystrophies

Dystrophinopathies (e.g., Duchenne muscular dystrophy, Becker muscular dystrophy)

Myotonic dystrophy

Facioscapulohumeral dystrophy

Limb-girdle dystrophy

Metabolic myopathies

Mitochondrial myopathies (e.g., ragged red fiber diseases)

Glycogen storage myopathies (e.g., McArdle disease)

Lipid storage myopathies

Congenital myopathies

Nemaline myopathy

Central core disease

Myotubular myopathy

Channelopathies

Myotonia congenita

Periodic paralysis

Malignant hyperthermia

Acquired diseases

Inflammatory myopathies

Polymyositis, dermatomyositis

Inclusion body myositis

Myopathies related to infection (e.g., HIV, HTLV-I, parasites)

Myopathies complicating systemic illness

Endocrine myopathies

Sarcoidosis

Critical illness myopathy

Toxic myopathies

Rhabdomyolysis

HIV = human immunodeficiency virus; HTLV-I = human T-cell lymphotrophic virus type I.

acute myopathy is rhabdomyolysis, often accompanied by myoglobin-uria. The most common causes for chronic myopathies are the muscular dystrophies, which are hereditary, and the inflammatory myopathies.

TABLE 11–4. CLINICAL DISEASE DETAILS OF MYOPATHIES

Condition	Features	Electrophysiologic Findings
Inherited diseases		
Muscular dystrophies		
Facioscapulohumeral dystrophy	Autosomal dominant, chromosome 4; onset 5–20 years of age; extremely variable expression from minimal facial weakness to severe disability; deltoids and forearm spared; Popeye arm appearance	Muscle biopsy shows myopathic changes. EMG shows non-myonecrotic myopathy (i.e., myopathic motor units without fibrillation potentials).
Limb-girdle dystrophy	Usually recessive, sometimes dominant; slowly progressive pelvic and shoulder girdle weakness, deltoids involved; variable expression, heterogeneous disorder; CK elevated 5–10 times normal	Muscle biopsy shows myopathic changes. EMG shows myonecrotic myopathy (i.e., myopathic motor units plus fibrillation potentials).
Metabolic myopathies		
McArdle disease (myophosphorylase deficiency)	Exercise intolerance; cramps and stiffness precipitated by brief, high-intensity exercise; onset second to third decade; autosomal recessive, chromosome 11; male predominance; second-wind phenomenon; no rise in venous lactate; occasional rhabdomyolysis; fixed proximal weakness with advancing age in one-third of patients; variants include late-life progressive proximal weakness and a fatal infantile form	Muscle biopsy shows PAS-positive vacuoles and an absence of phosphorylase. EMG shows electrically silent painful contractures induced by exercise.

(*continued*)

TABLE 11–4. CLINICAL DISEASE DETAILS OF MYOPATHIES (*CONTINUED*)

Condition	Features	Electrophysiologic Findings
Carnitine palmitoyltransferase deficiency	Recurrent attacks of rhabdomyolysis beginning in adolescence; precipitated by prolonged exercise or fasting; myalgia and stiffness common but no true cramp; no second wind; normal examination findings between attacks	Muscle biopsy is normal for routine stains; metabolic analysis may reveal the defect. EMG is normal between attacks, and shows a picture of rhabdomyolysis during acute episodes.
Mitochondrial myopathies	Includes Kearns-Sayre syndrome (progressive external ophthalmoplegia); MERRF and MELAS	Muscle biopsy shows myopathy with ragged red fibers.
Congenital myopathies	Includes entities such as nemaline myopathy, central core disease, myotubular myopathy, and many others; clinical picture variable	Muscle biopsy shows aberration (e.g., nemaline rods) that leads to the name.
Channelopathies		
Myotonia congenita; occurs in a dominant form (Thomsen disease) and a recessive form (Becker disease)	Characterized by generalized stiffness and myotonia, with little or no weakness and sometimes striking muscle hypertrophy	Muscle biopsy shows absence of type 2B fibers. The dominant form is probably caused by an abnormality of sodium channel function and the recessive form is probably caused by an abnormality of chloride channel function. EMG shows widespread, profuse myotonic discharges.
Periodic paralysis	Several different forms, all characterized by attacks of generalized weakness (similar attacks can occur with aberrations of serum	Hypokalemic, normokalemic, and hyperkalemic periodic paralyses are the classic subtypes; the first is precipitated by

(*continued*)

TABLE 11–4. CLINICAL DISEASE DETAILS OF MYOPATHIES (*CONTINUED*)

Condition	Features	Electrophysiologic Findings
	potassium in otherwise normal individuals)	low potassium, and the latter two are precipitated by administration of potassium (K+ sensitive). The familial forms are caused by an abnormality of membrane channel function.
Acquired diseases		
Inflammatory myopathies		
Polymyositis	Symmetric, progressive, predominantly proximal weakness; dysphagia; increased CK (5–10 times); myalgias uncommon; no skin lesions; increased risk of malignancy likely	Muscle biopsy shows fiber necrosis and inflammatory infiltrates. Nerve conduction studies are normal. Needle EMG shows variable findings depending on the stage and activity of the disease.
Dermatomyositis	Symmetric, progressive, predominately proximal weakness; dysphagia; increased CK; characteristic skin rash; disease is a vasculitis in childhood dermatomyositis; increased risk of malignancy in adult dermatomyositis	Muscle biopsy and electrodiagnostic findings are the same as in polymyositis.
Inclusion body myositis	Older patients; male predominance; slowly progressive/indolent, painless; often asymmetric weakness of proximal and distal muscles of arms and legs; weakness of wrist and finger flexors > deltoid and quadriceps > hip flexors; CK < 12	Muscle biopsy findings are the same as in polymyositis plus characteristic rimmed vacuoles are present. Electrodiagnostic findings are the same as in polymyositis.

(*continued*)

TABLE 11–4. CLINICAL DISEASE DETAILS OF MYOPATHIES (*CONTINUED*)

Condition	Features	Electrophysiologic Findings
	times normal; relatively resistant to immuno-suppressant treatment; ESR usually normal; not associated with malignancy	
Myopathy complicating systemic illness		
Hypothyroidism	Weakness; stiffness; cramps; myalgias; associated carpal tunnel syndrome; myoedema; muscle enlargement in some cases; marked elevation of CK; hung up reflexes	Muscle biopsy is usually normal. Minimal changes appear on EMG.
Steroid myopathy	Proximal weakness; mild atrophy; normal reflexes; normal or low CK; greatest risk is with high-dose, daily halogenated steroids in women	Muscle biopsy shows characteristic selective type 2 muscle fiber atrophy. EMG is usually normal.
Sarcoidosis	Young adults; muscle involvement common but rarely symptomatic; progressive weakness and wasting occur in some cases.	Muscle biopsy shows inflammatory myopathy with noncaseating granulomas. EMG findings usually indicate myonecrotic myopathy.
Critical illness myopathy	Prolonged paralysis in association with critical illness; usually after prolonged neuromuscular blockade, with or without concomitant steroids; variable CK elevation; occasional rhabdomyolysis	Muscle biopsy shows severe atrophy and selective lysis of thick filaments, especially in type 2 fibers. Electrodiagnostic findings are variable.

CK = creatine kinase; EMG = electromyogram; ESR = erythrocyte sedimentation rate; MELAS = mitochondrial encephalomyopathy, lactic acidosis, and stroke-like episodes; MERRF = myoclonic epilepsy with ragged red fibers; PAS = periodic acid Schiff.

Steroid Myopathy (see Table 11–4)

Excessive endogenous or exogenous corticosteroids can produce myopathy. Only rarely does a patient presenting with myopathy prove to have Cushing disease, but the possibility of steroid myopathy arises frequently when a patient receiving steroids as treatment for inflammatory myopathy develops increasing weakness. It may be difficult to distinguish an exacerbation of the underlying inflammatory myopathy from increasing weakness due to the development of steroid myopathy.

Rhabdomyolysis or Myoglobinuria

Breakdown of skeletal muscle (rhabdomyolysis) releases myoglobin into the circulation, which is then excreted in the urine to produce myoglobinuria. Patients with normal muscles can develop rhabdomyolysis or myoglobinuria under conditions of extremely vigorous exertion, such as military basic training, status epilepticus, prolonged immobility, or exposure to certain drugs (Enrichment Box 11–7). Patients who have underlying metabolic defects of their muscle may develop rhabdomyolysis or myoglobinuria with relatively low levels of exertion. Myoglobinuria can lead to acute renal failure. A common clue to its presence is urine showing a positive test for blood but no red blood cells on microscopic examination. The malignant hyperthermia syndrome is an important cause of rhabdomyolysis (see Enrichment Box 11–7).

Duchenne Muscular Dystrophy

Most of "Jerry's kids" have Duchenne muscular dystrophy (DMD), which is a progressive syndrome of muscle weakness beginning in childhood. Rapid growth and acquisition of normal motor milestones usually mask the presence of the disease until the patient is about 3 or 4 years of age and clearly begins to fall behind his peers. An inexorably downhill course follows. Patients are usually nonambulatory by about 10–12 years of age, and dead by 18–22 years of age. In addition to the progressive proximal weakness, patients with DMD typically develop muscle pseudohypertrophy, wherein fat and fibrous tissue replacement of damaged muscle lends the appearance of hypertrophy (Figure 11–2). This process most commonly affects the calf muscles. A host of other abnormalities occur as minor features of the disease (see Enrichment Box 11–7).

Myotonic Muscular Dystrophy

Although common, myotonic dystrophy often goes unrecognized. It is an autosomal dominant disease with extremely variable penetrance. The resulting manifestations are occasionally so subtle that families may not recognize that they are affected. In the typical case, there is

ENRICHMENT BOX 11-7

Rhabdomyolysis

A number of enzyme defects and other metabolic derangements of muscle metabolism can be responsible for episodes of rhabdomyolysis; the most common are phosphorylase deficiency (McArdle disease) and carnitine palmitoyltransferase deficiency (see Table 11–4). A common cause of rhabdomyolysis is pressure necrosis of muscle. In fact, the rhabdomyolysis syndrome was originally described during the bombing of London during World War II when victims were trapped under heavy debris for many hours, and after rescue were found to be passing red urine. More common in the modern era is pressure necrosis due to prolonged coma. It is common to find evidence of rhabdomyolysis in patients who have been "found down," having lain for hours or days immobile on a hard surface.

Duchenne muscular dystrophy

Other features of Duchenne muscular dystrophy (DMD) include cardiomyopathy, progressive scoliosis, and cognitive impairment. The pathogenetic basis of this condition was recently unraveled after an extremely long struggle. DMD is an X-linked disorder, with the defective gene on the short arm of the X chromosome at the Xp21 locus. Because of the genetic abnormality, affected patients fail to make dystrophin, a protein central to the integrity of the muscle membrane. The lack of dystrophin results in muscle membrane necrosis, damage to the membrane with ordinary mechanical forces, and failure of normal repair mechanisms.

Myotonic muscular dystrophy

Other manifestations of myotonic dystrophy include insulin-resistant glucose intolerance, progressive heart block, sleep apnea, and early cataracts. The etiology of myotonic dystrophy in some way relates to an unstable DNA fragment with pathological reduplications of a three-nucleotide sequence on the long arm of chromosome 19.

Malignant hyperthermia

Malignant hyperthermia refers to the development of extreme body temperature elevation, as high as 110°F-112°F, during general anesthesia, frequently accompanied by rhabdomyolysis and with a high morbidity and mortality rate. Some patients suffer from an underlying myopathy, often previously unrecognized, but malignant hyperthermia most often occurs with no previous intimation of neuromuscular pathology. An abnormality of calcium metabolism involving the sarcoplasmic reticulum precipitated by anesthesia induces extreme muscular rigidity with resultant hyperthermia and rhabdomyolysis.

distal muscle weakness coupled with myotonia (difficulty relaxing a muscle once contracted). Grip myotonia produces a characteristic sticky handshake, from which both shaker and shakee extricate themselves with difficulty, the patient using a telltale fanlike release. The frontal balding, hatchet face, droopy eyelids, and temporal wasting are so distinctive that experienced neurologists can recognize the disease at a glance, because affected individuals all tend to look like brothers and sisters (see Enrichment Box 11–7; Figure 11–3).

Other Common Muscular Dystrophies

Other muscular dystrophies include facioscapulohumeral dystrophy and limb-girdle dystrophy. See Table 11–4 for a brief overview.

POLYMYOSITIS

PM and adult dermatomyositis (DM), both forms of inflammatory myopathy, differ in the presence or absence of skin involvement. PM and DM most often occur in isolation, but can complicate other connective tissue disorders such as systemic lupus erythematosus, scleroderma, or mixed connective tissue disease. DM, and possibly PM, that develops in adults (but not children) may presage an occult neoplasm. Patients develop insidious proximal muscle weakness. Muscle pain and tender-

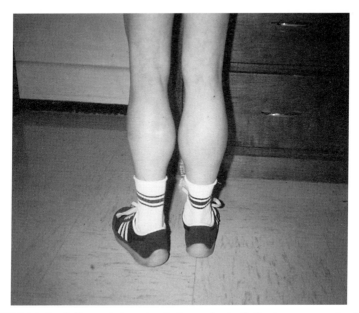

FIGURE 11–2. ■ Calf muscle hypertrophy in a patient with Duchenne muscular dystrophy.

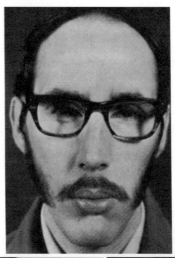

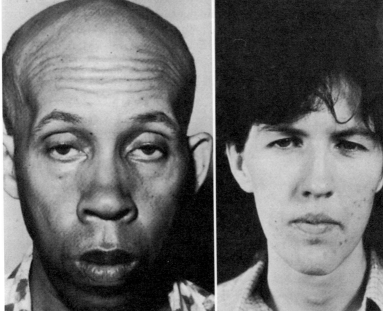

FIGURE 10–3. ■ Three patients with myotonic dystrophy, demonstrating the typical facies (hatchet face, temporal wasting, balding, bilateral ptosis). (From Dyken PR, Miller MD: *Facial Features of Neurologic Syndromes.* St. Louis, Mosby, 1980, p 304.)

ness are uncommon. Severe cases may develop dysphagia, pulmonary involvement, and rarely cardiac complications. Serum CK is elevated in most cases.

Initial treatment of inflammatory myopathy is usually with steroids. Childhood DM differs in important ways, clinically and immunopathogenetically, from the adult inflammatory myopathies. HIV infection predisposes patients to an inflammatory myopathy that is difficult to distinguish from the toxic effects of some antiretroviral agents.

12

Evaluation of Common Symptom Complexes

Many patients, especially those seen in neurologic outpatient clinics, have prominent complaints but a normal neurologic examination. Seldom does further workup reveal identifiable, structural disease, and it is difficult to define the process more completely than as a symptom or collection of symptoms. Common examples of such symptom complexes include headache, dizziness, and sleep disorders. Managing such problems, particularly headache and dizziness, is a large part of clinical practice.

Headache

Only a lucky few among us fail to suffer at least the occasional headache. A very unlucky minority have persistent, recurrent, or severe enough headaches that drive them to seek medical attention. Fortunately, effective therapy is available for most patients. The small cadre of patients with hard core, refractory headache can frustrate the therapeutic efforts of even the most skilled neurologist. Most headaches are benign, but occasionally headache is the presenting complaint in a patient with a serious and even life-threatening condition (e.g., hemorrhage, mass lesion, central nervous system infection). Table 12–1 lists clues in the patient's presentation that may indicate a potentially serious pathological condition.

CLINICAL SYNDROMES

The following are commonly seen headache syndromes.

Migraine

The pathophysiology of migraine is complicated. Migraine is generally divided into two large categories: with aura (classic migraine)

TABLE 12–1. CLINICAL FEATURES OF HEADACHE THAT SUGGEST A SERIOUS PATHOLOGICAL CONDITION

Presentation	Clinical Features
Age at onset	Childhood; > 50 years of age
History	Abrupt onset; first, worst, or atypical headache; worse at night or first thing in the morning; associated with loss of consciousness, visual disturbance, change in behavior or personality, fever, or vomiting without nausea; occipitonuchal or interscapular pain; associated with focal neurologic complaints, altered mental status, or history of recent head trauma (no matter how trivial); progressively severe pain; immunocompromised state; history of cancer; family history or personal history of conditions associated with subarachnoid hemorrhage/aneurysm (autosomal dominant polycystic kidney disease, Marfan syndrome, Ehlers-Danlos syndrome, fibromuscular dysplasia, pseudoxanthoma elasticum, neurofibromatosis type I)
Physical examination findings	Meningismus, fever, focal neurologic abnormalities, soft neurologic signs (pronator drift, asymmetric nasolabial fold, or plantar responses), clumsiness, drowsiness, altered mental status, papilledema

and without aura (common migraine). It is overly simplistic, but still useful, to think of migraine as having a vasoconstrictive component, which produces neurologic symptomatology, and a vasodilatory component, which produces the headache. Migraine is the most common type of vascular headache, and the terms are often used interchangeably. When the vasoconstrictive component of migraine precedes the vasodilatory component, the result is the syndrome of migraine with aura or classic migraine. Sometimes the vasodilatory component occurs in isolation, without preceding neurologic phenomenology, producing the syndrome of migraine without aura or common migraine. Sometimes transient neurologic accompaniments are much more prominent than the headache, causing acephalgic migraine or migraine without head pain. Sometimes major temporary or permanent neurologic deficits occur, the syndrome of complicated migraine.

Migraine Without Aura (Common Migraine)

Patients with common migraine have generally holocephalic, pulsatile head pain with accompanying nausea, vomiting, photophobia, and sonophobia. The headaches begin without aura or warning, generally last 2–3 days, are often perimenstrual, and affect women much more often than men.

Migraine With Aura (Classic Migraine)

Patients with classic migraine experience a well-defined aura or forewarning that presages the onset of the headache. The aura most often involves visual phenomena (scintillating scotomata, fortification spectra, flashing lights, wavy lines) but may consist of somatosensory dysfunction (hemi-numbness or hemi-tingling), hemiparesis, or other focal cortical aberrations such as aphasia. Symptoms may spread from one body part to another. Paresthesias involving the thumb and the corner of the mouth are particularly common. The aura typically lasts approximately 30 minutes, and is followed by a severe, unilateral (usually contralateral to the neurologic manifestations), throbbing headache associated with nausea, vomiting, photophobia, and sonophobia. The headache usually lasts only 4–6 hours, much shorter in duration than that of common migraine. Triptans or ergots taken during the aura phase can frequently prevent the headache phase (abortive therapy). Commonly used prophylactic agents, given daily for headache prevention, include beta-blockers, calcium channel blockers, and tricyclic antidepressants. Female preponderance persists in classic migraine, but less so than in common migraine.

Acephalgic Migraine

Sometimes the vasoconstrictive component occurs in relative isolation, producing neurologic symptomatology with little or no headache; this is the syndrome of acephalgic migraine. The neurologic symptoms are sometimes referred to as migrainous accompaniments. Older patients may sometimes begin to have episodic attacks of neurologic symptomatology with minimal or no headache, so-called late-life migrainous accompaniments; distinguishing these accompaniments from transient ischemic attacks may be difficult. More than one patient with "transient ischemic attacks refractory to therapy," with repeated episodes of transient neurologic deficit, has had the symptoms resolve when placed on antimigraine treatment.

Complicated Migraine

Sometimes the vasoconstrictive component is unusually severe or prolonged, causing prominent neurologic phenomenology, with or without a headache. When the neurologic dysfunction is the most prominent part of the migraine episode, the condition is referred to as complicated migraine. The aura that accompanies classic migraine is an expected part of that condition, and does not rise to the level of being considered complicated migraine. Examples of complicated migraine include hemiplegic migraine, ophthalmoplegic migraine, and basilar artery migraine. Patients with neurologic deficits due to complicated migraine may or may not give a history of past episodes of migraine (Enrichment Box 12–1). Table 12–2 lists the syndromes of complicated migraine.

Cluster Headache

In contrast to other headache syndromes, cluster headaches most often affect men. The pain associated with cluster headaches is steady, boring, aching, and relentless (not pulsatile) and is located in a periorbital or retro-orbital distribution. Cluster attacks are frequently associated with tearing of the eye or stuffiness of the nose on the side of the headache.

ENRICHMENT BOX 12–1

In hemiplegic migraine, the patient develops a prominent hemiparesis that is prolonged much longer than would be considered an aura. The hemiparesis may outlast the headache by hours or days, and occasionally the patient develops a fixed neurologic deficit, sometimes with a corresponding infarction visible on imaging studies. With ophthalmoplegic migraine, the patient develops extraocular nerve palsy, third, fourth, or sixth, with or without a headache. The ophthalmoplegia may be transitory or persistent. The syndrome of basilar artery migraine refers to patients who develop signs and symptoms typical of vertebrobasilar insufficiency (VBI), but are due to migraine. The attack of migraine-induced brainstem symptoms may or may not be followed by a headache.

The terms hemiplegic and ophthalmoplegic migraine refer to specific types of neurologic deficits. In fact, patients with complicated migraine may develop a focal deficit involving any part of the brain, and could easily have focal deficits such as aphasia, visual field deficits, or the like.

Patients with complicated migraine have, in the majority of instances, had vascular headaches in the past. However, they may not have recognized them as migrainous episodes. It is common for patients to deny a history of migraine, stating that they have "sinus" headaches, and when pressed go on to describe typical attacks of migraine. The vast majority of so-called sinus headaches are in fact migraine. It is worth delving into the headache history in patients, particularly young patients, who develop focal neurologic deficits for no apparent reason.

TABLE 12–2. COMPLICATED MIGRAINE TYPES

Hemiplegic migraine

Ophthalmoplegic migraine

Basilar artery migraine

Migrainous confusional state

Abdominal migraine

Late-life migrainous accompaniments

Cluster headaches seem particularly prone to occur at night, often 1–2 hours after falling asleep. A Horner syndrome may occur during the attacks and occasionally persists between attacks. The headaches are typically brief (about 30 minutes) and usually occur on a daily basis (sometimes several times a day) for a finite period of time (several weeks or several months). The patient may then enjoy long symptom-free intervals, sometimes lasting years. This "clustering" over time gives the syndrome its name. The pain of cluster headaches is extremely severe, and has led to suicide. Patients with cluster headaches often try to remain active during the headache episode, in contrast to patients with migraine headaches who seek quiet and stillness.

Tension Headache

Tension headache, now referred to as tension-type headache, is a grab-bag term used most often to describe head pain judged nonmigrainous in origin. It includes the ordinary headache occurring at the end of a stressful day in otherwise normal individuals, as well as the chronic, all day, everyday headache frequently seen in depressed patients. Another school of thought holds that tension headache merely constitutes another facet of the migraine syndrome, lying on the benign end of a vascular headache continuum that ranges from mild, nonpulsatile head pain without accompaniments through the common migraine syndrome to classic migraine. Occasional patients with clear-cut migraine have much more frequent but milder headaches that they ascribe to tension and stress ("mixed headache syndrome"), but they improve markedly with institution of prophylactic therapy for the migraine component. In the past, the term "muscle contraction headache" was used more or less synonymously with tension headache, although there was at best scant evidence that excessive muscle contraction was involved.

Chronic Daily Headache

Some patients have headache all day, every day for weeks, months, or years on end, unresponsive to any therapy. Many such patients consume prodigious amounts of analgesic medication, which begins to exert a paradoxical effect, exacerbating the headaches ("chronic painkiller headache" or "analgesic rebound headache"). Patients with "transformed migraine" have a history of episodic migraine that gradually evolves into a pattern of chronic daily headache, having features of both migraine and tension-type headache. Patients with chronic daily headaches seem to respond best to serotonin-elevating tricyclics and analgesic withdrawal. There is often a positive family history and a tendency to depression.

Temporal Arteritis (Giant Cell Arteritis)

Any new headache developing in an elderly patient should prompt consideration of temporal arteritis. Patients are usually older than 70 years of age, with a recent onset of headache that is characteristically unilateral, dull, boring, worse at night, and associated with scalp tenderness. They may have a history of weight loss, myalgias, arthralgias, fatigue, and a generally unwell feeling (the syndrome of polymyalgia rheumatica). Jaw claudication is a common accompaniment. Elevated sedimentation rates typify the condition. Inflammation of the ophthalmic artery may lead to ischemic optic neuropathy, with attacks of amaurosis fugax, central or cecocentral scotoma, disc edema, and a high likelihood of severe and permanent visual morbidity. Take new headaches in old patients very seriously. When the sedimentation rate equals the age in an elderly patient with headache, temporal arteritis is very likely.

Pseudotumor Cerebri

Patients with pseudotumor cerebri (also known as benign intracranial hypertension or idiopathic intracranial hypertension) develop diffusely increased intracranial pressure for reasons that remain obscure. The typical patient is a young, obese female who has menstrual irregularities. The primary symptom of pseudotumor cerebri is headache, which itself has no particular distinguishing features. Patients also develop papilledema, which may ultimately lead to visual loss. The visual loss is often preceded by episodes of visual obscuration, which consist of brief, fleeting episodes of grayout or brownout of vision involving one or both eyes, particularly provoked by standing. Another common clinical feature is tinnitus, sometimes pulsatile, due to transmission of the increased intracranial pressure to the middle ear through communications between the subarachnoid space and the cochlea.

Drug-Induced Headache

Many commonly used medications can produce headache as a side effect. It is not rare to help a headache patient to a greater degree by stopping a medication that is inducing headache than by adding yet another drug to an existing regimen. Caffeine use and abuse is ubiquitous and can contribute significantly to headache. Over-the-counter medications often contain caffeine. Other frequently problematic medications include calcium channel blockers, proton pump inhibitors, H_2 receptor antagonists, nitrates, sympathomimetics, xanthines, selective serotonin reuptake inhibitors, nonsteroidal anti-inflammatory agents, and oral contraceptives.

TREATMENT OF HEADACHE

Once serious pathological conditions have been excluded, the management of headache is generally symptomatic. Many therapeutic agents are available (Table 12–3). Details on the use of these drugs is beyond the scope of this discussion. For further information, see the Web sites *www.aafp.org/afp/971115ap/moore.html* and *www.aafp.org/afp/971200ap/noble.html,* or visit the JAMA Migraine Information Center at *www.ama-assn.org/special/migraine/treatmnt/drugtreatmnt. htm.* A recent practice parameter analyzed the evidence supporting the effectiveness of various antimigraine drugs [Silberstein SD: Practice parameter: Evidence-based guidelines for migraine headache (an evidence-based review). *Neurology* 55:754, 2000.]

Other Pain Syndromes

Patients with unexplained pain are seen frequently in the practice of most medical specialties, with only the site of pain varying. A neuro-

---

TABLE 12–3. MEDICATIONS FOR THE TREATMENT OF MIGRAINE

Triptans (serotonin$_{1B/1D}$ receptor agonists): sumatriptan and similar agents

Ergot alkaloids and derivatives: dihydroergotamine and similar agents

Antiemetics: phenothiazines

NSAIDs

Combination analgesics: aspirin, acetaminophen, caffeine, and bulbital in various combinations

Opiates

Other agents: steroids, isometheptene

NSAIDs = nonsteroidal anti-inflammatory drugs.

logic origin for many types of unexplained pain is commonly sought after other obvious etiological factors have been excluded. Pain problems frequently seen in neurologic practice include back and neck pain, facial pain, and total body pain. Back and neck pain are discussed in Chapter 11, DISORDERS OF THE SPINE AND SPINAL CORD.

FACIAL PAIN

Patients with trigeminal neuralgia or tic douloureux have sudden brief attacks of pain in the distribution of one of the branches of the trigeminal nerve, most often the mandibular. The attacks of pain are very brief and lancinating but may occur many times a day. Such an intermittent, lancinating, paroxysmal character is the defining feature of "neuralgic" pain in general, such as in glossopharyngeal, postherpetic, and other types of neuralgias.

The primary or idiopathic form of trigeminal neuralgia is most often due to an aberrant arterial loop arising from the vertebrobasilar system and impinging on the trigeminal nerve in the posterior fossa. Secondary or symptomatic forms of trigeminal neuralgia may occur with other types of underlying pathological conditions, such as neoplasm or multiple sclerosis. Demonstrable facial sensory loss or other abnormalities on neurologic examination suggest a symptomatic form of trigeminal neuralgia. The initial treatment is usually with carbamazepine.

Patients with atypical facial pain have more persistent discomfort in the face. They do not have the paroxysmal, lancinating attacks typical of trigeminal neuralgia; hence the pain is atypical. It is rare to identify an underlying etiological factor, and emotional factors are often suspected.

REGIONAL PAIN SYNDROMES

Patients often develop pain in regions of the body, sometimes for obvious reasons and sometimes not. Complex regional pain syndrome (CRPS) is a condition in which there is chronic pain and hypersensitivity, usually with features of autonomic dysfunction, in a certain body part, typically one extremity or a part of one extremity. The pain typically has a burning, dysesthetic quality. CRPS is divided into CRPS I, in which the syndrome follows a soft tissue injury, often seemingly minor, or a medical condition such as stroke or myocardial infarction, and CRPS II, in which the syndrome follows a peripheral nerve injury. Reflex sympathetic dystrophy, causalgia, and sympathetically mediated pain syndrome are older terms used for these conditions.

TOTAL BODY PAIN

Most patients who complain of total body pain suffer from fibromyalgia. Chronic fatigue syndrome is a similar, perhaps identical, disorder.

Fibromyalgia is a common condition, said to affect 2% of the population of the United States. It produces diffuse, often seemingly total body, aching pain, stiffness, and fatigue. The pain is particularly prone to occur in the neck, shoulders, upper back, lower back, and hip regions. Etiological factors remain obscure; emotional factors are often suspected of playing a major role. A disrupted sleep pattern is an accompanying feature in most patients. The pain seems to originate primarily in muscles and soft tissues, but there is little or no objective evidence of inflammation or other abnormality. Patients characteristically have multiple tender points in specific areas. The diagnosis is appropriate when there is chronic widespread pain, tenderness over at least 11 of 18 points at specific locations, and no evidence of any underlying disease process. Management is frequently difficult, despite many proposed cures.

Dizziness and Syncope

Dr. W.B. Matthews, a British neurologist, said, "There can be few physicians so dedicated as to not experience a slight sinking of spirit on learning their patient's complaint is dizziness." The conditions that may present as dizziness range from trivial to life threatening, and are often difficult to evaluate and manage. The nebulousness of the patient's description of dizziness often produces frustration on the part of the clinician, yet in few other conditions are the historical details so pivotal in making a correct diagnosis. Fortunately, the truly serious conditions that present as dizziness are rare.

An important step in evaluating a patient with dizziness is to have the patient describe what he means by "dizziness." The term true vertigo describes the sensation of environmental motion (spinning, whirling, lateropulsion) experienced by patients with peripheral vestibular disease. Indeed, patients with true vertigo nearly always have a peripheral vestibulopathy, but the absence of true vertigo does not exclude peripheral vestibular disease, especially if bilateral pathology exists, such as in ototoxicity due to drugs. Some serious conditions may present as dizziness without true vertigo, such as cardiac dysrhythmias and dysautonomic orthostasis (see GLOBAL CEREBRAL HYPOPERFUSION AND SYNCOPE). Because of the slow, indolent development of the vestibular nerve pathology, patients with acoustic neuroma usually present with vague imbalance and unsteadiness (plus hearing loss), not vertigo. Physicians should not make too much of the presence or absence of true vertigo in judging how seriously to take a patient's complaint of dizziness.

CLINICAL SYNDROMES ASSOCIATED WITH DIZZINESS

The following are commonly seen syndromes associated with complaints of dizziness or vertigo.

Peripheral Vestibulopathy

Peripheral vestibulopathy is the most common final diagnosis in patients with dizziness, where a specific condition can be identified. Typically, the patient describes whirling vertigo with a sense of environmental motion, often with accompanying nausea and occasional vomiting. In benign positional vertigo (BPV), the most common type of peripheral vestibulopathy, vertigo is induced by assumption of a particular head position or by rapid head movement. Classically, such patients experience vertigo when first lying down in bed at night. BPV attacks are brief, generally 10–30 seconds, and frequent, occurring many times in the course of a day. BPV probably results from degenerative, age-related changes in the otoliths, perhaps with fragmentation of an otolith particle on one side. In so-called vestibular neuronitis (also known as viral labyrinthitis, for which no firm evidence of viral infection exists), a more severe attack prostrates the patient for several days. Mild, brief attacks of vertigo similar to BPV may then plague the patient for months to years after seeming recovery. In Meniere disease, attacks of vertigo typically last several hours and patients describe other symptoms, either along with the vertigo or independently, including hearing loss (classically fluctuating), tinnitus, and a sensation of vague pain or fullness in the ear.

Global Cerebral Hypoperfusion

Cerebral hypoperfusion produces a sensation of lightheadedness, drunkenness, or impending syncope without spinning, whirling, or any illusion of environmental motion. Such hypoperfusion may occur under a variety of circumstances and may lead patients to seek medical attention because of their dizziness. When it is more severe, global cerebral hypoperfusion results in loss of consciousness (see syncope). In hyperventilation syndrome (HVS), hypocapnia-induced cerebral arterial constriction and the resultant hypoperfusion induces lightheadedness along with other symptoms, such as chest pain; headache; numbness and tingling of the hands, feet, and circumoral region; and occasionally outright syncope. Frequently, patients with HVS are unaware of their overbreathing, but the high minute volume of respiration produces dryness of the mouth, which patients may describe spontaneously or respond to on specific questioning. Orthostatic hypotension due to drugs, prolonged standing, dehydration, or dysautonomia likewise may present as lightheadedness or faintness. Accompanying symptoms are few, and only a careful history eliciting the relationship of the dizziness to posture makes the diagnosis.

Multisensory Defect Dizziness

Elderly patients "deafferented" because of separate disease processes affecting different sensory systems may present with complaints of vague dizziness, unsteadiness, and difficulty with balance. Patients can apparently compensate for and tolerate dysfunction of any one afferent system, but when multiple systems are involved imbalance and dizziness result. Thus, patients typically suffer from various combinations of poor vision (e.g., cataracts, macular degeneration), poor hearing (presbyacusis), mild peripheral neuropathy, and cervical spondylosis.

Vertebrobasilar Insufficiency

Although patients with vertebrobasilar insufficiency (VBI) usually have dizziness, it is rare for VBI to present as dizziness alone, and the diagnosis is tenuous unless there are associated symptoms to suggest brainstem ischemia (see Chapter 10).

SYNCOPE

Syncope is one cause of episodic loss of consciousness (see Chapter 10, OTHER SEIZURE-RELATED ISSUES). The final common denominator in cases of syncope is a sudden fall of blood pressure resulting in loss of consciousness. When the decrease in blood pressure is not severe enough to cause unconsciousness, patients may suffer from the symptoms of global cerebral hypoperfusion (see GLOBAL CEREBRAL HYPOPERFUSION).

Causes of syncope are many, and range from simple faint or vasovagal syncope, to life-threatening cardiac arrhythmias (Table 12–4). About 3% of the population experience at least one episode of syncope during their lifetime. The incidence of simple syncope is highest in late adolescence. A clinical evaluation including history, physical examination with supine and standing blood pressure measurement, and a resting electrocardiogram reveal the cause of syncope in about 50% of patients. Although neurologists see many patients with syncope, rarely is the cause actually neurologic. The most common cause of syncope in a neurologic setting is orthostatic hypotension, most often due to overuse of antihypertensive medications, sometimes due to dysautonomia. The most important consideration is to exclude serious underlying cardiac disease. There is a substantial risk of sudden death in older patients with cardiogenic syncope.

Sleep Disorders

Patients with disturbed nocturnal sleep frequently present complaining of excessive daytime sleepiness or extreme fatigue rather than nighttime insomnia. In contrast, most patients who complain of insomnia have depression or a misperception of inadequate sleep. Over the past 25 years, the study of sleep disorders has grown into a recognized med-

TABLE 12–4. ETIOLOGY OF SYNCOPE

Cardiac disease

  Arrhythmia (Stokes-Adams syndrome)

    Bradycardia or asystole

    Sick-sinus syndrome

    Supraventricular or ventricular tachycardia

  Hemodynamic obstruction

    Hypertrophic subaortic stenosis (HSS)

    Aortic stenosis

  Coronary artery disease

  Cardiomyopathy

Neurally mediated

  Vasovagal reaction

  Carotid sinus hypersensitivity

Orthostatic (postural) hypotension

ical subspecialty with its own certifying board. This text attempts to convey only the bare essentials of this topic.

NARCOLEPSY

The full syndrome of narcolepsy includes attacks of excessive daytime sleepiness, cataplexy (sudden collapse without loss of consciousness produced by laughing or other strong emotion), sleep paralysis (spells of inability to move during sleep/wake transitions), and hypnagogic or hypnopompic hallucinations (extremely vivid dreams during sleep/wake transitions). Diagnosis in the absence of the fully developed tetrad can be difficult. The most common and troubling aspect is usually the excessive daytime sleepiness, which can occur without the other features. Sleep apnea is prominent in the differential diagnosis.

SLEEP APNEA

Besides narcolepsy, sleep apnea is the other major condition causing excessive daytime sleepiness. Patients with sleep apnea suffer from chronic sleep deprivation due to innumerable awakenings because of apneic episodes occurring through the course of a night's sleep. Patients are seldom aware that they are having these awakenings, and merely present complaining of excessive daytime sleepiness and fatigue.

Two forms of sleep apnea are recognized: obstructive and central.

With obstructive sleep apnea, patients are usually obese and have a condition that causes hypotonia of the palatal and pharyngeal muscles. During deep sleep, these muscles collapse and obstruct the airway, leading to hypoxia, which then leads to awakening. Loud, raucous, obnoxious snoring is a common associated feature of obstructive sleep apnea. In central sleep apnea, an abnormality of the medullary respiratory centers leads to intermittent spells of apnea. Patients with central sleep apnea are not necessarily obese or loud snorers.

Index